BRAIN METABOLISM
AND
CEREBRAL DISORDERS

By

HAROLD E. HIMWICH, M.D.

Chief, Clinical Research Branch, Medical Division,
Army Chemical Center, Maryland

BALTIMORE

THE WILLIAMS & WILKINS COMPANY

1951

COPYRIGHT, 1951

HAROLD E. HIMWICH, M.D.

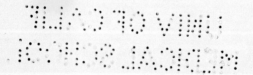

PRINTED AT THE
WAVERLY PRESS, INC.
BALTIMORE 2, MD., U. S. A

To my wife

To my wife

PREFACE

After arrangements for the publication of this volume had been completed I was asked to write a short preface to include some information on the contents and the group of readers for which it was intended. The subject of brain metabolism, in its various facets, is reviewed in this book. The time seems ripe for such a review. Definite gains have been made and it is well to consolidate them as an aid in giving direction to future research, research which has already begun to throw new light on some disease processes. The application of this knowledge to disease awaited the laborious, if brilliant, collection of fundamental data. First the extention of our knowledge of cellular physiology to include the cerebral cells. Next the quantitation of the metabolic rate of the brain *in vivo* made possible by blood flow methods such as that of Kety and Schmidt and finally, the application of this knowledge to disease as well as to such distortions of normal functions as are seen, for example, during anesthesia.

In a way I have been living with certain aspects of this work since their inception. Starting my investigations as a pupil of Graham Lusk and therefore imbued with the importance of carbohydrate metabolism as examined in the intact organism, I went to the laboratory of Otto Meyerhof where for the first time, I employed excised tissues in such studies. It was therefore natural to form a synthesis of these two different points of view and to study the metabolism of individual organs functioning normally within the body. This was made possible by collecting samples of their arterial and venous blood for the analysis of oxygen and other constituents. Using this method I stumbled on the observation indicating that the brain utilized carbohydrate chiefly for its foodstuff. Then when Sakel came along with his insulin hypoglycemia therapy for schizophrenia the opportunity was offered to test this conclusion. Once it was shown that the diminution of cerebral metabolic rate was the mechanism underlying the treatment, one thing lead rapidly to another. The symptomatic progression, successive constellations of neurological signs, and electroencephalographic changes disclosed additional evidence for Hughlings Jackson's hypothesis of the functional organization of the central nervous system, namely that of cephalad dominance over caudad activities. This led to a further study of metabolic changes during early postnatal growth, a period when cephalad dominance is approaching completion. Then came a host of data based on enzymatic studies from many laboratories, all supporting this conception which is also a cornerstone of the edifice built by Sir Charles Sherrington. Now we have come to a place where we can look back to see what we have accomplished before going on to the real work of the future namely to apply, more and more, our growing body of exact knowledge, to the study of disease.

When it occurred to the author to undertake this book he dictated what proved to be a small sized monograph, hardly more than an outline, covering some of the data presented in most of the chapters of this book. But when it became necessary to fill in supporting data, the tome grew to its present size. Dr. E. F. DuBois read the chapter on cerebral metabolic rate, the present Chapter 8, and asked why a description of cerebral circulation was not included, and then it seemed obvious that such a discussion was necessary in the consideration of certain disturbances, arteriosclerosis and arteriovenous aneurysm, to mention but two instances. The first draft of that chapter was sent to Dr. Harry Forbes for criticism, but he can not be held accountable for its present form. Similarly an early draft of Chapter 2, foodstuff of the brain, was criticized by Dr. Ephraim Racker and one of Chapter 9, the autonomic nervous system, by Professor Otto Loewi. I am grateful for their cooperation. My first introduction into the clinical aspects of this problem was guided by Dr. J. P. Frostig and it was with his cooperation that the subject of disease was broached. But I can not, for want of space, present the names of the many friends who have been buttonholed at meetings or importuned by letters in order to help elucidate debatable points. Even more am I indebted to my coworkers and their names are spread over the bibliography. We all try to be objective but we can see only through our own eyes. While we may disagree with some authorities in this field at least we try to explain why we have come to our conclusions and also attempt to marshal the facts on both sides of the question. I can not close this preface without saying that one of the two reasons that this book is dedicated to my wife is that next to me she suffered most in its production. A constant topic of conversation at our home was one or another aspect of this volume. It is hoped that the various parts of this book will be of aid to all those involved in the study of the brain, normal and abnormal: the neurologist and neurosurgeon, the psychiatrist and expert in mental deficiency, the psychologist and anesthesiologist, the workers in the various fundamental neurological sciences and the pediatrician and internist as well.

ACKNOWLEDGMENTS

Appreciation is expressed here for the fine cooperation of the authors and to the publishers for the use of the following figures:

FIG. NOS.	PUBLICATION	PUBLISHER	AUTHOR
6 14	Am. J. Med. Sci.	Lea & Febiger Pub. Co.	H. F. Root and T. M. Carpenter F. A. Gibbs
15, 16, 17, 42	Atlas of Electroenceph-alography	Addison-Wesley Press, Inc.	F. A. Gibbs and E. L. Gibbs (396)
18	J. Comp. Neur.	The Wistar Institute of Anatomy and Biology	H. S. Dunning and H. G Wolff (259)
20, 24	Am. J. Physiol.	American Physiological Society	S. W. Britton and R. F. Kline (116)
21			D. B. Tyler and A. van Harre-veld (953)
40			H. Hoagland, M. A. Rubin and D. E. Cameron (530)
46			M. B. Bender (75)
25	Principles of Human Physiology	J. & A. Churchill, Ltd.	Starling
26			Adapted from data by Potter (798)
29	Univ. of Missouri Research Bulletin	Dr. Samuel Brody	S. Brody and H. H. Kibler (117)
32	J. Neurophysiol.	Charles C Thomas	D. Nachmansohn (757)
34			M. A. Kennard and L. F. Nims (586)
43			D. B. Lindsley (667), L. H. Schreiner & H. W. Magoun
47			M. B. Bender and M. A. Kennard (76)
36	Proc. Soc. Exp. Biol. & Med.	Soc. for Experimental Biology & Medicine	R. E. Scammon, 20: 114–117, 1922–23
45	J. Exp. Biol. & Med.	Soc. for Experimental Biology & Medicine	E. Gellhorn (374)

Also the author is indebted to the *American Journal of Physiology* for permission to use Figs. 1, 22, 23, 27, 28, 31, 33, 41; to the *Archives of Biochemistry* for Fig. 30; to the *Archives of Neurology and Psychiatry* for Figs. 35, 48, 49, 50; to the *American Journal of Medical Science* for Fig. 37; to the *American Journal of Psychiatry* for Fig. 38; to the *Psychiatric Quarterly* (**18**: 357–373, 1944) for Fig. 39; to the *Journal of Neurophysiology* for Fig. 44; and to the *Journal of Anesthesiology* for Fig. 51. All of the above figures appeared in papers prepared by the author.

Finally the author is grateful to Dr. Emerson Crosby Kelly for the portrait of John Hughlings Jackson, which is reproduced with the permission of Richard Pennington, of the Redpath Library at McGill University, Montreal.

CONTENTS

PART I

ENERGETICS

PART II

PATTERNS OF NERVOUS ACTIVITY

PART I

Energetic

CHAPTER 1
INTRODUCTION

The functions of the central nervous system have been studied for many years. Probably the earliest data were furnished by clinical observations; accidental injury to the brain and forms of cerebral disease were the incentive for these inquiries. Later, a second source of information was uncovered when experimental investigation came into use. Functions of each part of the brain were explored by observing the effects of their stimulation, whether by mechanical, electrical or chemical means. The opposite experimental procedure was to examine the component parts of the brain by noting the effects of their extirpation on behavior and adaptive responses. Along with the development of the fundamental sciences, the chemical analysis of cerebral constituents took its place beside other experimental methods. More recently, recording of electrical potentials of brain, spinal cord and nerve, whether spontaneous or induced, has yielded information of significant value.

The biochemical analysis of the brain is perhaps the youngest of all research technic, and involves the analysis of the oxygen and carbon dioxide exchanges in the brain, commonly referred to as *respiratory metabolism*. Cerebral tissues freshly excised from the living organism are studied with the aid of appropriate apparatus. It is also possible to examine the brain with all its anatomic and physiologic connections by analyzing cerebral blood samples for their gaseous exchange. In animals the usual procedure is to trephine the skull (519) so that venous blood may be collected from the longitudinal sinus. The credit for developing the technic whereby cerebral blood can be withdrawn from the brain of a human being belongs to Dr. Myerson, the late Director of Research at Boston State Hospital. By tapping the internal jugular vein (756), he was able to collect samples of blood returning from the brain, and their analysis gave added information about the cerebral metabolic processes. Dr. Myerson's contribution is of particular importance to the physician because it has made the brain of the living patient available for biochemical research. Another step forward, the quantitative determination of cerebral blood flow, was subsequently achieved independently by two groups of investigators: Drs. S. S. Kety and C. F. Schmidt (596, 598), the University of Pennsylvania, and Dr. and Mrs. F. A. Gibbs and Dr. H. P. Maxwell (400), the University of Illinois. The data obtained by their methods enhance the significance of results made available by Dr. Myerson's technic.

The material of the text falls into two distinct divisions. We have called

3

the first part "Energetics", the methods by which energy is elaborated, as well as distributed to support nervous' activity. The second part, entitled "Patterns of Nervous Activity", explains energetics in terms of behavior. Though the emphasis in Part I is laid on cellular physiology and biochemistry, whereas the second part is more concerned with the integrated action of the various portions comprising the central nervous system, still each is dependent upon the other; the first part describes the processes necessary to support nervous activity, and the latter handles the problem of how the nervous system carries on at the expense of the energy elaborated within it.

The material on energetics is presented in the eight chapters which constitute the first part of the book. The subject of Chapter 2 is foodstuffs of the brain, carbohydrates and carbohydrate-split products, an advantage for the biochemist since these substrates, unlike the more difficult lipids, lend themselves well to quantitative analysis. Because of the importance of carbohydrate in the subsistance of the brain, we considered it wise to devote an entire chapter (3) to the neuroendocrine regulation of the foodstuff of the brain, blood sugar; and another (4) to explain why the brain does not cease functioning immediately when hypoglycemia befalls. In Chapter 5 it is suggested that all bodily oxidations, including those of the brain, have experienced a phyletic development whereby new enzyme systems arose in accordance with the need for a more rapid liberation of energy to sustain the ever-growing complexity of life. At this point, a chapter on cerebral circulation (6) was incorporated to broaden the background for subsequent metabolic discussion.

The cerebral metabolism of warm-blooded animals as they grow from the embryo to the newborn infant and finally into adulthood embodies Chapter 7, and here we meet the first opportunity to co-ordinate cerebral metabolism and phylogenesis. The eighth and ninth chapters are probably of greatest practical interest to the clinician since they are devoted to observations on the human being. Herein, the normal cerebral metabolic rate is computed and the variations in this rate wrought by disease are estimated. Our discussion is necessarily limited to those diseases which have been subjected to analysis of respiratory metabolism. Among them are included several of the psychoses, various mental deficiencies and certain forms of avitaminosis. Chapter 9 deals with the modifications of energetics by various therapeutic measures, in the hope of emphasizing for the clinician the effects of his treatments upon the brain.

The processes underlying our behavior can be analyzed in their simplest form in terms of elementary reflexes, whose arcs ramify in the central nervous system. When working together, these reflexes form a functionally organized and integrated unit. But, to study each component performing its part in this vast system separately is another problem, a great deal more complicated, and this analysis is the purpose of the second part of the book, "Patterns of Nervous Activity". Scientists have found that by closely examining persons whose brain has been temporarily depressed or permanently injured, they were able to unveil the specific contributions of each integral part. Any condition whereby the brain is deprived of energy, whether it be through therapeutic measures such as insulin hypoglycemia and anesthesia, or whether it be an anoxic deprivation resulting from an accident, gives us an opportunity to allocate some elements of behavior to their respective areas of representation in the brain. Of cardinal importance in accomplishing this task is the concept of neurophylogenesis, employed repeatedly throughout the book, and applied to the human brain in the concluding four chapters. Chapter 10 deals with the somatic division of the central nervous system, the patterns of activity mediated by the cerebral centers governing the neuromuscular adaptations of the body. In a further analysis of these cerebral centers, Chapter 11 singles out the visceral division of the central nervous system, and the patterns of activity modulated by the autonomic centers situated therein. The phenomenon of narcosis is considered in Chapter 12 and the phyletic generalization is applied to a symptomatic analysis of barbiturate action. Once we appreciate this theory of "levels of function", the advantages accruing to the physician in understanding the normal and treating the abnormal nervous system are manifold. A few of the immediate objectives and future problems are outlined in Chapter 13.

* * *

In all medical research the underlying motive in the mind of the investigator is to find knowledge which may be used either to help the diseased individual or to prevent the inception of ill health. The scientist may be stimulated by some preconceived idea which he wishes to put to test. Or, he may work without a guiding hypothesis but with the hope of uncovering new information. The former working philosophy was utilized in Chapter 7 on animal brain metabolism, and also in Part II, in its entirety. The latter motive finds fruition in the material of Chapter 2 on the foodstuff of the brain; also in observations on human cerebral metabolism in health and disease (Chapters 8 and 9).

Outstanding in its influence on the author is the theory of Hughlings Jackson (558) on the phyletic organization of the central nervous system[1].

[1] Hughlings Jackson wrote of three levels: the lowest consisting of the spinal cord, medulla and cerebellum, an intermediate one including the motor cortex and striatum and the highest formed partly of the pre-frontal cortex. In this volume we are concerned with Hughlings Jackson's conception of levels of function rather than his specific anatomic delimitation of these levels.

For purposes of clarity and also because of its import in the composition of this book and in the interpretation of experimental results, the theory of Hughlings Jackson is rehearsed as follows:

The brain of man as we see it today looks like a static structure which has existed unchanged for eons. But when it is examined more closely in the light of the phyletic conception, we see that it has come to its present construction as a result of a long series of accretions, beginning with the spinal cord and medulla oblongata and spreading in a cephalad direction, layer upon layer, until the cerebral hemispheres form the greatest mass of the brain. It is not to be supposed that each level is independent of its predecessors, but rather that it exists with a specific relation, both anatomically and physiologically, to the phyletically older portions (944). Owing to this relation, the central nervous system may function as a unit, but a unity which is brought to a higher plane of integration with each successive step. The human brain is undoubtedly the latest arrangement of the central nervous system, but not necessarily the final one.

Probably the earliest aquatic vertebrate, as far as organization of the central nervous system is concerned, was chiefly a bulbospinal animal, and irrespective of the subsequent development of the brain, the bulb always remained an important center especially for viscero-somatic integration. In the course of evolution, each additional part of the brain did not accrue in a haphazard fashion but took root directly in front of the pre-existing part, and always toward the oral end of the animal. Sir Charles Sherrington (876) has expressed vividly Hughlings Jackson's conception.

"That leading end, the head, has receiving stations signalling from things at a distance, things which the animal in its forward movement will next meet. A shell of its immediate future surrounds the animal's head. The nerve-nets in the head are therefore busy with signals from a shell of the outside world which the animal is about to enter and experience. The brain has thus arisen where signalling is busiest and is fraught most with the germ of futurity. Small wonder then that the brain plays a great role in the motor management of the muscle. Nerve management of muscle resolves itself largely into management of nerve by nerve, especially by brain, more and more so as evolution proceeds. With no greater equipment of muscle the superimposed amount of nerve becomes greater and greater; each new nerve-growth seems to entail further nerve-growth. Fresh organization roofs over prior organization. Brain is an example. 'So on our heels a fresh perfection treads.' But were it a government office we might be suspicious. This brain of ours is a perfect excrescence although our endowment of muscle remains but moderate".

To climb the phyletic ladder from our remotest ancestors through the fish, amphibia, reptiles and mammals, would entail a tremendous volume of description, which is not the point of this treatise. The general trend of this process of cephalization, or concentration of neural functions in the oral end of the animal, may be described briefly: as far back as the fish the brain is divided into five portions as it is in man, but in the fish and amphibia the chief site of integration for sensory and motor impulses lies in the midbrain. In these species the highest portion of the brain consists chiefly of the olfactory bulb, and the cerebral cortex which becomes all-important in man, is represented only by a thin layer of cells. On further ascending the phyletic scale to reptiles and birds as well as mammals, the subcortical structures immediately anterior to the midbrain become more prominent, as the organism achieves greater coordinating control. Lastly, the cerebral cortex, though getting off to a late start, gradually attains more complexity of structure and diversity of function until in the lower mammals it surpasses all other regions, and in the primates, especially in man, forms the largest and most complex part of the cerebral tissue.

Similar phyletic relationships are seen within the segments themselves as well as in the brain as a whole. Close examination of the most recent layer of the brain shows that it is divided into two portions—the phyletically newer cerebral hemispheres and the more primitive subcortical basal ganglia. These motor ganglia, in turn, are made up of the neostriatum and paleostriatum. Such a division is also found in the thalamus, the midline nuclei being comparatively ancient sensory centers, while the other nuclei developed along with the cerebral hemispheres, and served as way-stations for sensory impulses relayed on to the cortex. The cerebellum may likewise be divided into parts of different phyletic origin (250). The paleocerebellum makes connections with the cord and the vestibular nuclei of the medulla, while the neocerebellum was developed simultaneously with the motor and sensory areas of the cerebral cortex.

Though each part of the brain is capable of subserving special functions, the brain acts as an integrated unit because of the anatomic and functional relationships existing among its constituent parts. It would seem that once a section is formed, it is never scrapped, but is retained and combined with the next succeeding phyletic layer, continuing to play its part under the guidance of this newer layer.

Evidence for such a conception is found not only anatomically but also physiologically. Each portion of the central nervous system, even the lowest—the spinal cord—retains within it the centers for functional integration. The spinal animal (875), a decapitated preparation kept alive by artificial respiration, still responds to stimulation with an appropriate muscular action. Though these primitive reflexes are preserved even in the highest animals, they are nevertheless modified by the newer layers. The motor expression of their activities can take place only "with the permission" of the higher centers. In a word, the recent levels preside over and dictate to the older and less specialized ones, holding them in check. It is necessary to have such an hierarchy of organization because the newer parts bring to the central nervous system a more delicate sensory discrimination and a finer execution of motion. In this connection, not only are tactile sensation and perception of pain more accurately appreciated and localized when the cerebral hemispheres are active, but motor responses are better adapted to stimuli. For the organism, however, to take advantage of these improved capacities, the behavior of the lower portions must be subjected to the control and regulation, the inhibition and reinforcement of the higher planes. Examples of inhibition and reinforcement are legion and many are presented in the present text, but a most convincing experimental proof for inhibition comes from the work of Marion Hines (528a) who demonstrated that stimulation of a strip on the anterior border of the motor cortex (4s) in the monkey suppresses current activity, in this instance tonic extension of an extremity, and that ablation of that strip results in spasticity due to removal of inhibitory influences.

We are all familiar with Charles Darwin's work which has established the theory of evolution of species (222). Hughlings Jackson's conception is a special application of Darwin's theory to the central nervous system. The importance of this interpretation appears not only in the analysis of normal physiology as indicated by the fact that the caudad sections of the brain function only under the guidance of the more cephalad ones, but it is also of practical value in explaining the origin of pathologic phenomena. An abnormal clinical manifestation may arise either from stimulation of some part of the brain, or constitute a release phenomenon as a superior part of the brain gives way, permitting the unrestricted activity of a lower and more primitive area. This segregation of the regions in the brain and their interactivity is of extreme consequence in seeking a diagnosis and treatment for cerebral disease. Because complexity of organization is accompanied by susceptibility to deprivation of cerebral energy, the changes observed in anoxia, hypoglycemia, and anesthesia, for example, are a mixture resulting from failure of the newer parts of the brain and hyperactivity in the older portions. Much of the work in this book bears an intimate relationship to the theme on neurophylogenesis, and much of our evidence not only supports this hypothesis, but extends its usefulness into biochemical, morphologic and clinical fields.

CHAPTER 2

FOODSTUFF OF THE BRAIN

I. INTRODUCTION

The life of an organism is maintained and its work is performed by the expenditure of energy liberated in the oxidation of foodstuffs. This energy builds energy-rich phosphate bonds[1] which in turn support, among other cerebral functions, perception of environmental changes, co-ordination of perceptions with physical responses, memory and thinking. Cerebral performance, unlike that of muscle, cannot be estimated simply in terms of physical equivalents, such as foot pounds or kilogram meters but it is related, as is the work of other organs, to the volume of oxygen used or the amount of foodstuffs consumed. The quantity of work performed depends upon efficiency; for secretory organs it is between 2 and 10 per cent (34) and for muscle 20 and 25 per cent (467). Similarly the energy required for the conduction of the nervous impulse may be only a part of the total energy metabolism of the brain. To understand why this is so, we shall discuss briefly the turnover of energy in a portion of the nervous system which has been subjected to close scrutiny, namely, peripheral nerve. It must be emphasized that some of the energy elaborated by nerve is not involved in conduction but is diverted to trophic functions, including the maintenance of structure. When this energy support is withdrawn, as occurs after the axon is severed from the cell body, the portion cut away from the cell body degenerates. On the other hand, the conduction of the nervous impulse possesses a basis in energy, as indicated by a gaseous exchange and a heat production which increase with frequency of stimulation. To return to our chief interest, the work of the brain requires energy and it has been demonstrated that the oxygen intake of that organ rises with its activity (856). But in the brain, as in peripheral nerve, energy is also necessary for trophic purposes. It is difficult to separate completely the energy demands of structure and of activity, since the latter are built upon the former and their functions merge on the neuronal surface.

Conduction is a surface phenomenon, characterized by an electrical potential, as well as by chemical changes, all however concentrated near the neuronal surfaces (758). But trophic processes are also involved in surface activities. When nerve or any other tissue dies, it loses its semipermeability and permits the rapid diffusion of substances through its cell walls. At

[1] For discussions of energy-rich phosphate bonds as the immediate source of energy for the maintenance of cellular structure and functional activity, See Chapter 4 page 55 and Chapter 5 page 71, footnote 5.

rest energy metabolism maintains permeability at a minimum for certain ions, i.e., sodium and chloride. During activity, the surface becomes more permeable at the same time energy supports the conduction of the impulse. Thus a good share of the energy made available in peripheral nerve, and presumably in the synapse which connects neurons, as well as in the brain, is spent upon surface integrity.[2]

Not all substances can be utilized by the brain as sources of energy. In general, there are three ways to determine whether substances may be so utilized: (1) the ability of foodstuff to support cerebral metabolism, (2) the respiratory quotient, which is an indicator of the foodstuff oxidized by the brain, and (3) a quantitative comparison of the oxygen intake and the absorption of a given foodstuff. These methods will now be considered in the above order.

II. Methods for determining foodstuffs used by brain

A. *Ability of foodstuff to support metabolism and other functions of the brain*

When a specific foodstuff serves as a sole source of energy for any organ, the oxygen intake is a measure of the utilization of that substance by the organ. Our problem is to determine what foodstuffs the brain oxidizes and this has been studied by three general methods.

Excised cerebral tissues. By the first method, the oxygen consumption and carbon dioxide output of thinly sliced or minced tissues are measured after insertion into a Warburg respirometer (973) or any similar apparatus. The addition of various carbohydrates and non-carbohydrates to the fluids in which the excised cerebral tissues are suspended, and the determination of the gaseous exchange makes it possible to ascertain which substances support metabolism *in vitro*. In many of these experiments, the stimulating effect of a given substrate on respiration was singled out from others as the substrate was not added until the intrinsic food supplies of cerebral tissues were exhausted.

Among the carbohydrates which were found to be oxidized in the brain, glucose is most potent, and in decreasing order of effectiveness are fructose (674, 805, 237, 607), mannose (805) and galactose (805, 871), hexose diphosphate and hexose monophosphate.[3] Pentoses are practically inert

---

[2] The discussion on the surface activities of peripheral nerve is extended to include the brain because the excitable properties of the central neurons are similar to those of the peripheral nerves; some of the peculiarities of the synapse can be demonstrated on fibers and the synapse may not differ, except quantitatively, from the peripheral axon (365, 285).

[3] Huszak (547) notes differences between the preferential foodstuffs of the slowly oxidizing white and the more rapid grey: the former utilizes glycogen and phosphorylated hexoses, the latter, unphosphorylated hexoses and chiefly glucose. In both

(805). The non-carbohydrates tested include lactic acid (674, 24, 738, 739) and pyruvic acid (674, 24, 805, 788, 789, 570, 271) which sustain the steady rate of oxygen intake as well as does the carbohydrate, glucose. Succinic acid (805, 788, 271, 36, 629) and alpha-ketoglutaric acid, (628, 725, 565) are oxidized more rapidly than alpha-glycerophosphate (788, 565, 804) and phosphoglyceric acid (570). Glutamic acid[4] (608, 805, 623, 624, 985, 570) and alcohol (1029, 826, 520) in small concentrations may also undergo some oxidation. Despite the fact that the brain is formed chiefly of lipid material, the oxidation of fat by the brain has not been demonstrated. All evidence indicates that the brain does not oxidize fatty acids (569) nor is it able to obtain energy from the oxidation of ketone substances (569, 407). Acetoacetic acid, an apparent exception (877), is of little practical importance because of its slow oxidation rate in the brain (803). Some of the substances which are readily oxidized by the excised cerebral tissues such as succinic acid, for example, do not occur in the blood in significant amounts. It may be concluded from these observations on excised tissues, therefore, that among the foodstuffs of the brain, only glucose, lactic acid and pyruvic acid are of practical importance. In accordance with this specialization in the type of foodstuff the rate of cerebral utilization of glucose is faster than that observed in hepatic, cardiac or renal slices (779a).

Brain IN SITU during insulin hypoglycemia. We will next examine the respiratory response to glucose, lactic and pyruvic acids for the intact animal in order to determine whether these substrates are as necessary for the brain *in situ* as for excised cerebral tissues. The effect of glucose will be examined first.

The insulin treatment for schizophrenia (845), a treatment which involves the use of large doses of insulin to reduce the level of blood sugar, affords an opportunity for such an examination. This method permits us to study not only the effects of removing this physiologic sugar from the body, but also the results of administering glucose to the hypoglycemic individ-

---

tissues, however, the breakdown occurs in accordance with the Embden-Meyerhof scheme (see schema, page 68, Chapter 5).

[4] It has been known for some time that glutamic acid is the only amino acid oxidized by the brain, and more recently it has been found to increase the rate of formation of acetylcholine (671) acting as coenzyme to choline acetylase (762), the enzyme which aids the formation of acetylcholine. Perhaps this reaction furnished the suggestion for the therapeutic use of glutamic acid in petit mal epilepsy (799). In fact, this reagent was first employed in the treatment of this disease on the hypothesis that the slow brain waves which characterize the petit mal attacks are in some way connected with an impaired formation of acetylcholine. (See footnote page 71, Chapter 5, for discussion of the part played by energy-rich phosphate bonds in the synthesis of acetylcholine). Further work however makes it improbable that glutamic acid penetrates the blood-brain barrier (see pages 117–119 and 123).

ual.[5] If glucose is the important foodstuff of the human brain, the rate of brain metabolism should fall sharply directly following a decline of blood sugar. The determination of brain metabolism *in situ* involves two factors: (1) the cerebral arterio-venous oxygen difference per 100 cc. of blood, obtained by analyzing samples of arterial and venous blood of the brain for oxygen, and (2) the rate of blood flowing through the brain per minute. If brain metabolism remains constant, these two factors bear an inverse relationship to each other: that is, a faster blood flow makes for a smaller arterio-venous difference; a slower blood flow, a larger arterio-venous difference, this being true as long as the oxygen intake of the brain remains unchanged. A fall of brain metabolism, on the other hand, is indicated in one of three ways: (a) a constant blood flow with a decrease in arterio-venous oxygen difference, (b) a decrease in blood flow with a constant arterio-venous oxygen difference, or (c) a diminution of both variables. We can rule out the second and third possibilities in studies of insulin hypoglycemia because no great changes of blood flow were observed as a result of this treatment. This conclusion is based on observations (681) (477) made with the aid of thermocouples on human subjects, as well as on rabbits (646). In neither case were there any hypoglycemic convulsions to disturb the blood flow. More recently similar observations (316) were obtained on patients using an entirely different method depending upon the response of cerebrospinal fluid pressure to compression of the jugular veins. (For further discussion of more accurate methods see Chapter 8).

The relative constancy of cerebral blood flow during hypoglycemia (600) facilitated the evaluation of the second factor required for estimation of brain metabolism, namely, arterio-venous oxygen difference (492, 202, 481, 512, 508). In a typical example (Fig. 1) of a patient receiving the insulin treatment for schizophrenia (512), a normal level of blood sugar, 89 mg. per cent, fell to 25 mg. per cent[6], after the injection of insulin, while the initial normal arterio-venous oxygen difference of 7.0 vol. per cent decreased to 4.4 vol. per cent.[7] This low value (4.4 vol per cent) was reached at approximately the time when the patient lost contact with the environment, that is, intentional acts were no longer observed and the patient could not be aroused. As the hypoglycemia continued, the arterio-venous oxygen difference decreased further to a value of 1.3 vol. per cent. After this level was reached, sugar was administered by stomach tube to terminate the treat-

---

[5] It should be pointed out that the experiments performed on human and animal subjects in hypoglycemia simulate those in which excised cerebral tissues were permitted to exhaust their intrinsic food supplies until oxygen intake fell to a low level before the addition of substrate (805).

[6] mg. per cent = milligrams per 100 cc. of blood.

[7] vol. per cent = cc. per 100 cc. of blood.

ment. As the patient aroused, the cerebral oxygen utilization increased first to 4.0 and then to 6.3 vol. per cent, while blood sugar rose to 70 and 111 mg. per cent. These data indicate that removal of sugar from the blood is followed by a decrease in brain metabolism, a decrease which is restored to

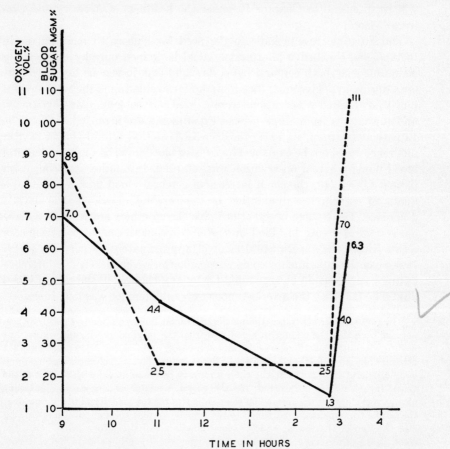

TIME IN HOURS

Fig. 1. The effects of the administration of glucose during hypoglycemia on the cerebral arterio-venous oxygen difference and the level of blood sugar.

normal by the administration of glucose. Substantiating these conclusions are nine more observations (512) of five patients taking the same treatment. The average initial difference between the oxygen content of their arterial and venous blood was 6.8 vol. per cent. At the time they lost environmental contact, the average arterio-venous oxygen difference had fallen to 2.6 vol. per cent, and during deepest depression the oxygen difference fell further to 1.8 vol per cent. After the administration of glucose, samples of blood drawn as soon as contact with the environment was re-established revealed an average arterio-venous difference of 5.1 vol. per cent. Complete restoration of the arterio-venous oxygen difference to the initial value was somewhat delayed. The factors responsible for this delay will be discussed in Chapter 10 under the headings of *Recovery* and *Protracted Shock*.

Though these results indicate the need for glucose to maintain brain metabolism, conclusive information could be gained only by determining simultaneously both cerebral blood flow and arterio-venous oxygen difference during hypoglycemia. (See footnote for evaluation of data on cerebral blood flow). Such observations were carried out on a number of patients, and the figures from three typical experiments are arranged in Table 1. In patient Br, 6/21/40, (477) the decreased cerebral arterio-venous oxygen difference could not be explained by a faster blood flow, because the cerebral blood flow by actual observation was retarded. In another experiment on patient C, 7/1/40, the small increase of cerebral blood flow was not adequate to explain the diminution of the cerebral arterio-venous oxygen difference. These three observations plus eleven others not tabulated show an average decrease in blood flow of 7 per cent during hypoglycemia, a result within the experimental error of approximately 10 per cent (512). In none of the experiments[8] could the small arterio-venous oxygen difference during hypoglycemia be accounted for by any changes in the rate of blood flow. The fact that the arterio-venous oxygen difference was low, therefore,

[8] In these experiments the thermoelectric blood flow recorder was used, an apparatus by which the change in blood flow from the original pre-insulin value, but not the absolute blood flow, was determined. Gregg and Shipley (418) point out that this method is valid if: (1) provisions are made for detecting changes in blood and body temperature; (2) the needle tip is known to be immobilized with respect to the vessel into which it is inserted; (3) the vessel diameter undergoes no significant change; (4) clots are not formed on the needle tip; (5) the velocity of blood flow over the needle tip remains proportional to the velocity of flow throughout the remaining cross section of the vessel; and (6) blood flow is at all times forward. When these conditions are observed, changes in galvanometric deflection should indicate correctly directional changes in flow.

In the present experiments, the needle, after being inserted into the internal jugular vein, was immobilized by strips of adhesive. The lumen of the needle was filled with an obturator which was removed only to collect a sample of blood or to insert the thermocouple. Clot formation was signaled by a noticeable deflection of the galvanometer, whereupon the clot was broken up by pushing the obturator somewhat beyond the tip of the needle. As far as we know, all of the criteria of Gregg and Shipley were observed, save the first—concerning the temperature of the patient. It should be noted that the results obtained with the thermoelectric blood flow recorder are in general agreement with others determined by the nitrous oxide technic (600).

affords proof that a fall in blood sugar finally makes for a reduced brain metabolism.

Another way to determine the necessity of glucose for brain metabolism

TABLE 1

Effect of glucose on arterio-venous oxygen difference and cerebral blood flow during insulin hypoglycemia

1 PATIENT AND DATE	2 TIME	3 OXYGEN DIFF. VOL. %	4 GLUCOSE ART. MG. %	5 6 BLOOD FLOW		7 REMARKS
				Observed (1)	Calculated (2)	
Br	8:10	6.1	83			110 units insulin at
6/21/40	10:40	4.1	19	−10%	+49%	8:40
	11:40	2.2	15	−30%	+177%	
	12:40	2.3	17	−10%	+170%	
	1:40	1.3	13	0%	+369%	
C	9:30	6.7	97			500 units insulin
7/1/40	1:25	4.6	43	+10%	+51%	9:37. 25 gm. glu-
	2:30	4.2	39	+20%	+60%	cose 2:39. 2:43
	3:33	5.7	22	0%	+18%	aroused
Br	10:54	1.5	34			25 gm. glucose
6/27/40	11:15	5.3	117	−20%	−72%	10:56. 10:59 aroused

(1) The first cerebral blood flow was taken as the control and the following changes were expressed in terms of percentage of this standard.

(2) $\dfrac{\text{Control AVO}_2 \text{ diff. minus observed AVO}_2 \text{ diff.}}{\text{observed AVO}_2 \text{ diff.}}$ = per cent change of cerebral

blood flow if brain metabolism remains unchanged. i.e. $\dfrac{6.1 - 4.1}{4.1} = 49\%$

Br, 6/21/40, exhibited an initial arterio-venous oxygen difference of 6.1 vol. per cent and a blood sugar value of 83 mg. per cent. After the injection of insulin, his blood sugar fell during a period of five and one-half hours to 13 mg. per cent. Meanwhile his arterio-venous oxygen difference decreased gradually to 4.1, 2.2, 2.3, and 1.3 vol. per cent. If these differences had been caused by more rapid blood flow, the *calculated* increases in velocity would have been, as seen in column 6, 49, 177, 170 and 369 per cents, respectively. The *observations* of blood flow, however, (column 5) made by a modification of Gibbs' thermostromuhr method (325, 271) revealed the reverse changes. The blood flow was not faster but slower: −10, −30, −10, and 0 per cents. In the experiment on C, 7/1/40, the *calculated* increases of blood flow were 51 and 60 per cents, while the *observed* increases were less, 10 and 20 per cents, respectively. In the second experiment on Br, 6/27/40, the blood flow would have been reduced by 72 per cent if brain metabolism had remained constant. Actually, blood flow slowed down only 20 per cent and brain metabolism increased with the injection of glucose and the arousal of the patient.

is to inject glucose during hypoglycemia, and in this condition to ascertain whether brain metabolism is raised (477). The metabolic changes following such an injection can be seen in the second observation on Br 6/27/40 (Table 1). The arterio-venous oxygen difference rose from 1.5 to 5.3 vol. per cent, while blood sugar increased from 34 to 117 mg. per cent following the intravenous administration of glucose. In this observation, a decrease of 72 per cent in blood flow would have been necessary to cause such a change in arterio-venous oxygen difference if brain metabolism had remained unchanged. Actually, blood flow decreased only 20 per cent. The greater arterio-venous oxygen difference after the administration of glucose was thus caused by a higher metabolic rate of the brain rather than by a diminished cerebral blood flow. This striking increase in cerebral metabolism was reflected in the clinical condition of the patient. Within three minutes after receiving 25 gm. of glucose intravenously, he aroused from his coma. These crucial observations demonstrate that blood sugar is an important factor in determining the rate of brain metabolism. When the supply of glucose is inadequate, brain metabolism decreases below the normal value, but it can be restored by the administration of glucose. Four gm. of glucose injected intravenously is the minimum which will arouse a patient from hypoglycemic coma (1028). The passing of the coma follows a return of the cerebral arterio-venous oxygen difference to approximately 5 vol. per cent. For patients in more profound hypoglycemia, however, a somewhat larger dose, 8 gm., is required. For example, a patient with this dosage temporarily regained contact with his environment as his cerebral arterio-venous oxygen difference rose from 1.3 vol. per cent to 5.0 vol. per cent (477). In view of the fact that the intravenous administration of glucose does not significantly influence cerebral blood flow, the increased arterio-venous oxygen difference is a sufficient indication of a corresponding rise of brain metabolism.

Hypoglycemia, because it deprives the brain of glucose, affords the proper conditions for testing the availability of any other foodstuff to support the energetic demands of the human brain. The results with 4 gm. and 8 gm. of glucose were used as standards, to appraise the effects of the injections of lactic and pyruvic acids. In order to make a thorough evaluation of brain metabolism, observations of cerebral blood flow were made simultaneously with arterio-venous oxygen difference, before and after the injection of lactate or pyruvate. From Table 2 we see that the injection of 20 gm. of racemic sodium lactate in patient Br, 7/8/40, (477) while in hypoglycemic coma produced no significant change either in arterio-venous oxygen difference or cerebral blood flow. On another occasion, the administration of 7.5 gm. of pyruvate to Br, 7/10/40, (477) also failed to alter arterio-venous oxygen difference and blood flow beyond the experimental error. The administration of 10 gm. of pyruvate in an experiment not included in the table also did not change the character of the results. In none of these instances was brain metabolism stimulated sufficiently to arouse the patient though the pyruvate was equivalent and the lactate more than equivalent to the dosage of glucose (8 gm.). The implications of these experiments speak for themselves. They demonstrate what was merely suggested in a much larger series of experiments (1028) where only arterio-venous differences were estimated. In these observations, the average arterio-venous oxygen difference was increased by only 1.3 vol. per cent from 5 to 20 minutes after the injection of 20 gm. of racemic sodium lactate, and 2.2 vol. per cent, 25 to 50 minutes after injection. This increase in arterio-venous oxygen difference, less than that produced by the injection of 8 gm. of glucose, (3.7 vol. per cent) was not adequate to arouse the patients from coma (477). Sodium pyruvate (409) raised the average cerebral arterio-

TABLE 2

Effect of lactate and pyruvate on arterio-venous oxygen differences during insulin hypoglycemia

1 PATIENT AND DATE	2 TIME	3 OXYGEN DIFF. VOL. %	4 GLUCOSE ART. VEN. MG. %		5 LACTIC ACID ART. VEN. MG. %		6 PYRUVIC ACID ART. MG. %	7 REMARKS
Br 7/8/40	12:30 12:44	1.6 1.9	17 17	12 14	13 40	10 43		20 gm. sodium lactate 12:35
Br 7/10/40	11:30 11:50	2.1 2.6	19	24 25	14 31		1.50 2.86	7.5 gm. sodium pyruvate 11:37

venous oxygen difference by only 1.2 vol. per cent and also failed to arouse the patient. The results on the brain *in situ*, therefore, fail to confirm those obtained on excised cerebral tissues, for in the latter, glucose, lactic and pyruvic acids were equally effective, whereas the *in situ* experiments place glucose far above either pyruvate or lactate in availability to the brain.

The reasons for the failure of lactic and pyruvic acids to raise brain metabolism sufficiently to arouse the patient are not entirely clear. This phenomenon may involve at least two factors: (1) ability of the brain to oxidize the various foodstuffs after they have entered the cerebral cells, and (2) permeability of the brain to the foodstuff. It might be assumed that lactate and pyruvate are consumed too slowly to support cerebral function adequately. Excised cerebral tissues, however, are capable of oxidizing lactic (674, 24, 738, 739) and pyruvic acids (674, 24, 805, 788, 789, 570, 271) as rapidly as glucose, and this should be expected to hold for the brain *in vivo* since the same oxidative enzymes are present in both preparations. On the other hand it is probable that the pressure of oxygen is not the same throughout the brain and that areas not immediately adjacent to capillaries may suffer a partial deprivation of oxygen. Nevertheless, the results obtained on the brain *in vivo*, instead of being due to the difference in oxidative rates, may be ascribed to a greater permeability of the brain *in situ* to glucose than to lactate and pyruvate. A cause for the differential permeability may be the capillaries and especially their epithelial coat, through which the substances must pass before entering the brain *in vivo* (347). In excised cerebral tissues the substances may enter the brain without previous passage through these structures. The question of cerebral permeability and the part played by the surfaces of the brain cells is considered in pages 117–119 and 123.

The observations on lactate reveal that *in situ* the brain is relatively impermeable to that substance (915). Unlike glucose, which is readily absorbed by the brain, lactate reveals no such exchange at normal concentrations (481). A comparison of the resting concentrations of lactate in the arterial and venous blood of the brain does not disclose utilization even during hypoglycemia (481) when recourse must be had to some other foodstuff than glucose. In those patients who exhibit hypoglycemia without convulsions, there is no rise in the level of lactate because of the absence of violent muscular exercise. Though the absorption of lactic acid by the brain cannot be demonstrated at resting levels, yet that organ is not entirely impermeable to this substance, as can be proved when the level of this acid in the blood is considerably elevated. This phenomenon has been observed in the normal (724) animal. Some absorption of lactate (1028) was also noted after its injection in hypoglycemic patients. These observations are in accord with the conclusion of Stone (915) that the diffusion rate of lactate between blood and brain is slow. The failure of the injected lactate to raise cerebral metabolism sufficiently to arouse the patients may be attributed therefore to a sluggish rate of cerebral penetration. The slight clinical effect of pyruvate (409) may similarly be ascribed to a slow transfer from blood to brain (610). Yet the possibility of a retarded oxidation cannot be ruled out in view of the fact that the brain releases small but definite amounts of lactate (391) and pyruvate (524) to the blood.

Alcohol has also been administered to patients in hypoglycemia. Goldfarb and Wortis (408) gave 200 cc. of 25 per cent alcohol by mouth to each of 10 patients and 50 cc. of 10 per cent alcohol, intravenously to an 11th. The average cerebral arterio-venous oxygen difference (AVO$_2$ difference) was 3.0 vol. per cent before alcohol and 3.1 vol. per cent after alcohol, and this in spite of the fact that the brain is permeable to that agent (388). Since the administration of ethyl alcohol failed to raise the cerebral AVO$_2$ difference and to reestablish contact with the environment of patients in hypoglycemic coma, it is probable that the metabolic processes of the brain cannot be supported adequately by the oxidation of ethyl alcohol.

(See Chapter 12 discussion of the narcotic effects of alcohol and an evaluation of its ability to depress cerebral oxidation).

Finally, glutamic acid (716) has been reported to be efficacious in restoring environmental contact during insulin hypoglycemia. This restorative action may be attributed to the oxidation of glutamate by the brain. But before coming to a final conclusion other factors should be considered: for example the cerebral impermeability to glutamate (606) and the ability of the body to convert that substance to carbohydrate, an action which probably occurs chiefly in the liver. In that way glutamate may afford an indirect source of glucose.

According to Mayer-Gross and Walker (716) and Weil-Malherbe (785a) the restorative action of glutamic acid can not be attributed either to its direct utilization as fuel for the brain cells or to its conversion into glucose by the liver. The latter has calculated that the rise in blood sugar produced by minimal effective doses was four times greater than could be accounted for by the amount of glutamic acid injected and concludes that its action is due to adrenergic stimulation causing the mobilization of hepatic glycogen. That investigator points to the similarity between the results of injection of glutamic acid and those of adrenaline not only on blood sugar but also on blood pressure and pulse rate. He also suggests that adrenergic stimulation may account for the therapeutic effects of glutamic acid in mental deficiency.

Except for glutamate the patient with hypoglycemia has not been used to study the availability of substrates other than glucose, lactate and pyruvate and alcohol for brain conditions. The opportunity for testing other foodstuffs is available, however, as long as patients with schizophrenia are treated with insulin hypoglycemia.[9]

Brain IN SITU of a hepatectomized preparation. In the last section the effect of the removal and injection of glucose on the oxygen utilization of the brain was stressed, and the clinical results on the mental status of the patient were also mentioned. Additional observations of cerebral activities other than oxidative, i.e., maintenance of life, and the normal electroencephalogram (see Chapter 6, p. 106), are afforded by study of an animal deprived of its liver under surgical operation, known as the hepatectomized preparation. The results obtained with this preparation are of interest to us because the substances which maintain life in the hepatectomized animal must do so largely by supporting the functions of the central nervous system. Following the removal of the liver, which is the chief endogenous source of blood sugar, continued utilization of this

[9] Acetopyruvic acid exhibits a protective action in rats against death by insulin hypoglycemia. Probably the pyruvic moiety of the acetopyruvic molecule contributes to the carbohydrate metabolism of the animal (643).

substance soon brings on a state of hypoglycemia. Only the brain is deprived of energy by this rapid fall of blood sugar because the other organs can still carry on their functions by the oxidation of fat. The disappearance of blood sugar therefore creates the condition whereby the effects of glucose and other substrates of the brain may be studied. It is well known that the liver absorbs the various hexoses, transforms them into glycogen and returns them in the blood in the form of glucose (see Chapter 3). For that reason, it is significant that fructose[10] does not sustain the hepatectomized preparation (705, 706), this being one of the hexoses which is transformed to glucose in the liver. Even in the absence of the liver, some carbohydrates are converted to glucose by enzymes in the blood, while other carbohydrates remain stable. Carbohydrates which retain their structure, and are not changed to glucose in the blood, such as sucrose, lactose and inulin, cannot maintain the life of an animal after extirpation of the liver. There are other carbohydrates, according to Mann (705, 706), which can support the hepatectomized preparation because they are changed to glucose in the blood stream. These are mannose, maltose and glycogen. The possibility exists that mannose is oxidized by the brain directly without previous transformation to glucose (805). Among the non-carbohydrates which assume carbohydrate form as a result of the action of the liver, neither glycine nor lactic and pyruvic acids have any restorative effect after hepatectomy. The results with lactic (674, 24, 738) and pyruvic (805, 788, 789) acids are in striking contrast with those obtained on excised cerebral tissues, but in agreement with the observations on patients in insulin hypoglycemia (1028). Other non-carbohydrates such as ethyl alcohol and acetic acid are of no avail after hepatectomy.

[10] The fact that fructose supports the metabolism of excised cerebral tissues does not necessarily contradict the observation that the intravenous injection of fructose is of no avail to the hepatectomized preparation, because the observations of Klein and co-workers (609) disclose that fructose passes from blood to brain at a rate which is much slower than that of glucose.

It is also of some interest that the metabolism of fructose proceeds more slowly than that of glucose as can be concluded from the experiments of Meyerhof and Wilson (741). The less rapid glycolysis of fructose by brain extracts than that of glucose, observed by these workers, may be explained by their demonstration that the transfer of phosphate from adenosinetriphosphate to fructose proceeds at a slow rate in the presence of glucose. This difference in rates of transphosphorylation is a result of the greater affinity of glucokinase for glucose than for fructose (883a). Brain in contradistinction to liver and muscle does not possess fructokinase as well as glucokinase. (See Chapter 5, Page 71 for a brief discussion of the enzymes catalyzing the phosphorylation of various hexoses). In addition to the handicaps of permeability and metabolism fructose is readily excreted by the kidney whenever its concentration rises in the blood stream, again rendering that substance less valuable than glucose for brain metabolism.

These observations on the ability of foodstuffs to maintain life agree, on the whole, with others in which the electroencephalogram was used as an indicator of the substrates which supported the brain of a hepatectomized preparation (701). The electroencephalogram (EEG), which undergoes changes characteristic of hypoglycemia following hepatectomy, was restored to normal by glucose, mannose and maltose, but fructose and galactose, pyruvate, hexose diphosphate, glyceric aldehyde, succinate and glutamate were without restorative action. Thus glucose and substances which may change to glucose in the blood stream are efficacious in sustaining the hepatectomized preparation, as judged by either of the above criteria. Comparing the results obtained with excised cerebral tissues, human subjects in insulin hypoglycemia, and the hepatectomized animal, the weight of evidence points to glucose as the substance of prime importance in supporting brain metabolism.

B. *The respiratory quotient as an indicator of the foodstuff used by the brain*

One of the most useful indicators of the foodstuffs oxidized in the body is the respiratory quotient. This quotient is a ratio between the volume of carbon dioxide produced and the volume of oxygen consumed in metabolism, and is obtained by analysis of the inspired and expired air for oxygen and carbon dioxide. This ratio has been widely employed to determine the energy exchanges of the entire body because each foodstuff possesses a characteristic respiratory quotient, and differentiation can be made between the various foodstuffs oxidized by the resting subject.

The oxidation of fat produces a quotient of 0.7, and of protein, 0.8, while the combustion of carbohydrate yields a respiratory quotient of 1.0. After the ingestion of mixed diets, values between 0.7 and 1.0 are generally observed. When computing the respiratory quotient of a single organ, samples of its arterial and venous blood are analyzed for carbon dioxide and oxygen content, per 100 cc. of blood traversing the organ. This technic has been applied to the brain, and in 1929 (519) it was first disclosed that the brain of anesthetized or unanesthetized dogs possesses an average respiratory quotient of 1.0 under a wide variety of conditions (519).[11] This value was also observed in the brain of anesthetized cats (196) and monkeys (856). For the dog, cat and monkey brain, then, carbohydrate is the chief source of energy.

In 1931 (650), an average respiratory quotient of 0.95 was found in 120

[11] In these experiments the analyses of the blood gases probably reflected accurately the gaseous contents of the blood *in vivo*. The samples were collected without contact with air and kept over mercury in specially constructed glass containers so there could be no interchange of gases between blood and air. Oxalate and fluoride were used to inhibit coagulation and glycolysis and the blood samples were analyzed soon after collection.

observations of the brain of human beings. The small deviation from unity may be attributed to chance variations, and to the error inherent in the method. These fluctuations became less significant in a larger series of more than 250 observations (1025) which yielded an average of 0.98. In another series of observations of 50 intelligent, healthy, electroencephalographically normal young men, the average respiratory quotient was 0.99 (392). Because of the (64, 389) different sources of the blood in the right and left internal jugular veins of most individuals (see Chapter 6) the bilateral similarity of the cerebral respiratory quotients in resting man (399) indicates that the respiratory quotient is the same throughout the brain. Though the extracerebral source of a fraction of the internal jugular venous blood must be taken into consideration, probably the chief factor in the distortion of an individual respiratory quotient is the discomfort that may attend the collection of the blood samples. Any interference with the normal respiratory pattern may temporarily alter the gaseous exchange. Increased respiratory efforts, consequent to fear or pain, may not only alter the carbon dioxide and oxygen content of the arterial blood, but also cause an excessive loss of carbon dioxide from the body, as well as retard the cerebral blood flow, both of which may influence the carbon dioxide and oxygen content of the cerebral venous blood (770, 390). Despite these technical obstacles, the average ratio remains sufficiently close to 1.0 to indicate that the human brain is supported in its function chiefly, if not entirely, by the energy obtained from the combustion of carbohydrate,—in this case, the glucose obtained from the blood. This conclusion renders it improbable that fat and protein provide significant amounts of energy for cerebral metabolism in normal conditions. Fats and proteins, however, do play their part in the structure and function of nervous tissues (384).[12] The proteins are found most abundantly in the grey matter, and along with vitamins and minerals, make up the cerebral enzyme systems (Chapter 5). The grey matter also contains some lipids, but the greatest part of the lipids is used for the formation of the myelin sheaths.

[12] Hydén and Hartelius (550) employed the ultra violet microscope and demonstrated the utilization of protein substances both with motor activity and sensory stimulation. Restitution of these substances occurs with the assistance of polynucleotides. Malononitrile, $CH_2 (CN)_2$, exerts a potent effect on the nucleoprotein metabolism and in the rabbit stimulates the large nerve cells to increased production of nucleic acids and protein substances.

Patients suffering from severe psychic disorders reveal low nucleoproteins in the pyramidal cells of the frontal cortex (Lamina III). On this basis malononitrile was injected into patients with schizophrenia or depression, most of whom had failed to respond to other treatments. The results were construed to be in the nature of a favorable stimulation and it was concluded by the authors that psychic functions correlated with the neucleoprotein metabolism of the nerve cell.

The cerebral respiratory quotient may be obtained not only from the brain *in situ* but also by an examination of surviving (excised) cerebral tissues. The respiratory quotient of such tissues in the presence of glucose is unity according to most observers (674, 240, 1029, 237), confirming the conclusion for the brain *in situ*, and emphasizing the importance of glucose in particular as a foodstuff for the brain. Quotients approaching 0.9 (489, 32, 270, 272), and indicating the oxidation of some non-carbohydrate food-stuffs along with carbohydrates, have also been reported. In the absence of any substrate the respiratory quotient of excised cerebral tissues is still lower. Such values however may be a result of artifactual processes which do not occur *in vivo*. Even though non-carbohydrate foodstuffs may supply energy for excised cerebral tissues, the energy so obtained in the presence of glucose is adequate to maintain only a small part of brain metabolism.

C. *Quantitative comparison of cerebral oxygen intake and carbohydrate utilized*

So far, the experimentation leads us to believe that of all the possible foodstuffs of the brain, glucose is the most important. Additional evidence in support of this conception can be obtained by a quantitative comparison of the glucose consumed and the oxygen utilized by the brain. In one series of experiments (32) on excised cerebral tissues of rats, the glucose utilized accounted for approximately ¾ of the oxygen consumption. In another series of such experiments the glucose disappearance accounted for the entire oxygen intake. The oxidation of glucose, therefore, accounts for the greatest part of the oxygen intake of excised cerebral tissues.[13]

Although these carbohydrate balances of excised tissues afford information on fundamental energy exchanges, only a study of the brain *in situ* can reveal the energy requirements of the functioning brain. Such balances were obtained for human beings by analysis of cerebral arterial and venous blood samples for glucose and oxygen. Because no significant differences were noted in the results obtained from schizophrenic patients and from normal subjects, values for both will be considered together. The average figure for the arterio-venous oxygen difference in the normal unanesthetized human being has been reported as 6.4, 6.7, and 6.9 vol. per cent by three groups of observers (392, 391, 1025). A value of 6.7 vol.

[13] A comparison can be made between the oxygen and glucose utilization because 3 cc. of oxygen are required for the combustion of approximately 4 mg. of glucose. In the first series of experiments the glucose utilization of excised cerebral tissues *calculated* from the oxygen intake, according to the above relationship, was 2.1 mg. per 100 mg. dry weight of tissue per hour, and the *observed* utilization, 1.6 mg. In the second series of experiments, both the *calculated* and *estimated* utilizations of glucose coincided with a value of 1.1 mg.

per cent may therefore be regarded as the resting cerebral arterio-venous oxygen difference. This amount is close to those reported on patients with schizophrenia, 6.7 (1025), 6.8 (508) (512), and 7.0 vol. per cent (480) (481). The average glucose intake may be taken as 10 mg. per cent, the result of carefully controlled experiments on a series of normal young men (392). This value concurs with that of two other series of normal human beings whose averages were 9 mg. per cent (1025) and 10 mg. per cent (392), and also with observations of 10 mg. per cent (1025) and 12 mg. per cent (481) on two series of schizophrenic patients. An oxygen consumption of 6.7 vol. per cent is satisfied by 8.9 mg. per cent of glucose. The small difference between the latter figure and the observed one, 10 mg. per cent, is accounted for by the conversion of glucose to lactic and pyruvic acids, for the brain releases 1.6 mg. per cent of lactic acid (391) and 0.22 mg. per cent of pyruvic acid (524). In the dog, a similar ratio of a slight excess of glucose utilization in relation to oxygen intake is observed (492). The consumption of oxygen is 9 vol. per cent and of sugar, 14 mg. per cent. This ratio, noted both in human beings and in dogs indicates that the energy requirements of the brain *in situ* may be fulfilled entirely by the sugar removed from the blood.

III. SUMMARY

A review of the data on the foodstuffs used by the brain reveals that the oxidation of various carbohydrates, especially glucose, as well as of non-carbohydrates, including lactic and pyruvic acids, maintains the steady oxygen consumption of excised cerebral tissues.

The evaluation of the role of glucose, lactic and pyruvic acids for the brain *in situ* was studied on patients subjected to insulin hypoglycemia. Lacking glucose, brain metabolism was diminished as evidenced by a decrease of the arterio-venous oxygen difference while blood flow remained relatively constant. Following the administration of glucose, brain metabolism was restored towards normal levels. Lactate and pyruvate were less effective than glucose in augmenting brain metabolism possibly because of relative impermeability of the blood-brain barrier to substances carrying negative charges.

These conclusions obtained from the study of the human brain were confirmed by observations that the hepatectomized animal could be sustained by some carbohydrates but not by non-carbohydrate substances. Glucose, and carbohydrates which may change to glucose in the blood, were effective. Lactic and pyruvic acids were of no avail.

Further evidence on the foodstuff used by the brain may be obtained by determining its respiratory quotient. *In vivo* the cerebral respiratory quotient of the human being, the monkey, the dog, and the cat is 1.0

within the limits of the experimental error, indicating that carbohydrate is oxidized exclusively. The respiratory quotient of cerebral tissues excised from various mammals may be lower than 1.0, but approaches unity in the presence of glucose. This evidence indicates that the oxidation of the carbohydrate, glucose, supplies most, if not all, of the energy required to maintain cerebral functions.

The conclusion that glucose is the chief substrate of the brain is supported by additional evidence obtained from glucose balances and oxygen utilizations. For excised tissues of the rat, the greatest part of the oxygen taken in by the brain is consumed in the combustion of glucose. In man and dog, the oxygen consumption of the brain *in situ* can be accounted for entirely by the oxidation of glucose absorbed from the blood passing through the brain. In view of this function of glucose, blood sugar assumes a role of special importance in sustaining brain metabolism.

CHAPTER 3

MECHANISMS FOR MAINTAINING THE CARBOHYDRATE SUPPLIES OF THE BRAIN

I. FUNDAMENTAL FACTORS OF CARBOHYDRATE METABOLISM

In the previous chapter, the relationship of the level of blood glucose to the maintenance of brain metabolism was presented. The data reviewed indicate that hypoglycemia causes a diminution of the cerebral metabolic rate and that the reestablishment of the normal concentration of blood sugar restores brain metabolism. Because of this metabolic relationship, it becomes necessary to examine the factors controlling the level of blood sugar as well as the fundamental processes involved in carbohydrate metabolism.

Although glucose may be formed from both protein and the glycerol fraction of fat after they have been processed in the body, the only readily available source is carbohydrate. All forms of carbohydrate except glucose must also go through several preliminary steps before they become "blood sugar". When carbohydrates are ingested, they are split by the enzymes of the gastro-intestinal tract to their proximate principles which are hexoses, compounds containing six carbon atoms; for example, sucrose is split to glucose and fructose, and lactose to glucose and galactose. After a meal containing carbohydrate, these hexoses are absorbed from the intestines into the blood stream where they increase in concentration before they pass to all body fluids. This excess of hexoses throughout the body is termed *inundation* (146). From the body fluids the hexoses enter the cells of the various organs: brain, liver, muscle, heart and kidney. When the concentration of any particular hexose in the blood exceeds the renal threshold, it is excreted in the urine (Fig. 2). Glucose, for example, is excreted when its concentration rises to approximately 180 mg. per 100 cc. of blood. A portion of the hexoses retained in the body is oxidized in the various organs. The hexoses not immediately oxidized may be either converted to glycogen and stored, chiefly in liver (340, 405, 38) and muscle (189, 87, 381), or they may be transformed to fat (254).

The liver has an important role in carbohydrate metabolism. It not only converts the various hexoses to glycogen (185), but also exerts a similar effect on certain 3-carbon compounds, such as lactic acid, pyruvic acid,[1]

[1] Studies with tagged carbon atoms show that carbon dioxide and 4-carbon compounds are intermediary substances in glycogen formation. This reaction may take place through pyruvate (957, 1019).

and the glycerol fraction of fat. The liver, in addition, possesses the ability to form glycogen from some of the deaminized amino acids.[2]

The liver is the chief organ, though not the only one (841, 818), which

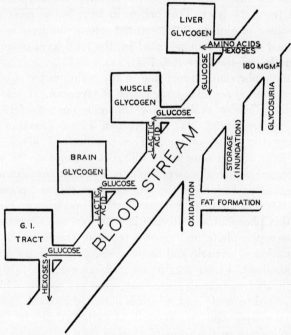

Fig. 2. The changes of carbohydrate metabolism produced by the activities of the various organs of the body. After a meal the hexoses, products of carbohydrate digestion in the gastro-intestinal tract, are absorbed into the blood stream where they increase in concentration. From there they are absorbed by all the tissues of the body as indicated for the liver, muscle, and brain, and back again to the gastro-intestinal tract, but for the latter only in the postabsorptive state to maintain its metabolism until the next meal. If the concentration of the hexoses exceeds 180 mg. per cent, they are eliminated through the kidneys (glycosuria). Otherwise, they may be either stored as such (inundation), or in the form of glycogen, they may be transformed into fat, or oxidized. It should be noted that whereas liver glycogen is broken down to glucose before entering the blood, muscle and brain glycogen must first be transformed to lactic acid.

converts these various substances to glycogen. Formation of glycogen (glycogenesis) augments hepatic glycogen stores and makes possible two other important functions of the liver: the breakdown of hepatic glycogen to glucose (glycogenolysis) and the subsequent release of this glucose to the blood stream. No matter from what substance the hepatic glycogen is

[2] See Peters and Van Slyke (786) Table 8, pg. 140 for list of compounds that can be converted to glycogen.

synthesized, it is converted to only one form of hexose—glucose—before it is released into the blood stream. In the post-absorptive period, the period following completion of digestion, the various hexoses are no longer absorbed from the intestines. The source of blood sugar therefore is the glucose freed from the liver. This organ, in fact, is the most important endogenous source of glucose. The essential role of the liver in the maintenance of blood sugar is demonstrated by the fatal hypoglycemia which follows extirpation of the liver (98, 705).

Skeletal muscle plays an indirect role in the maintenance of blood sugar level. Like the liver, it contains large stores of glycogen. Muscle glycogen, however, is not directly available for the maintenance of blood sugar because, like the brain (392, 524), its glycogen is transformed to lactic acid before entering the blood stream. The products of glycogen breakdown in the liver and in muscle are different because of the manner in which these organs handle glucosephosphate. The liver contains an enzyme (186), phosphatase, which frees the glucose from this compound so that it can enter the blood stream without further breakdown. Muscle does not contain this phosphatase. Glucose is therefore not liberated, but instead the glucosephosphate undergoes a series of transformations ending with the formation of pyruvic and lactic acids. (See Chapter 5 for carbohydrate metabolism). Under conditions such as exercise (516) and adrenalemia (188, 189), muscle glycogen may serve as a source of blood sugar by being converted to lactic acid, which is liberated into the blood stream, absorbed by the liver and reconverted to carbohydrate in that organ. Hepatic carbohydrate in the form of glucose then returns to muscle via the blood stream from which it is absorbed and stored as glycogen. The cycle (516, 189) may be diagrammed as follows:

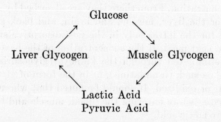

This glucose-lactic acid cycle is made possible by the differences in the enzyme systems which facilitate the formation of glucose in liver and lactic acid in muscle (186). The liberation of glucose from the liver and absorption of that substance by muscle is a continuous phenomenon. Lactic acid, however, is liberated from muscle only after it accumulates in that organ. A high concentration of lactic acid in the blood is one of the two requisites for the absorption of lactic acid by the liver. The other is a low concentration of glycogen in the liver (163, 506). Pyruvate, in general, follows the pattern of lactate (527) and the hepatic absorption of pyruvate is facilitated by hyperpyruvemia and a fasted nutritional status.

The glucose-lactic acid cycle is the mechanism whereby a hypoglycemic depression is lightened, sometimes to the point of regaining contact with environment, after convulsions have enveloped the body. Such violent muscular activity accelerates the energetic demands of the muscle and at the same time decreases the oxygen supply by interfering with the respiratory movements. Lactic acid released to the blood stream as a result of the convulsions is absorbed by the partially depleted liver and then *made available in the* form of glucose. The brain receives a portion of this additional glucose and thereby metabolic depression is either lessened or dispelled completely for a short while.

II. The neuroendocrine regulation of blood sugar level

A. *Anatomical components*

We have discussed some of the processes which are responsible for the presence of glucose in the blood. During post-absorptive conditions, however, additional mechanisms maintain the blood sugar within the normal limits of 70 to 110 mg. per cent.[3] These regulatory mechanisms usually prevent blood sugar from rising above 180 mg. per cent even after the ingestion of one to two grams of carbohydrate per kilogram of body weight.

The maintenance of blood sugar within these narrow limits is complicated and involves both neural and hormonal elements. The hormonal element consists of the principles of the islands of Langerhans, the adrenal medulla, anterior pituitary, adrenal cortex, thyroid gland, ovary, and perhaps the posterior pituitary. The neural element is formed of the two branches of the autonomic nervous system, the sympathetic and parasympathetic. The sympathetic branch influences the level of blood sugar

---

[3] The exact value in the healthy individual varies with the method employed for determining blood sugar. But in patients with disease of endocrine glands, of the autonomic nervous division or of the liver, the blood sugar level may be abnormally altered as discussed elsewhere in this chapter. Gildea, Mailhouse and Morris (402) report that the psychotic patient, even when in greatest excitement, fails to exhibit the hyperglycemia which is a usual accompaniment of intense emotional stress in the non-psychotic individual. On the other hand according to Braccland, Meduna, and Vaichulis (106) the administration of the two-dose glucose tolerance test to patients in an acute schizophrenic episode reveals an abnormally high level of blood sugar. The results of these two groups of workers are not necessarily contradictory since their experimental conditions were not the same. The reader is referred to the original papers for further discussion. Hoskins (541a) reveiws the regulation of blood sugar level in schizophrenia and includes it as part of the pattern of a defective homeostasis which he concludes characterizes that disorder.

by regulating the hormonal element, adrenaline. This hormone limits a dangerous fall in blood sugar. The parasympathetic branch changes the level of blood sugar by controlling the hormonal element, insulin. This hormone acts to prevent a rise of blood sugar which might result in the renal elimination of glucose.

For both branches of the autonomic division of the nervous system there are suprabulbar and medullary centers which are connected with each other. (See Chapter 11 for further discussion on this subject). The medullary parasympathetic centers send out efferent impulses by way of the vagus nerve to the islands of Langerhans situated in the pancreas. The medullary sympathetic centers transmit impulses through fibers to the lateral horn cells of the spinal cord, and from them to the peripheral sympathetic efferents of the adrenal medullae (158, 159, 160, 161, 545). In the final analysis, the action of the parasympathetic is dependent on the ability of the islands of Langerhans to release insulin; while the activity of the sympathetic rests partly on the ability of the adrenal medulla to release adrenaline. The reason that this branch does not depend entirely on the adrenal medulla is that the sympathetic axons also elaborate adrenaline. In addition to adrenaline, nor-adrenaline (arterenol) is released both by the adrenal medulla and by adrenergic nerves. Nor-adrenaline (149) differs somewhat from adrenaline physiologically (295) and is demethylated adrenaline, chemically.

B. *Parasympatho-insulin apparatus*

That one of the peripheral portions constituting the parasympathetic branch of the autonomic division, the right vagus nerve, carries impulses which can stimulate the island of Langerhans has been shown in experiments by Britton (114) and La Barre (634). Both experimenters stimulated the vagus directly with a tetanizing electric current. La Barre demonstrated an increased insulin content of venous blood returning from the pancreas; and Britton, a fall of blood sugar in this same kind of experiment. The usual stimulus for the vagal activity on the islands of Langerhans is a high level of blood sugar acting upon the cerebral centers of the parasympathetic system. Using an entirely different preparation, Zunz and La Barre (1036, 1037) perfused the head of a dog, making it independent of its own blood but not of its nerve supply. Though their experiments were not confirmed by another group of workers (368), still their conclusions are essentially sound, namely, that: a fall in systemic blood sugar is the response to the perfusion of the brain with hyperglycemic blood. These conclusions are supported by the observations of Hoet and Ernould (532) who observed a more persistent and higher level of the hyperglycemic curve in the vagotomized than in normal rabbits. The normal response may be ascribed to the influence of the high level of blood sugar on the parasympathetic centers situated in the hypothalamus and the bulb, and to the subsequent increased flow of insulin. The bulbar centers, since they give rise to the vagus nerve, are essential for the increased reflex insulin secretion. Recently Gellhorn (374) has presented new data on the role of the vagus on insulin secretion and some of this evidence is reviewed in Chapter 11, pages 314–316 of this volume.

The insulin apparatus may be stimulated directly (12) as well as by nervous reflex. The influence of direct stimulation has been observed by Gayet and Guillaumie (366, 367) who first removed the pancreas of a dog, and then grafted the same animal with the pancreas of another dog. The transplanted pancreas was deprived of all its nervous connections; nevertheless, the level of blood sugar was regulated by this denervated organ (12). Though by this direct response the level of blood sugar is reduced without nervous intervention, the latter may render the insulin apparatus more sensitive to a small rise of sugar in the intact organism.

It is probable that in post-absorptive periods, the islands of Langerhans are in continuous operation at a comparatively low level of activity in response to slight direct and reflex stimulation. This activity is increased by any rise of blood sugar above the normal levels; such, for example, as occurs after each meal containing carbohydrate. In a person taking the usual three daily meals, blood sugar may be expected to mount after each meal. This hyperglycemia facilitates an increased activity of the parasympathetic centers situated in the hypothalamus and the bulb. Impulses arising from these centers then go on through the vagus to the islands of Langerhans, increasing the secretion of insulin. The rise of blood sugar also acts directly on the island apparatus. As a result of the two sources of stimulation, the amount of insulin liberated by the pancreas is increased and the extent to which blood sugar can rise is limited. The reader is referred to Chapter 5 for a more detailed description of fundamental reactions by which insulin prevents the rise of blood sugar. In brief, however, one action of insulin is to overcome an hormonal inhibition which prevents the initial reaction in the utilization of blood glucose by the tissues. The anterior pituitary (178) halts the use of glucose by blocking this first metabolic step (800) and in this regard the adrenal cortex plays only an accessary role to reinforce the anterior pituitary (801). With the aid of insulin these inhibitory effects are lifted and the initial threshold is successfully passed as blood sugar falls. Insulin not only facilitates the entrance of glucose into the metabolic machinery but subsequently affects the metabolic processes by accelerating the reaction governing the rate of glycogen formation in the liver. By influencing the enzyme phosphorylase hepatic glycogen is stored more rapidly (927)[4] during glucose plethora. When glucose is available to the non-nervous tissues the results of insulin are diverse and two of the foremost are: the promotion of carbohydrate oxidation in non-nervous tissues[5] (185, 37, 86, 87, 39), the acceleration of glycogen storage in liver (381, 847, 92) and muscle (189). In the depancreatized animal[6] however the oxidation of carbohydrate decreases in all organs except the brain (see Chapter 5, Sect. III), and the carbohydrate stores of the body, particularly those of the liver, are depressed. The injection

[4] Insulin when injected into the intact animal may raise blood sugar temporarily and also causes glycogenolysis by its action on liver cells (929). The portion of the insulin preparation which causes these paradoxical results, unlike insulin, does not arise in the beta cells of the islands of Langerhans but appears as a contaminant in some commercial preparations of insulin. One source of this contaminant is the alpha cells of the islands and the physiological role of that substance is yet to be elucidated. The acceleration of glycogenolysis therefore can not be regarded as characteristic of endogenous insulin.

[5] The anterior pituitary principle does not retard carbohydrate metabolism in the brain perhaps, as suggested in Chapter 5, because it does not penetrate that organ. Thus the brain appears to be the exception to the general rule that the anterior pituitary hormone and insulin regulate the initial reaction in the utilization of glucose. These hormones however play important parts in cerebral carbohydrate metabolism due to their influence on blood sugar level, the theme of this chapter. Insulin affects the brain indirectly not only by lowering blood sugar but also by influencing other blood constituents (557, 448) and the contents of the cerebrospinal fluid (263, 898, 899). Phosphorus, potassium and amino acids are among some of the substances altered following insulin injection. In this chapter we are specifically concerned with the neuroendocrine control of the cerebral food supply, but it must be remembered that the endocrine glands exert manifold effects on the brain. They may modify the cerebral metabolic rate, as in the case of thyroxin, by accelerating the general metabolic rate. (See Chapter 9 for description of thyroid action). Androgen on the other hand may act on brain oxidations directly. Eisenberg, Gordan and Elliott (269) have been able to show that the presence of testosterone, whether *in vitro* or *in vivo*, depresses the oxygen intake of cell suspensions from the cerebral hemispheres of rats. These authors believe that testosterone functions as a metabolic brake upon the oxidation of glucose by rat brain. It would seem that testosterone, a steroid, unlike the protein anterior pituitary hormone, penetrates the blood-brain barrier. The studies of Weil and co-workers have revealed that the chemical constitution of the brain may be modified by the action of the male and female sex hormones (982) thyroxin (989, 980) and the principles of the adrenal cortex (983).

[6] Pancreatectomy in dog and cat produces severe derangements similar to those observed in the clinical picture of diabetes in man. Far milder changes however, occur after pancreactetomy in rabbit (415) and goat (695) and in duck (750) and owl (768). Even in man surgical removal of the pancreas causes a relatively mild type of diabetes with the low daily insulin requirement of 30-50 units (823). Though the role of the pancreas in diabetes is not well understood the therapeutic action of insulin and the ability of that hormone to increase the oxidation of carbohydrate are well established (786).

of insulin in such a preparation restores normal carbohydrate metabolism (38).

Insulin exerts additional effects and one of these is to retard the transformation of protein to carbohydrate (748) and thus to diminish glycogen storage in the liver. According to Drury (254) insulin also accelerates the formation of fat from carbohydrate, an action which is of greatest quantitative importance during carbohydrate plethora. (See Chapter 4 for further discussion on the action of insulin).

C. *Sympatho-adrenaline apparatus*

In contrast with the parasympathetic member of the autonomic division which, as we have said, limits a rise of blood sugar, the sympathetic member counteracts a fall of blood sugar. Macleod (699) demonstrated that this action to antagonize a fall of blood sugar is caused by impulses passing through the splanchnic nerves to the adrenal medullae and liver. The splanchnic impulses to the liver mobilize hepatic glycogen so that greater amounts of glucose are discharged into the blood stream. The impulses to the adrenal medullae then stimulate the liberation of adrenaline to the blood stream (148, 544), which in turn, acts synergistically with the splanchnic nerves to enhance hepatic glycogenolysis and thus raise blood sugar (635).

Claude Bernard (83) presented the first evidence for the existence of sympathetic centers in the medulla oblongata when he found that puncture of the floor of the fourth ventricle of the brain is followed by hyperglycemia. Since this very effect can be prevented by splanchnectomy, the hyperglycemia must have been caused by sympathetic impulses passing from the medulla oblongata through the splanchnic nerves. A rise of blood sugar is caused not only by medullary centers belonging to the sympathetic division (119), but also by suprabulbar centers. Donhoffer and Macleod (249), by making lesions in various parts of the brain were able to demonstrate a center located in the pons capable of mediating a rise of blood sugar. Hyperglycemia has also been observed when the hypothalamus has been injured, and this holds true regardless of whether the injury is accomplished experimentally by lesions in the brain of animals (843), or whether it occurs in patients as a pathologic degeneration of the cells in and near the hypothalamus (961). A tetanizing current on the hypothalamus achieves the same hyperglycemic effect (515). This rise of blood sugar seems to be peculiar to the hypothalamus because stimulation of other parts of the brain does not bring about such a reaction. Application of the tetanizing current to the cerebellum, for example, does not result in an increase in concentration of blood sugar (515).

Just as the sympathetic centers can be excited by injury, or by a tetanizing current, a third stimulus to these centers is a low blood sugar. First, as a result of the hypoglycemia, the cerebral hemispheres are depressed, and this depression dispenses with the regulatory action of the hemispheres imposed on the subcortical sympathetic centers, which heretofore had been kept in check. These centers thus released facilitate a reflex rise of blood sugar. The action travels along this path: Impulses pass through the hypothalamic, pontine and bulbar centers down to the lateral horn cells of the spinal cord, the lateral ganglia, and finally through the splanchnic nerves to the adrenal medullae and liver. Hepatic glycogenolysis is increased and blood sugar raised.

Adrenaline not only promotes the breakdown of glycogen in the liver but also in the muscle. As adrenaline is liberated into the blood stream,

TABLE 3

Effects of injection of adrenaline on glycogen stores and blood sugar

EFFECT	MUSCLE GLYCOGEN	LIVER GLYCOGEN	BLOOD SUGAR	LACTIC ACID	REMARKS
1.	−	−	+	+	
2.	−	+	+	+	Secretion of insulin

Effect 1. The primary effect of the injection of adrenaline is a depletion of glycogen stores of muscle and liver, and increase in concentration of glucose and lactic acid in the blood.

Effect 2 consists of a redeposition of liver glycogen made possible not only by the previous depletion of hepatic glycogen and increase in lactic acid, but also by the accelerated formation of insulin in response to the high level of blood sugar (171).

the glycogen of liver and muscle is split into glucose and lactic acid, respectively. Later, however, there is a secondary rise of hepatic glycogen which occurs as the lactic acid liberated by muscle is reconverted to glycogen in the liver (847), a process facilitated by the insulin secreted in response to the high blood sugar (171). Adrenaline, by building up the blood lactic acid, accelerates the activity of the glucose-lactic acid cycle and in this way makes muscle carbohydrate available for maintaining blood sugar level. Adrenaline, moreover stimulates the anterior pituitary gland (684a) and thus assures the simultaneous cooperation of the anterior pituitary and the adrenal cortex in combatting hypoglycemia as discussed in the next section.

This review indicates how the two branches of the autonomic division, in conjunction with the two hormones they regulate, act to maintain blood sugar level. Any rise above normal values is counteracted by increased activity of the parasympatho-insulin apparatus, and any fall, by acceleration of the sympatho-adrenaline function.

III. Effect of Hormones, other than Insulin and Adrenaline, on the Level of Blood Sugar

A. *Anterior pituitary*

The neuroendocrine balance of the parasympatho-insulin and sympatho-adrenaline systems is influenced by the principles of the anterior pituitary, adrenal cortex, thyroid and posterior pituitary glands. The responses of these four glands to changes in the level of blood sugar are not results of reflex nervous control but, at least for the anterior pituitary are direct reactions to a low concentration of glucose in the blood as well as indirect responses to the adrenaline evoked by hypoglycemia (684a). In this way, the secretions of these glands regulate the amount of sugar available to the tissues.

The action of the anterior pituitary gland is next in importance to insulin and adrenaline in the control of blood sugar level. The anterior pituitary gland influences blood sugar level not only by virtue of its own product which prevents the initiating reactions required for the metabolism of glucose but also through its relations with other endocrine glands (543), such as the adrenal cortex, thyroid, the gonads and islands of Langerhans, which also determine blood sugar level. The anterior pituitary releases trophic hormones which stimulate the other endocrine glands to activity. When the anterior pituitary cuts down the elaboration of trophic hormones, the activities of these ductless glands subside. Normally a balance is maintained between the products of these glands and their trophic hormones for a reciprocal relationship exists between them. For example the endogenous adrenocorticotrophic hormone production is hampered by a rising titer of adrenal cortical steroids (684a). But with a faster utilization of steroids their production is accelerated by additional adrenocorticotrophic hormone. Any condition of stress, such as hypoglycemia, arouses the anterior pituitary which in turn stimulates its dependent glands including the adrenal cortex. Extirpation of the anterior pituitary results in the complete loss of trophic hormones, finally producing a secondary degeneration of the remaining glands. It has also been suggested that the anterior pituitary gland accelerates the mobilization of liver glycogen and acts synergistically with adrenaline (133, 193, 97, 98). The evidence on this point, however, is controversial (840).

The actions of the anterior pituitary gland have been studied both in the laboratory and in the clinic.[7] Both methods of investigation lead to

[7] The administration of adrenocorticotrophic hormone, for example in rheumatoid arthritis, leads to changes of various types with however, restoration to normal pat-

similar conclusions. They reveal that the anterior pituitary gland is always functioning, though not at a constant rate, to increase the level of blood sugar, partly directly (543, 91), and also with the aid of the adrenal cortex (461). Hypophyseal activity probably depends a great deal upon the level of blood sugar: weakened when the blood sugar is high and diabetogenic action is not required (468, 124); more intense when blood sugar is low. The anterior pituitary, therefore, tends to raise blood sugar during hypoglycemia. Thus, the chief mechanism by which this gland counteracts a fall of blood sugar is by preventing its utilization (800) in non-nervous tissues and a sign of this prevention is a diminution in carbohydrate oxidation. Such a depression is observed following the injection of anterior pituitary extracts when the respiratory quotient falls (838). Glycogen accumulates in muscles perhaps because of the greater utilization of fat as their fuel. In the absence of the anterior pituitary gland, there is the reverse physiologic response: blood sugar falls, the respiratory quotient rises (328, 329, 837), and muscle glycogen stores are reduced. Because of the removal of the diabetogenic effect which occurs with hypophysectomy, an animal thus prepared becomes sensitive to both injected and endogenous insulin. Even in the depancreatized animal, extirpation of the anterior pituitary will ameliorate the diabetic condition as indicated by a fall of blood sugar, and by an increase of respiratory quotient (154). The removal of the inhibitory influence of the anterior pituitary is, however, not adequate to restore completely the ability to utilize glucose. Since the adrenal cortex is regarded as acting only to reinforce the anterior pituitary (801) the entire inhibitory effect might be expected to be eliminated, if this were the only point of insulin attack. The cause for this incomplete restoration in the depancreatized hypophysectomized preparation, known as the Houssay animal (543), must therefore be sought elsewhere than in the initial hormone controlled reaction and may be attributed, in part, to the loss of the effect of insulin upon hepatic phosphorylase, an action not controlled by the anterior pituitary. The resultant retardation of hepatic carbohydrate transformations impedes the ability of the liver to satisfy adequately the tissues' needs for carbohydrate.

The principles of the anterior pituitary exert other complex effects on carbohydrate metabolism (338, 893, 710). In addition to the direct inhibition of glucose utilization, the anterior pituitary through the lactogenic, adrenocorticotrophic, and growth hormones influences carbohydrates indirectly. Here we are not referring to the trophic actions exerted on their

---

terns on cessation of medication. The changes induced include a diabetic condition, Cushing's syndrome and in some instances a psychosis with excitement, hallucinations and delusions.

respective receptors but to the effects of the trophic hormones upon the islands of Langerhans. Crude extracts of the anterior pituitary gland diminish the insulin content of the pancreas, but the purified lactogenic and adrenocorticotrophic hormones cause its accumulation (339). The effect of the latter two to increase the islet content, however, is not adequate to counteract the other anterior pituitary factors so that when crude extract is injected, the insulin concentration within the island apparatus is depressed. The continued injection of large amounts of anterior pituitary extract finally leads to degeneration and atrophy of the beta cells of the islands of Langerhans, the cells which presumably secrete insulin (10, 440, 85).

A suggested (246) mechanism for the destructive action takes into consideration the rise of blood sugar caused by the anterior pituitary injections and the responses of the islet tissue to the long enduring hyperglycemic stimulus: first hyperactivity and then exhaustion. After degeneration of the island apparatus, the anterior pituitary diabetogenic action exerts its depressant effect on glucose utilization unopposed by insulin, and complete diabetes follows (245).

Clinical observations (215) of the effects of excessive secretion of the anterior pituitary gland have been made on patients with acromegaly who may exhibit high blood sugar levels and other symptoms of diabetes. Conversely, Wilder observed patients with hypopituitarism who suffered from severe hypoglycemic attacks (1000).

The action of the anterior pituitary gland to slow carbohydrate utilization is accomplished directly by depressing the glucokinase reaction; indirectly, by stimulating the adrenal cortex as discussed in the next section, pathologically in large doses by causing insular degeneration and lastly by stopping the secretion of insulin at its very source in the pancreas (13).

B. *Adrenal cortex*

The secretion of the adrenal cortex strengthens the effect of the anterior pituitary gland to impede the utilization of glucose by non-nervous tissues (800, 839). The experimental data reveal that injections of adrenal cortical extracts (1038) and synthetically prepared steroids (838, 685, 553) raise blood sugar and depress carbohydrate oxidation (578). Corticosterone, 11-dehydrocorticosterone, 17-hydroxycorticosterone (Kendall's Compound F) (767a) and 11-dehydro-17-hydroxycorticosterone (Kendall's Compound E) also known as cortisone possess diabetogenic activities. Desoxycorticosterone, however, exhibits little effect in comparable doses (685, 553, 943, 660, 989, 414).[8] In contrast to the results from injections

---

[8] These products have been isolated from the adrenal cortex, and also synthesized in the laboratory. In general, their structure resembles that of dehydrocorticosterone

of anterior pituitary extracts, the carbohydrate not oxidized after injection of adrenal cortical compounds is stored in liver (685) instead of in muscle, because of an accelerated transformation of protein to carbohydrate in the liver (838, 685). On the other hand the extirpation of the adrenal cortex reduces the blood sugar level (828, 454, 115, 932), increases the oxidation of carbohydrate, and depletes the carbohydrate stores of the body, particularly those of the liver (187, 188, 683, 299).

Either adrenalectomy (685, 453, 686) or ligation of the adrenal veins (504) ameliorates pancreatic diabetes as the cortical reinforcement of the inhibition emanating from the pituitary gland is eliminated (801). Both operations reduce the blood sugar level and the glycosuria. Although the respiratory quotient has not been computed in adrenalectomy, ligation, at least, results in an increase of the respiratory quotient from the diabetic level of 0.7 to 0.79, indicating the oxidation of some carbohydrate. This improved ability to consume carbohydrate is limited, however, since the administration of carbohydrate results in no further rise of the respiratory quotient. The inhibitory powers of anterior pituitary are still active and account for the remaining depressant effect on carbohydrate oxidation in the depancreatized adrenalectomized dog.

The clinic presents evidence similar to that produced in the laboratory. McQuarrie and Johnson (728) were the first to report symptoms of diabetes requiring insulin in a patient suffering from hyperfunction of the adrenal cortex (904). In contrast, patients with destructive changes in the adrenal cortex, for example in Addison's disease, reveal spontaneous hypoglycemia. In addition to an accelerated oxidation of carbohydrate, the development

DEHYDRO CORTI COSTERONE

whose structural formula is diagrammed below. Only the members of this group which have an oxygen atom on the eleventh carbon atom influence carbohydrate metabolism significantly. Desoxycorticosterone, for example, does not contain an oxygen atom on this carbon.

of hypoglycemia is facilitated by a diminution in the rate of gluconeogenesis from protein. The chief conclusion to be drawn in regard to the influence of the adrenal cortex on the level of blood sugar is that, like the anterior pituitary, the adrenal cortical hormone works to overcome a fall of blood sugar by inhibiting the processing of glucose by non-nervous tissues. Hypoglycemia not only excites the production of adrenocorticotrophic hormone but also of adrenaline. That hormone in turn reinforces the influence of hypoglycemia upon the anterior pituitary gland, thus additional cortical steroids are released into the blood stream (684a).

The hormonal influence of the anterior pituitary and adrenal cortex to diminish the utilization of glucose is neutralized by insulin. The amount of carbohydrate consumed in the body, therefore, depends upon a balance between these two opposing influences. The non-nervous organs of the body possess an intrinsic capacity to metabolize glucose, which may be either accelerated or retarded by shifts of this endocrine balance. The brain, however, oxidizes carbohydrate readily and probably does so independent of hormonal regulation perhaps because the blood-brain barrier (see Chapter 6) is impermeable to the anterior pituitary hormone. Nevertheless, indirectly the islands of Langerhans, anterior pituitary and adrenal cortex do affect cerebral oxidation by their influence on the level of blood sugar.

C. Ovary

The activities of the anterior pituitary and adrenal cortical glands to raise blood sugar level are not only stimulated by hypoglycemia but also by some naturally occurring estrogenic substances such as estradiol and estriol, as well as the artificially produced diethyl-stilbestrol (423, 247, 560, 552). The effects of the estrogens to raise blood sugar level and increase liver glycogen (551) are exerted chiefly through the combined activities of the anterior pituitary gland and the adrenal cortex. In hypophysectomized or adrenalectomized animals (684, 561), the female sex hormones do not produce these results or are less effective (554). In the intact organism, these hormones start a chain of reactions by stimulating the anterior pituitary gland to release the adrenocorticotrophic hormone. The latter then acts upon its specific glandular receptor to cause the liberation of the adrenal cortical hormone which, in turn, influences carbohydrate metabolism. The primary effect of the estrogens, however, is exerted on the anterior pituitary.

Testosterone, the internal secretion of the testicle, unlike the ovarian secretion, probably does not affect carbohydrate metabolism in physiologic concentrations. In distinction to the powerful influence of small doses of stilbestrol, massive ones of testosterone and methyl testosterone are only weakly diabetogenic (658, 720, 552).

D. *Thyroid*

It is important for the regulation of the blood sugar level that the secretion of the thyroid gland is under the control of the anterior pituitary. Hypoglycemia, as well as its attendant adrenalemia, stimulate the anterior pituitary gland and cause the production of the thyrotrophic hormone (684a). The latter evokes the activity of the thyroid gland and its manufacture of thyroxin. Thyroxin like adrenaline accelerates the breakdown of hepatic glycogen. There is reason to believe that both organs act synergistically in this way to combat hypoglycemia. The belief for their synergistic effects is based upon their similarities both in chemical structure and physiologic activity. They both stimulate the sympathetic centers in the brain (378). Additional evidence indicates that the presence of the thyroid gland is necessary for the peripheral action of adrenaline (53), or at least that it sensitizes organs to the stimulating effects of the sympathetic nerves (26). The hyperglycemia induced by adrenaline is increased in the presence of thyroxin when the hepatic glycogen stores are adequate (137). If, however, due to an excessive secretion of thyroxin, glycogen stores are depleted, then adrenaline hyperglycemia will be diminished in comparison with the normal response. Unlike the influence of adrenaline, that of thyroxin on blood sugar level is a prolonged one. Thyroxin does not induce transitory changes in the level of blood sugar because of the comparatively slow development and slow decay of thyroxin activity (632).

E. *Posterior pituitary*

Our knowledge of the effect of the posterior pituitary gland on carbohydrate metabolism has been obtained chiefly by observing the effects of injection of the hormone of that gland. There is little evidence that extirpation of the posterior pituitary gland affects carbohydrate metabolism in a significant manner. An early important experiment was made by Burn (133) who noted that injections of posterior pituitary extract counteracted the low blood sugar level produced by insulin. Rather surprisingly, this extract also exerts the reverse effect as it diminishes a high blood sugar caused by injection of adrenaline (133). At present we have no adequate explanation for the inhibiting effect of injections of pituitrin on adrenaline hyperglycemia. However, the ability of the posterior pituitary extract to combat insulin hypoglycemia may lie in its power to raise blood sugar by mobilizing liver glycogen (371). The hormone of the posterior pituitary gland also produces lactacidemia by breaking down muscle glycogen (514). Thus, posterior pituitary extract accelerates the glucose-lactic acid cycle between liver and muscle. The probable mechanism for this action is a general depression of metabolism (513) which impairs the energy required for glycogen synthesis and therefore favors glycogenolysis both in liver and muscle (371). (For further analysis of the pituitary-insulin antagonism, see Wislicki (1015)).

This review on the endocrine control of blood sugar discloses that only one hormone, insulin, acting under parasympathetic influence lowers the blood sugar level. The chief antagonist of insulin is the sympatho-adrenaline apparatus. The thyroid and posterior pituitary, like adrenaline, act antagonistically to counteract hypoglycemia by mobilizing liver glycogen, while the anterior pituitary, adrenal cortex, and ovary counteract low blood sugar by inhibiting the utilization of glucose in non-nervous tissues. These two kinds of responses do not operate separately. On the contrary, their joint activity is assured by the unifying effect of a single exciting factor as well as the ability of adrenaline to stimulate the anterior pituitary.[9] That gland in turn not only liberates adrenocorticotrophic hormone to act on the adrenal cortex but also thyrotrophic hormone to arouse the thyroid gland. These four glands, at least, are bound together in a hormonal alliance to oppose hypoglycemia. Nature apparently takes great care to halt any fall of blood sugar, as can be seen by the multiplicity of factors which act to prevent such a catastrophe. This multiplicity of defense against hypoglycemia assures the maintenance of a fairly normal level of blood sugar despite the failure of one or another component in the defense.

EFFECTS OF HORMONES ON THE LEVEL OF BLOOD SUGAR
Insulin
(Islands of Langerhans)
↓
Blood Sugar Level
↗   ↖
Anterior Pituitary   Adrenal Medulla
Adrenal Cortex   Thyroid
Ovary   Posterior Pituitary

FIG. 3. Only one endocrine element, insulin, acts to lower blood sugar. The hormones counteracting the effect of insulin may be divided into two groups: those arising from the anterior pituitary, adrenal cortex and ovary, which diminish the rate of oxidation of glucose, and others from the adrenal medulla, thyroid and posterior pituitary which accelerate hepatic glycogenolysis.

IV. FUNCTION OF THE NEUROENDOCRINE BALANCE IN PREVENTING THE FALL OF BLOOD SUGAR

The fact that only one hormone acts to lower blood sugar while, there are several hormones whose duty it is to prevent a fall, seems to indicate

[9] There is also evidence for another viewpoint which however may not be contradictory but rather complementary namely that the hypothalamus liberates a hormone which activates the anterior pituitary (446a) and that adrenaline stimulates the hypothalamus. From this viewpoint the hypothalamus is a link not only in the neuronal segment of the neuroendocrine chain but also in the hormonal segment.

that the significance in maintaining the blood sugar level does not lie in limiting a rise in the sugar, but in averting a disastrous decline. The physiologic function subserved by this prevention of hypoglycemia is the continuous supply to the brain of its chief foodstuff. Except in the case of the brain, the intrinsic ability of most organs to oxidize carbohydrate is limited (878, 255), and depends upon the neuroendocrine balance for any change in their rates of oxidation. When the supply of carbohydrate in the body is ample, the neuroendocrine balance acts in such a way as to permit all the organs to share in this plethora and to consume increased amounts of glucose. In any condition in which the body is deprived of carbohydrate, the neuroendocrine balance diminishes the ability of all organs except the brain to use glucose and thus saves all available carbohydrate for the brain (88). The utilization of blood sugar by the non-nervous tissues is therefore regulated in such a way that the brain is always provided with sufficient carbohydrate. In addition, whenever hypoglycemia threatens, some of the components of the neuroendocrine balance accelerate hepatic glycogenolysis and thus counteract the fall of blood sugar.

A. Glucose tolerance test

The concept that the neuroendocrine balance functions to continuously supply the brain with its foodstuff is partly based upon the results of the glucose tolerance test. An analysis of these results discloses the integrated actions of the various components. In general, there are two types of glucose tolerance tests: the one-dose test and the two-dose test. In the one-dose test, glucose is administered intravenously or orally in one dose of 1 to 2 grams of glucose per kilogram of body weight. Blood samples are drawn at various intervals, $\frac{1}{2}$ hr., 1, 2, 3, and 4 hours after administration of carbohydrate. A curve is plotted (see Fig. 4) with the blood sugar levels in mg. per cent as ordinates, and time as abscissae. In the two-dose test, the usual amount of glucose is divided into two doses given at least one half-hour apart (300). Since the two-dose test is a more sensitive indicator of the activities of the various factors composing the neuroendocrine balance, that test shall be used for our analysis.

Before the administration of glucose, blood sugar is usually at a postabsorptive level of approximately 90 mg. per cent. Following the first dose of carbohydrate, blood sugar rises at the half-hour to approximately 140 mg. per cent, or at the most to 180 mg. per cent. The second dose is dispensed at this time. The subsequent reaction observed in the one-hour sample is different from that of the half-hour sample. Instead of a decided rise in the level of the curve, there is either a slight rise, not exceeding 5 mg. per cent (95), no rise at all, or a fall. This improved utilization of carbohydrate following the second dose is called the Staub-Traugott

(912, 950), or Hamman-Hirschman (441) phenomenon. Analysis of blood collected in the second hour reveals a rapid fall in the level of the blood sugar, which, at the third and fourth hours, may drop below the post-absorptive level. Finally, the curve ascends to the original value.

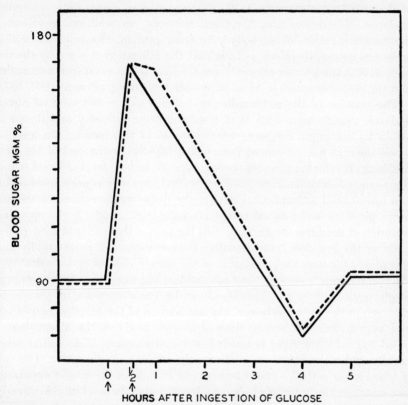

FIG. 4. In general, the changes of the endocrine balance are the same both in the one-dose (full line) and two-dose (broken line) glucose tolerance tests. The striking difference between the two tests is: that the second dose in the two-dose test is utilized more efficiently than either the first dose of this test, or the single dose in the one-dose test. The reason for this efficiency rests on the endocrine balance, which by the time of the second administration, has been shifted in favor of a faster carbohydrate metabolism. Arrows indicate administration of glucose.

The level of blood sugar at each point on this curve is determined by the neuroendocrine balance. Between meals, after the absorption of glucose from the gastro-intestinal tract has ceased, the neuroendocrine balance acts in such a fashion as to prevent the development of hypoglycemia. The work of Best, Haist and Ridout (88) suggests that secretion of insulin drops off after the stimulating effect of a raised level of blood sugar, due to the previous meal, has ceased. Such an adaptive decrease in the rate at which insulin is formed results in a dampening of the first step of glucose metabolism in the non-nervous tissues and therefore reduces their absorption of glucose. This reduction is intensified by a greater diabetogenic activity of the anterior pituitary (543, 91, 838) and adrenal cortex (82) to depress oxidation of carbohydrate. A cortical hormone, in addition, accelerates the new formation of carbohydrate from protein. The principle of this endocrine action, therefore, is to inhibit the utilization of sugar by the tissues, so that the glucose released from the liver becomes adequate to maintain the post-absorptive level at approximately 90 mg. per cent (894, 897).

The reaction of the neuroendocrine balance to the first dose of carbohydrate, though immediate is of slowly growing intensity and does not attain its maximum for some time. Because of this inertia, the level of blood sugar is not prevented from rising rapidly by the end of the first half-hour. By this time, under the influence of the high level of blood sugar, the neuroendocrine balance has been shifted, and this is accomplished by two interrelated accommodations: (1) the diabetogenic actions of the anterior pituitary and adrenal cortex are halted (82), and (2) the opposing secretion of insulin is stepped up (89). Because of these adaptations, called forth by the first dose, glucose enters the metabolic mill more rapidly and this makes for improved oxidation of the second dose of carbohydrate by the non-nervous tissues of the body, and at the same time favors storage of glycogen in liver and muscle. Once the transformation of glucose to glycogen in the liver has begun, the momentum of the reaction carries on, and by the time the second dose of glucose is given, the absorption of blood sugar by the liver is much faster and glycogen is deposited more rapidly under the influence of the newly released insulin (928). The rise of blood sugar with the first dose not only stimulates the insulin apparatus to counteract the anterior pituitary-adrenal cortex factors but also directly impairs their influence, for the Hamman-Hirschman (441) phenomenon has been observed in depancreatized animals receiving constant doses of insulin (895, 894), and in eviscerated preparations free of that hormone. Bergman and Drury (82) have compared the utilization of glucose in fasted and fed eviscerated animals and observed that glucose was utilized more rapidly in the animals that had been fed before the eviscerectomy. The improved management of carbohydrate by these animals must therefore be attributed to glands other than the pancreas and liver, probably to a diminished activity of the anterior pituitary and adrenal cortex. Direct evidence on the role of the anterior pituitary has been obtained by Himsworth and Scott (468), whose hypophysectomized rabbits failed to handle successive doses of carbohydrate with improving advantage. They concluded that the decreased function of the anterior pituitary gland was one of the factors necessary for the more rapid utilization of blood sugar following the second administration of carbohydrate. These changes in the activities of the various components of the neuroendocrine balance diminish the rise of sugar as observed in the second blood sample taken at the first hour.

At this time, the absorption of carbohydrate is completed but the endocrine balance is still set for the rapid utilization of blood sugar. As a result, blood sugar descends and may even reach hypoglycemic levels. However, during the third and fourth hours, the emergency action of the sympatho-adrenaline apparatus is brought into activity, the stimulus being the low level of blood sugar. As a result, hepatic glycogenolysis is accelerated and a hypoglycemia, dangerous to the brain, is averted. The thyroid can act synergistically with adrenaline (378, 53) but whether or not the posterior pituitary gland does so is unknown. An important part of the remedial effect of adrenaline is obtained by evoking the cooperation of the anterior pituitary and adrenal cortex which decrease the utilization of carbohydrate by non-nervous tissues. These emergency actions of the sympatho-adrenaline apparatus are necessary intermediaries until the post-absorptive neuroendocrine balance is reestablished. By the time blood sugar is raised above hypoglycemic levels, the activities of the insulin apparatus are diminished and those of the anterior pituitary and adrenal cortex are so modulated as to ensure the comparatively slower rate in the utilization of sugar which is characteristic of the post-absorptive period.

V. Summary

The fundamental processes of carbohydrate metabolism have been reviewed and the factors controlling blood sugar level have been analyzed in order to understand the mechanisms supplying the brain with its chief foodstuff. The level of blood sugar is regulated by a neuroendocrine balance which involves the activities of the parasympatho-insulin system, the sympatho-adrenaline system, the anterior pituitary gland, adrenal cortex, and the ovary, the thyroid and posterior pituitary glands.

The neuroendocrine equilibrium, in large measure, acts on the brain indirectly through its influence on non-nervous tissues. These tissues appear to have their glucose consumption adjusted in response to cerebral needs as reflected in the shifts of the balance. Thus, when there are ample supplies of blood sugar, its utilization by all non-nervous tissues is accelerated, permitting these tissues to share with the central nervous system in the carbohydrate plethora. On the other hand, when the carbohydrate of the diet is inadequate, its utilization by non-nervous tissues is depressed, preserving the available carbohydrate for the brain. Even with ample carbohydrate, after its absorption in the gastro-intestinal tract has been completed, hypoglycemia is imminent because the mechanisms which make for utilization of carbohydrate are still active. The low level of blood sugar, however, is itself a stimulus for increasing the activity of factors counteracting hypoglycemia.

The integrated action of the neuroendocrine balance is analyzed by the use of the two-dose glucose tolerance test. In the post-absorptive condition the rate of the insulin secretion is diminished while the activities of the anterior pituitary and adrenal cortex are correspondingly accelerated. As a result of these changes, less glucose is consumed by non-nervous tissues; the carbohydrate released by the liver is spared in this manner and remains available for the brain. The administration of carbohydrate and subsequent rise of blood sugar cause a shift in the neuroendocrine balance which permits the non-nervous tissues to initiate the utilization of more glucose, facilitating oxidations and glycogen storage, while the brain continues to employ its full requirement. The shift in the balance facilitating these changes requires some time for development. When the second dose is given one half-hour later, however, the shift may be completed. Blood sugar therefore does not rise to the extent to which it did following the first dose. After the absorption of carbohydrate is completed, the neuroendocrine balance again exhibits the characteristic of inertia to such an extent that hypoglycemia threatens because of the rapid absorption of carbohydrate by non-nervous tissues. However, in response to low blood sugar, the sympatho-adrenaline system is called into action, accelerating hepatic glycogenolysis, evoking the inhibitory actions of the anterior pituitary-adrenal cortex upon carbohydrate utilization, thus raising blood sugar and affording the brain additional supplies of carbohydrate. Finally, the post-absorptive balance is reestablished and the absorption of glucose by non-nervous tissues is again depressed.

The analysis of the two-dose glucose tolerance test discloses that many hormones combat a fall of blood sugar but that only one hormone, insulin, acting under parasympathetic influence, lowers the blood sugar level. Chief among the factors to support blood sugar is the sympatho-adrenaline apparatus which, like the thyroid and posterior pituitary glands, counteracts hypoglycemia by mobilizing liver glycogen. The anterior pituitary and its reinforcing adrenal cortex inhibit glucose consumption by non-nervous tissues, an inhibition neutralized by insulin. The multiplicity of the defense against hypoglycemia indicates the importance of preventing a fall in the blood sugar level. Hence, the brain is insured a continuous supply of its chief foodstuff, glucose, and this appears to be a cardinal function of the neuroendocrine balance of carbohydrate metabolism.

CHAPTER 4

MECHANISMS MAINTAINING BRAIN METABOLISM DURING HYPOGLYCEMIA

I. THREE MECHANISMS PROTECTING THE BRAIN DURING HYPOGLYCEMIA

Cerebral metabolism does not cease immediately in a state of hypoglycemia. Small amounts of glucose are still supplied to the brain and these serve to sustain the brain though at a lower metabolic rate than normal. This maintenance of cerebral metabolism is important for it makes possible the temporary continuation of cerebral function in the event of hypoglycemia. Complete recovery after a short period of metabolic depression is facilitated, and even during prolonged hypoglycemia, the extent of injury to the brain is limited.

In order to understand how these mechanisms act to maintain cerebral metabolism during this type of hypoglycemia, a knowledge of how insulin hypoglycemia is produced is first necessary. Observations of the glucose released by the liver reveal that larger amounts of glucose are poured into the blood stream during hypoglycemia than with normal levels of blood sugar (506, 207). These observations, which apply particularly to the early stages of hypoglycemia, also disclose that blood sugar continues to fall despite the accelerated production of hepatic glucose. The fact that blood sugar level is low therefore indicates that its utilization is more rapid than the release of hepatic glucose into the blood stream. Though glucose is removed by all the tissues of the body, the effect of insulin to promote the absorption of blood sugar is exerted only on the non-nervous tissues (800, 801).

That profound hypoglycemia is brought on because the glucose of the blood is utilized too quickly is illustrated in an experiment on a schizophrenic patient receiving the insulin treatment (508). Because the tissues are removing the sugar so rapidly, the intravenous injection of 8 grams of glucose, caused a rise of only 7 mg. per cent, from 22 to 29 mg. per cent in blood samples collected before the injection and a few minutes after. The injected glucose was absorbed by all of the tissues of the body including the brain as indicated both by the clinical change in the patient as he regained contact with his environment temporarily, and by the cerebral arterio-venous oxygen difference which increased from 1.3 vol. per cent to 5.0 vol. per cent. The more rapid removal of glucose prevents blood sugar from rising even though the liver continues to put out glucose. Because insulin hypoglycemia is caused chiefly by the accelerated absorption of blood sugar by non-nervous tissues, the activities of the mechanisms protecting the brain are directed to increasing the glucose supplies of the brain, and to diminishing the glucose used by the non-nervous tissues.

Two mechanisms act to procure additional glucose for the brain, and a third works to impede the amount of carbohydrate used by non-nervous tissues. The two mechanisms increasing the carbohydrate supplies to the brain are: (1) the formation of glucose from the glycogen stores of the brain, and (2) the continued liberation of hepatic glucose into the blood stream. The third mechanism decreases the carbohydrate used by non-nervous tissues by substituting the utilization of fat, thus sparing the available carbohydrate for the brain.

The possibility of a fourth mechanism comes from the work of Elliott Scott and Libet (272) who found that in the absence of glucose almost half the oxygen utilized by homogenized cerebral tissue was consumed by non-carbohydrate material. The authors, therefore, suggest that under conditions of severe hypoglycemia the brain *in vivo* may also oxidize non-carbohydrate material, but they point out that such oxidations are not adequate to support the brain during hypoglycemic coma.

The activities of the first and second mechanisms will be discussed together before describing those of the third.

II. COMPARISON OF THE FIRST AND SECOND MECHANISMS

A. *Effects on carbohydrate stores of the body*

Table 4 presents the changes of carbohydrate content in the various organs of the body resulting from the activities of the first and second mechanisms. The time relations of the third mechanism to the first and second mechanisms are also mentioned. The first effect of the administration of insulin and ample amounts of carbohydrate is to increase the carbohydrate stores of muscle (189, 87, 381) and liver (405, 340, 178, 38) above their typical values which may be about 500 and 5,000 mg. per cent, respectively. But sometimes hepatic glycogen may be diminished (184, 46) as the liver supplies glucose for the heightened carbohydrate requirements of the non-nervous tissues of the body. Brain glycogen is left unchanged (589).

The second effect starts with the fall of the level of blood sugar. Responsible for this decrease is the glycogenesis in liver (340) and muscle (381), together with the acceleration of carbohydrate oxidation by all non-nervous tissues. Both mechanisms supplying glucose to the brain cerebral (590) and hepatic (189) glycogenolysis, become more active as soon as blood sugar begins to diminish. As a result of this diminution, less sugar is available, and the brain absorbs sugar from the blood in amounts which are not adequate to maintain the high rate of cerebral metabolism. The small intrinsic store of cerebral glycogen is then utilized as an additional source of carbohydrate (first mechanism). The fall in brain glycogen (590, 164) is a direct response to hypoglycemia and is uninfluenced by

TABLE 4

Approximate values for the glycogen content (mg. per 100 gm. of tissue) of various organs during prolonged insulin hypoglycemia

EFFECT	BLOOD SUGAR	GLYCOGEN OF CEREB. CORTEX	SKELETAL MUSCLE GLYCOGEN	LIVER GLYCOGEN	REMARKS
1.	90	90	500 (+ increment due to insulin & CHO)	5000 (+ increment due to insulin & CHO)	Insulin and carbohydrate administered simultaneously
2.	50	50	400 (ref. 185, 192)	3500	Hyperactivity of the sympatho-adrenaline system
3.	20	30	300 (no convulsions; ref. 185, 192. may go to 0 with convulsions ref. 86.)	500	Hyperactivity of adrenal cortex and anterior pituitary

Table 4 summarizes the progressive changes in the glycogen content of the various parts of the animal body during profound hypoglycemia.

Effect 1 portrays characteristic values for the postabsorptive state and in addition indicates the increases of liver and muscle glycogen resulting from administration of insulin and carbohydrate. The dose of insulin, however, is excessive in relation to the carbohydrate, and because of this excess hypoglycemia ensues.

Note that Effect 2 pictures the glycogen content of the organs at the time when the central nervous system first reacts to hypoglycemia. The susceptibility of brain glycogen to hypoglycemia is outstanding. The resistance of muscle glycogen to hypoglycemia, uncomplicated by convulsions (185, 192) is in direct contrast to liver and cerebral glycogen stores, both of which sustain relatively greater losses.

The third effect, the greatest depression of the glycogen deposits, is seen only in most profound hypoglycemia, but even here, because fat oxidation is speeded up, the organism is not entirely stripped of carbohydrate. In this table the figures for glycogen of the cerebral cortex and the liver are those obtained from the observations of Kerr and his co-workers (589, 590). With a somewhat different biochemical method, Chesler and Himwich (164, 168) arrived at values which were approximately 20 mg. per cent less for cerebral cortical glycogen in all three values (70, 30 and 10 mg. per cent). The normal muscle glycogen (737) is depleted completely only in the event of convulsions (86).

hormonal changes, unlike the second mechanism which is accelerated by the hormone adrenaline (847, 189, 188).

Despite the activities of these mechanisms, the glucose supplied to the brain is inadequate. The first part of the brain to be depressed by lack of foodstuff is the cerebral cortex, which may possess a higher rate of metabolism than other cerebral regions (523, 528, 488, 495, 953) since it is among

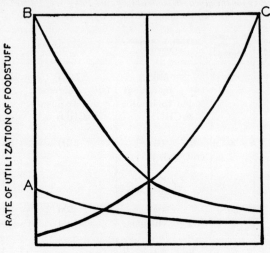

DURATION OF HYPOGLYCEMIA

Fig. 5. Quantitative and temporal relationships of the maximum activities of the three mechanisms protecting the brain during hypoglycemia. A represents breakdown of brain glycogen (Mechanism I). B represents liver glycogen converted to glucose and utilized by brain (Mechanism II), and C, fat utilization (Mechanism III). The first mechanism begins activity as soon as hypoglycemia develops. The second commences simultaneously with the first, and functions at a more rapid rate. Later the rate of the second mechanism also decreases, thereby affording less hepatic glucose to the blood stream. With less glucose available, the oxidation of carbohydrate is replaced by that of fat, until non-nervous tissues oxidize fat chiefly, if not entirely.

the first to lose its glycogen in the adult organism (164). The hypothalamus, then, with its autonomic centers is released from cortical control (508, 350). Consequently, sympatho-adrenaline activity is stepped up and the adrenaline is poured into the blood stream (459, 939, 635). In response to this adrenalemia the liver puts out more glucose than under normal concentrations of blood sugar (second mechanism (506, 207)), leaving hepatic glycogen supplies reduced. Muscle glycogen is relatively resistant in the face of rapid glucose oxidation. The outpour of sugar from the liver, however, is not adequate to keep up with the speed at which non-nervous tissues are consuming the glucose. Blood sugar, therefore, continues to fall.

The third effect comes into play when hypoglycemia is prolonged. Liver glycogen is further decreased despite the transformation of portein to carbohydrate in the liver, a function promoted by the adrenal cortex (838, 685). The glucose given out by the liver becomes even smaller; and the non-nervous tissues resort to oxidation of fat in increasing amounts as a substitute for the glucose (third mechanism).

To summarize the sequence of events presented in the table: when blood sugar falls as a consequence of a large dose of insulin, the supply of brain glycogen dwindles as a result of the activity of Mechanism I, and the loss of liver glycogen begins, due to the function of Mechanism II, the latter process being stimulated by the secretion of the adrenal medulla. As the level of blood sugar continues low, liver glycogen decreases still more despite gluconeogenesis from protein. The carbohydrate available for the various organs is reduced, and for want of some foodstuff, the non-nervous tissues must oxidize fat in greater quantities (Mechanism III) (Figure 5).

B. *Duration of activities*

The second mechanism continues to function after the activity of the first has diminished quantitatively. At the time when approximately half of the cortical glycogen has been utilized, the liver retains as much glycogen as in the post-absorptive state (590). The material for the second mechanism to act upon is therefore present during hypoglycemia. Apparently the glycogen stores of the cerebral cortex are most sensitive to hypoglycemia (164). The activity of the liver protects the glycogen especially that of the lower portions of the brain and maintains the function of the vital medullary centers. The second mechanism, which is in continuous activity even with a normal level of blood sugar becomes most effective as blood sugar falls. At this time, the breakdown of liver glycogen, an intrinsic function of the liver (894), is accelerated by the sympatho-adrenaline apparatus. The initial high value of hepatic glycogen commences to diminish as the liver releases large amounts of glucose to the blood stream. Later, the hepatic release of glucose begins to subside as the depression of cerebral metabolism is extended from the cerebral cortex to include the hypothalamus (508, 350). The resulting cessation of sympatho-adrenaline activity and the reduction of the glycogen stores of the liver dampens the intensity of the second mechanism. This mechanism does not stop completely though sympatho-adrenaline over-activity has ceased. Even in the most prolonged hypoglycemia (506, 207), it operates though at a mild rate on the small amount of glycogen still present in the liver. This glycogen is newly formed from portein and also from lactic acid if convulsions supervene.

The presence of hepatic glycogen in this profound stage of hypoglycemia may be demonstrated by the injection of adrenaline (845) or metrazol (480), either of which raises blood sugar after a prolonged period of hypoglycemia. Further proof that the second mechanism sustains the brain against low blood sugar is shown by the consequences of extirpation of the liver, an operation which is followed by the rapid death of the organism in hypoglycemia (706).

C. Quantitative importance

The second mechanism not only acts over a longer period than the first, but is quantitatively more significant. This difference may be observed by two methods: (1) an estimation of the relative quantities of sugar absorbed by the brain from the blood, and of sugar resulting from the breakdown of brain glycogen, and (2) a comparison of the amounts of glycogen available in liver and brain.

First method. For the first method it is necessary to compare the oxygen and glucose utilized by the brain from the blood. The oxygen absorbed from the blood represents the volume of that gas required for all oxidations in the brain, and therefore includes the combustion of the glucose obtained as a result of the breakdown of brain glycogen, as well as that from liver glycogen.

[A] *Total cerebral O_2 intake* = [B] O_2 *utilized by glucose obtained from liver through blood* + [C] O_2 *utilized by glucose arising from brain glycogen.*

The blood glucose utilized by the brain can be used to measure hepatic contribution to brain metabolism. The oxygen necessary for the combustion of the hepatic component subtracted from the total oxygen consumption yields information on the cerebral component. Or, [C] = [A] − [B].

[A] is obtained by an analysis of cerebral blood for oxygen; [B], by a determination of the glucose absorbed by the brain from cerebral blood: In order to obtain [C], it is necessary to remember the theoretical relationship: that 3 cc. of oxygen are required for the combustion of approximately 4 mg. of glucose. With the aid of this theoretical relationship it can be shown that with normal levels of blood sugar the total metabolism of the brain is supported by the sugar derived from the blood, because the amount of glucose absorbed from the blood is in fact somewhat in excess[1] of that required to account for the total cerebral oxygen consumption; oxygen intake averages 6.7 vol. per cent (481, 1025, 512, 391) and glucose 10 mg. per cent (481, 1025, 391). The theoretical relationship is therefore fulfilled when the concentration of blood sugar is normal; hepatic glucose may be regarded as the support of cerebral metabolism, and brain glycogen remains

[1] The slight excess of glucose that apparently is not oxidized may be explained by its conversion into lactic (391) and pyruvic (524) acids as indicated by the small amounts of these substances liberated into the blood stream.

constant. Even during hypoglycemia most of the glucose for cerebral oxidations may be obtained from blood sugar. Evidence for this conclusion is the fact that the theoretical relationship between oxygen and glucose may exist despite the low blood sugar. In experiments reported by Himwich, Bowman, Wortis and Fazekas (481), the averages were reduced to 3.1 vol. per cent oxygen and 4.2 mg. per cent sugar. The total glucose used by the brain though less than normal is of hepatic origin in this case. In other instances, however, the glucose absorbed from the blood is relatively less than the oxygen intake, and one explanation for this disproportion is that the brain may have supplied a significant portion of the carbohydrate utilized by that organ. For example, in a series of observations made on a patient subjected to insulin hypoglycemia, the oxygen utilized from the cerebral blood was 3.3 vol. per cent, 4.1 vol. per cent, 5.4 vol. per cent and the corresponding glucose utilizations were 0 mg. per cent, 4 mg. per cent and 3 mg. per cent, all values less than the theoretical. The amount of glucose removed from the blood is too small to account for the cerebral oxygen consumption. That the brain can supply a portion of the carbohydrate utilized is demonstrated by the observation of Kerr, Hampel and Ghantus (590, 166) previously referred to, that brain glycogen had diminished when signs of hypoglycemia developed. These observations reveal that the brain usually receives most of its support from the glucose of hepatic origin (Mechanism II).

Second method. A more exact idea of the relative proportions of glucose obtained from the liver and from brain glycogen can be gathered by a comparison of the glycogen content of the liver and brain. From Table 4 we see that the glycogen stores of the liver are much greater than those of the brain. The glycogen content of the human cerebral cortex has not been determined, but examinations of the cerebral cortex of dogs, cats, and rabbits by Kerr and co-workers (589, 590) revealed average values of 98, 87, and 82 mg. per cent, respectively. Chesler and Himwich (166), using somewhat different biochemical methods, observed slightly lower values, 73 and 68 mg. per cent for the cortex of dogs and cats, respectively. The results of both groups of workers agree in regard to the small glycogen content of the brain. Kerr (590) noted symptoms of hypoglycemia when the glycogen values for cerebral cortex fell to 50 mg. per cent or less in all these species. This value is not the lowest he reported, for with a continuation of hypoglycemia, reductions to approximately 30 mg. per cent occur frequently.

Chesler and Himwich (164) found the glycogen content of the canine brain to vary in different parts with normal levels of blood sugar. The figures in mg. per cent ranged: cortex, 73; caudate nucleus, 58; thalamus, 62; colliculi, 50; cerebellum, 35; medulla, 39; and cord, 29, with perhaps 60 mg. per cent as a fair average. During hypoglycemia a progressive fall in the glycogen content was observed (166), starting with the caudate nucleus and, after including the cerebral hemispheres, extending down the brain stem, the medulla being most resistant. Since most parts of the brain were virtually depleted of glycogen in hypoglycemia of long duration, it was concluded that this form of carbohydrate (glycogen) may be regarded as a storage product to be drawn upon only in the emergency of hypoglycemia and perhaps anoxia. It should not be confused with the carbohydrates which are a part of the architecture of the brain, such as the galactose forming the structure of the cerebrosides, and which do not become available as energy unless the brain suffers destruction. A fall in human cerebral glycogen of 60 mg. per cent, similar to that above observed in dogs, would suggest that a brain weighing 1.3 kilograms yields 0.78 grams of cerebral glycogen as its content decreases from 1.17 grams to 0.39 grams. This fall in cortical glycogen would result from the activity of the first mechanism.

The glucose released from the liver is shared by all the organs of the body. The contribution of the liver to the brain metabolism may therefore be evaluated by calculating the total breakdown of hepatic glycogen and then estimating the fraction thereof obtained by the brain. The liver may weigh on the average 1.5 kilos with a concentration of glycogen of 3 per cent or 45 grams of carbohydrate before the injection of insulin. Even in profound hypoglycemia, the hepatic glycogen deposit is not completely depleted. About $\frac{1}{10}$ of the deposit may be retained in that organ. Nevertheless the total carbohydrate output of the liver may represent at least 45 grams of glycogen because the initial content is supplemented by the glycogen newly formed in the liver from protein and from lactic acid liberated by muscles. It is therefore probable that the amount of glycogen broken down in the liver during hypoglycemia is at least as great as the hepatic content before the injection of insulin.

Soon after the injection of insulin all the organs of the body are oxidizing carbohydrate chiefly, and the cerebral share will approach in value $\frac{1}{6}$ of the total carbohydrate released by the liver since the cerebral requirement is approximately $\frac{1}{6}$ of the entire basal metabolism. When the other organs begin to oxidize increasing quantities of fat, the brain probably absorbs much more than $\frac{1}{6}$ of the carbohydrate released by the liver. The brain may therefore receive from the liver, glucose arising from more than 7.5 grams of glycogen ($\frac{1}{6}$ of 45) and from the brain 0.78 grams of glycogen, a ratio of approximately 10:1. If the liver contains more than 45 grams of glycogen before the injection of insulin, as it may when replete, the ratio will be greater than 10:1.

The length of time brain metabolism can be maintained on these glycogen stores may be estimated by taking into consideration the rate of cerebral glucose utilization. If the brain absorbs 45 cc. of oxygen per minute (see page 178 Chap. 8) then $(45 \times \frac{4}{3})$ 60 milligrams of glucose per minute or 3.6 grams of glucose per hour are consumed in this process. A value of 1.8 grams of glucose per hour, however, is likely during hypoglycemia when cerebral metabolic rate is significantly reduced.[2] The hepatic quota of 7.5 grams of glycogen yields approximately 8.3 grams of glucose,[3] sufficient to support the brain for $4\frac{3}{5}$ hours (8.3/1.8). The cerebral glycogen quota of 0.8 grams produces 0.9 grams of glucose,[3] enough to sustain brain metabolism for an additional one half hour (0.9/1.8) and making a total duration of approximately five hours within which the brain can withstand profound hypoglycemia without irreversible damage to the nervous tissues. These calculations, admittedly only tentative, nevertheless indicate the comparative amounts of glucose obtained for brain oxidations from the breakdown of glycogen deposits in the brain and in the liver. The slight relative importance of the first mechanism in comparison with the second is thus evaluated on a quantitative basis.

Hypoglycemia not only diminishes cerebral glycogen but other carbohydrate products: glucose, lactate and pyruvate (776). The significance of the loss of carbohydrate to the brain can be better appreciated if it is considered in relation to the energy-rich phosphate bonds because the influence of carbohydrate oxidation is exerted through these bonds. The immediate source of energy to support nervous functions arises from the breakdown of adenosine triphosphate. Phosphocreatin is an additional source of energy-rich phosphate bonds which aid in the maintenance of adenosine triphosphate. Since the bonds are resynthesized at the expense of carbohydrate oxidation it is not surprising that with severe hypoglycemia the energy-rich phosphate bonds are exhausted as phosphocreatin and adenosine triphosphate are depleted while adenosine diphosphate accumulates (776). The energy-rich bond may be regarded as playing the role of the middle-man which transfers the energy obtained from carbohydrate oxidation for the support of the brain.

III. THIRD MECHANISM

A. *The shift from carbohydrate oxidation to fat*

The reduction in the level of liver glycogen as a result of Mechanism II not only hinders the efficacy of the second mechanism, but initiates the third mechanism, the accelerated utilization of fat. Because of the inade-

[2] In severe hypoglycemia, C.M.R. may be reduced to 1/4 normal, and for the present calculations a value of 1/2 normal C.M.R. may be taken as the average for the entire period of hypoglycemia.

[3] The relation of the weight of glycogen, $(C_6H_{10}O_5)n = 162n$, is to that of glucose, $n\ C_6H_{12}O_6 = n\ 180$, as 9:10.

quate supply of blood sugar, fat must be oxidized in increasing amounts in order to furnish the calories necessary for the maintenance of bodily function. If the oxidation of fat increases beyond the ability of the body to accomplish complete oxidation, ketosis occurs. This result of the third mechanism is to be attributed directly to the diminution of hepatic glycogen. To quote Burn and Ling (135), ". . . the amount of ketonuria is inversely proportional to the amount of liver glycogen."

The increased oxidation of fat by non-nervous tissues, initiated by a lack of carbohydrate supplies, is intensified by the gradual shift of the endocrine balance in response to a low level of blood sugar. This shift accelerates the third mechanism by two direct effects on the amounts of carbohydrate and fat oxidized: any remaining carbohydrate oxidation is inhibited and the oxidation of fat is further stimulated. The hypoglycemia may augment the diabetogenic effects of the anterior pituitary and the adrenal cortex, to inhibit the utilization of glucose and thus counteract, though unsuccessfully, the overpowering dose of insulin (543, 91, 838, 1038, 685, 553). Other activities of these two glands promote fat oxidation (809, 810) and cause the accumulation of ketone substances (136, 139, 93, 1034, 556).

The results of the hypoglycemia and the shift of the endocrine balance to change oxidations from carbohydrate to fat are evidenced by three biochemical signs: (1) decreased utilization of blood sugar by the organs, (2) fall of the respiratory quotient, and (3) ketosis, if fat oxidation becomes excessive. These three types of evidence will now be reviewed, and applied to non-nervous organs of the body: skeletal muscle, cardiac muscle, and liver. In these organs, unlike the brain, metabolism is not depressed by hypoglycemia because fat is oxidized in place of carbohydrate. This is not so for the brain since it oxidizes little, or no fat and therefore its oxygen intake must decrease during hypoglycemia (481). The oxygen used by canine muscle has been shown to be sustained even though the muscles seemed to utilize less carbohydrate in hypoglycemia (492). Muscle probably does not consume a large fraction of its intrinsic glycogen stores during hypoglycemia provided there are no convulsions (86). The only remaining source to be used by the muscle is the blood sugar. By analysis of the blood going to and from the muscle, it was found under normal conditions that muscle absorbed 7.6 mg. per cent of sugar, but that during hypoglycemia, only 1.9 mg. per cent was taken from the blood by the muscle. In contrast, the average intake of oxygen was not significantly different: 6.9 vol. per cent, with normal levels of blood sugar, and 6.0 vol. per cent in hypoglycemia (492). The oxidation of fat by muscle must have been increased in order to account for an unchanged oxygen intake.

Because the respiratory quotient is an indicator of the kind of food oxidized, it becomes important to follow the changes of this quotient during hypoglycemia. Cruickshank and Startup (211) studied cardiac metabolism by removing both heart and lung from the body of an animal, but keeping the vascular connections between these organs intact. In this way they could alter the conditions under which the heart pumps and the lungs oxygenate the blood without interference from other organs. In one crucial group of experiments in which their object was to study blood sugar level and its effect on the foodstuffs oxidized by the heart, they cut down the blood sugar concentration and observed that the respiratory quotient of

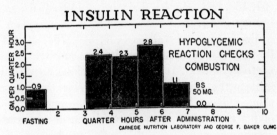

FIG. 6. Respiratory quotients of a patient whose diabetes had started two months prior to the observations (831). After 100 units of insulin were given to the fasting patient, he was oxidizing 0.9 gm. of carbohydrate per ¼ hour, with a respiratory quotient of 0.78. Intravenous injection of 50 gm. of glucose was followed by the combustion of 2.4, 2.3 and 2.8 gm. of carbohydrate per ¼ hour, while the respiratory quotient rose 0.90. After that, the carbohydrate oxidized diminished first to 1.1 gm. and finally to 0 gm. With the latter value, the respiratory quotient was 0.69 and blood sugar 50 mg. per cent, as a result of continued insulin action. At this time the patient suffered a hypoglycemic reaction, was uncomfortable, and sweating profusely.

the heart also fell; and when the blood was entirely devoid of sugar, the respiratory quotient was 0.7 (the quotient of fat). The total oxygen intake of this preparation was not changed significantly during the time that the quotient fell; the oxidation of fat was therefore substituted for that of carbohydrate. Root and Carpenter (831) observed similar changes of the respiratory quotient in a patient with diabetes who was given 100 units of insulin while in the post-absorptive state, and his respiratory quotient[4] was then found to be 0.78. Subsequently, 50 gm. of glucose were injected intravenously, and as the insulin began to act on this glucose, carbohydrate oxidations achieved a value of 0.90. After the glucose had been consumed, however, the quotient fell to 0.69. The body was forced to resort to the oxidation of fat because at that time the blood sugar level was 50 mg. per cent. In these observations, fat oxidation replaced that of

[4] These respiratory quotients were non-protein values depending upon the relative amounts of carbohydrate and fat oxidized and excluding the contribution of protein.

carbohydrate when the rapid utilization of glucose, stimulated by insulin, evoked hypoglycemia.

In addition to a diminished utilization of blood sugar and a fall of respiratory quotient, the accumulation of ketone substances is a sign of the predominant oxidation of fat. Ketonuria during hypoglycemia in animals has been reported by various workers (805, 177). Somogyi has observed this excretion of ketone substances in diabetic patients with overdoses of insulin (892) and in schizophrenics receiving the insulin therapy (891). Ketone substances, produced chiefly in the liver (276, 152, 511, 407, 905, 94) may be absorbed and oxidized by other organs of the body, for example, muscle (94, 152, 888, 346, 55, 266), heart (407, 979), gastro-intestinal tract (407), kidney (569), spleen and testes. The brain, on the other hand, does not utilize ketone substances (407, 569, 755) except for acetoacetic acid to a limited extent (803), and it can convert beta-hydroxy butyric acid to acetoacetic acid. It has been previously concluded that the brain cannot initiate the oxidation of fat, and since ketones are products of fat oxidation, it may now be added that the brain cannot complete the oxidation of fat even after it has been initiated by another organ. Because most organs can burn fat (905, 825), production of ketone substances is not necessarily limited to the liver but may occur in other non-nervous organs: skeletal muscle (407, 510), heart, gastro-intestinal tract, kidney, spleen, and testes (569). Again the brain is an exception (407, 569, 755), it does not produce ketone substances.

From these data it is apparent that the third mechanism protects the brain only because it spares for that organ any carbohydrate present in the blood stream. Brain destruction (143) therefore occurs finally despite the function of the third mechanism, when the glucose afforded by the liver and brain is not adequate to supply the foodstuff required for maintaining cerebral structure.

B. *Comparison of insulin hypoglycemia with diabetes*

An appreciation of the effects of the third mechanism may be obtained by comparing the changes in the metabolism of foodstuffs which occur during hypoglycemia with those which occur in diabetes. The utilization of glucose by non-nervous tissues is greatly slowed in diabetes,[5] carbohydrate oxidation is impeded, that of fat is substituted, and the transformation of protein to carbohydrate is accelerated. These changes are evidenced by a fall of the respiratory quotient, development of ketosis, and the in-

[5] This viewpoint of diabetes which has recently received strong support from the work of the Coris' laboratory((800, 801) Chapter 5) has been termed the under-utilization interpretation of diabetes mellitus i.e. most parts of the diabetic organism, with the exception of the brain, suffer an impairment in the use of glucose. A rival explana-

creased urinary excertion of nitrogen. During prolonged hypoglycemia, similar changes occur in carbohydrate, fat and protein metabolism as indicated by: the fall of the quotient (831), the accumulation of ketone substances (892, 891), and the increased protein metabolism, the last of which is described by Milhorat and Chambers (743) as well as Ingle and co-workers (555). The similarity between diabetes and prolonged hypoglycemia may be reduced to one common factor, a poor oxidation of carbohydrate.

Two factors are fundamental if carbohydrate oxidation is to be accelerated: insulin and ample amounts of carbohydrate. In diabetes, glucose utilization is retarded for want of insulin (800, 801). After prolonged hypoglycemia the absorption of glucose is slowed for want of carbohydrate supplies to the organs. In the presence of excessive doses of insulin, the function of that hormone to accelerate the use of glucose finally effects a diminution of hepatic glycogen. The hepatic release of glucose is accordingly reduced, and fat oxidation accelerated. During insulin hypoglycemia the non-nervous tissues of the body therefore pass from a condition in which they oxidize carbohydrate predominately to one which is similar to a diabetic episode. This diabetic reaction is not immediately reversed, despite complete activity of the injected insulin. After a series of hypoglycemic periods, carbohydrate oxidation continues to be depressed and carbohydrate production from protein is stepped up for some time. The impaired glucose tolerance of animals (555) and schizophrenic patients (688) following treatment with insulin hypoglycemia exemplifies this functional reorganization of carbohydrate metabolism. The endocrine balance of the body has been temporarily altered: insulin formation is dampened, both anterior pituitary and adrenal cortex exert their diabetogenic actions, and the latter gland exalts the transformation of protein to carbohydrate. This deviation of the endocrine balance is, however, transient and is readily terminated by repeated administrations of carbohydrate.

The similarities between insulin hypoglycemia and phlorhizin diabetes are striking. In both states the organs are deprived of their carbohydrate supplies by hypoglycemia. Both conditions can therefore be alleviated if the blood sugar is reinforced by administration of carbohydrate (998). The chief difference between these two unphysiologic states depends upon the manner in which the hypoglycemia is produced. In phlorhizin diabetes,

---

tion, the over-production theory, claims for its basis a hepatic supply of glucose so excessive that normal utilization fails to cope with it. Soskin (896), one of the leading proponents of the over-production conception, in association with Levine, presents his side of the question in the book, Carbohydrate Metabolism. Their book is suggested to those desiring an exhaustive and remarkably clear account of carbohydrate metabolism.

the blood is depleted of its sugar chiefly because the kidneys are rendered incapable of retaining the sugar of the blood (880), and the carbohydrates of the body are drained in the urine. With excessive insulin, the tissues are drawing on the blood sugar in amounts far above the hepatic supply.

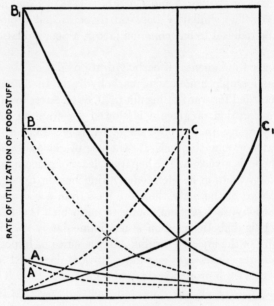

FIG. 7 illustrates the changes which occur in the functions of the three mechanisms as a result of well-filled glycogen stores being subjected to sympatho-adrenaline stimulation. The usual pattern is indicated by broken lines: A represents the breakdown of brain glycogen; B, the liver glycogen converted to glucose and utilized in the brain, and C, the oxidation of fat. The modifications produced by the large amounts of liver glycogen are drawn in with solid lines: A_1, B_1 and C_1 all represent the same processes as A, B and C except that the curves are changed in accordance with the increased glycogen stores of the liver. A longer interval is therefore required before the liver glycogen is reduced to low levels, and the brain absorbs more glucose of hepatic origin. Accordingly the brain glycogen is spared for a longer time, and the initiation of the accelerated oxidation of fat is postponed.

IV. Effect of large hepatic glycogen stores on the integrated action of the three mechanisms

The usual hypoglycemic pattern of metabolic activity is an integration of the functions of the three mechanisms. This pattern is modified when the second mechanism, the release of hepatic glucose, becomes quantitatively more important because of unusually large glycogen stores. The greater amount of carbohydrate freed by the liver delays the depletion of the glycogen stores of the brain (first mechanism) and postpones the accelerated utilization of fat (third mechanism).

The heightened activity of the sympatho-adrenaline apparatus upon well-filled hepatic stores, and the consequent augmentation of the hepatic glucose poured into the blood stream causes this retardation in the development of the usual hypoglycemic pattern. In all patients receiving the insulin treatment for schizophrenia, the over-activity of the sympathetic apparatus approches a maximum when the hypothalamus is first entirely released from cortical control (508, 350). At that time cortical function is suppressed and contact with the environment is lost.

If the hepatic glycogen stores are well-filled, the outpouring of glucose will be great enough to supply blood sugar to the brain, as well as to non-nervous tissues. In that case, the cerebral cortex will not become deeply depressed and contact with the environment will be retained for a much longer time. This phenomenon of resistance to coma is observed in patients who are given an opportunity for replenishment of liver glycogen, as a result of rest over the week-end from the daily insulin treatment. A dose of insulin adequate to produce coma on the preceding Friday may fail to do so on the succeeding Monday. The effect of over-activity of the sympatho-adrenaline system upon well-filled stores of liver glycogen produces such an increased release of hepatic glucose as to prevent the development of coma.

If this conception is correct, then this form of insulin resistance is not an absolute phenomenon but a relative one and should disappear as the glycogen stores of the liver are reduced. In that case, hypoglycemia sufficiently prolonged should finally result in the precipitation of coma. An example illustrating such a loss of insulin resistance over a period of time was observed in a patient who became comatose at the end of the fourth hour after he had maintained contact with the environment despite a low level of blood sugar throughout this period.

V. Summary

Three mechanisms function to prevent the complete cessation of brain metabolism during hypoglycemia: (1) the formation of glucose from cerebral glycogen. (2) The release of hepatic glucose to the blood stream. This intrinsic function of the liver is accelerated by the sympatho-adrenaline apparatus and is therefore maximal during the period when the cerebral cortex is depressed and the hypothalamus is released. The stimulating effect of the sympatho-adrenaline apparatus loses most of its power after the hypothalamus is included in the cerebral depression. (3) A change in utilization from glucose to fat by non-nervous tissues, saving the carbohydrate of the blood stream for the brain. The oxidation of fat increases as the second mechanism becomes less effective.

A comparison of the three mechanisms reveals the second to be of greatest value to the organism. It not only acts for a longer period than the first, but is quantitatively more important, perhaps in a ratio greater than 10:1. When the second mechanism does not afford sufficient foodstuff to maintain cerebral structure, the first and third mechanisms do not prevent brain destruction.

The efficiency of the second mechanism depends chiefly upon the amount of glycogen in the liver. When the hepatic glycogen stores are abundant, the second mechanism affords large amounts of carbohydrate to the brain and the activities of the first and third mechanisms are delayed. A schizophrenic who stuffs himself with food during the week-end rest from the insulin treatment illustrates how the brain may be sustained as long as the hepatic glycogen holds out, and thereby prevents loss of contact with environment. When hepatic glycogen stores are finally reduced, the second mechanism becomes less effective and the functions of the first and third mechanisms are expedited.

CHAPTER 5

THE OXIDATION OF CARBOHYDRATE
IN THE BRAIN

I. FUNDAMENTAL CONCEPTS OF CARBOHYDRATE OXIDATION

An exploration into the mechanisms of carbohydrate oxidation in the brain, or in any other tissue, demands the knowledge of various highly specialized branches of chemistry. In order that readers who are not so equipped may nevertheless obtain an appreciation of the fundamental concepts of carbohydrate oxidation, we will first describe briefly the contents of this chapter in non-technical language. We believe that such knowledge is of practical value in understanding both brain physiology and brain pathology. Once these ideas are explained simply, omitting chemical formulas and diagrams, the chemical basis for these ideas will then be described in more detail so that those who have the necessary background or wish to acquire it may obtain not only the general conception of carbohydrate oxidation in the brain, but also a more complete treatment of this subject.

* * *

Our knowledge of cellular oxidation of carbohydrate is based on observations of a large variety of cells not only of mammalian origin but also of lower animals, yeast and bacteria. The data thus accumulated will be examined in order to determine wherein they apply to oxidations of cerebral cells.

The three oxidative factors. In general, most oxidative processes occurring in living matter involve the interaction of three different factors: *enzymes, foodstuffs* and *oxygen*. In the final analysis, everything contained within the cell, including these three factors, is composed of materials brought from the outside world. The amount of any material which must be supplied to the cells depends upon its rate of utilization. The rate, however, is not the same for all substances. Enzymes, for example, are utilized slowly, and may be regarded as relatively constant cellular constituents, while foodstuffs and oxygen are consumed so rapidly that they must be replaced in large and continuous quantities. The supply of glucose is initiated in the digestive processes of the gastro-intestinal tract from whence it is absorbed into the blood stream and carried to the brain and all parts of the body. The third factor, molecular oxygen, diffuses from the air in the lungs to the blood in the pulmonary capillaries, and is transported by the blood to the body and brain cells.

Outside the body, foodstuffs are not oxidized unless the process is

63

brought about by catalysts, oxidizing agents or high temperatures; the heat of a flame facilitates the combination of hydrogen and carbon in the foodstuff with oxygen to form water and carbon dioxide respectively. Within the body, a catalytic function is fulfilled by enzymes which accelerate the same combinations at the body temperature of 37°C. The enzymatic oxidation of carbohydrate will constitute the main purpose of this chapter, since this substrate, as pointed out in Chapter 2, is the chief fuel of the brain.

Phylogenesis of carbohydrate oxidation. The process of oxidation, fundamental though it is, according to one suggestion is a comparatively modern development as a method for liberating energy to maintain life. Long before energy was obtained from the oxidation of glucose, organisms thrived by means of energy made available by the splitting of glucose (992, 58), and the ultimate forming of pyruvic and lactic acids. Later, in the course of evolution, a further and much greater release of energy was delivered to the cell when the energy of pyruvic acid was made available by its oxidation. About $\frac{1}{12}$ of the total energy liberated in the oxidation of carbohydrate is released in the formation of pyruvate, and the remaining $\frac{11}{12}$ during its subsequent oxidation.

The oxidation of pyruvic acid consists essentially in the giving up of hydrogen atoms from the carbon skeleton on which they are hung. During this process carbon dioxide is liberated. The hydrogen which is given up *could* combine with oxygen directly, but this would mean a sudden and uneconomic release of energy. Fortunately, intermediary substances evolved whose duty it was to carry the hydrogen from the foodstuff to the oxygen. By such a stepwise procedure the energy is liberated in a smoother, more continuous and efficient manner in the body. In view of this evolutionary conception, we have divided the description of glucose utilization into two stages: one in which glucose breaks down to pyruvic acid, and a later phyletic development whereby pyruvic acid is oxidized to water and carbon dioxide.

Various oxidative schemes and their application to the brain. The accumulated experience of Embden (275), Meyerhof (736), Parnas (783), Cori (190), Lardy and Ziegler (639), and others has yielded a definite conception of the steps involved in the formation of pyruvic acid from glycogen. These steps entail a series of reactions in which glycogen, with the aid of specific enzymes, breaks down to glucose. Glucose, in turn, under the catalytic action of other enzymes, is split into smaller compounds, finally giving rise to pyruvic acid.

The second part of this scheme whereby pyruvic acid is oxidized has likewise been elucidated. Workers in this field are now agreed on the reaction by which pyruvic acid is broken down to CO_2 and H_2O. In this process (626, 1018) pyruvic acid, after joining a carrier substance, undergoes further changes in the course of which the major energy made available during carbohydrate oxidation is finally released. Agreement also exists on another point; that diphosphothiamin (vitamin B_1) plays an essential role in the oxidation of pyruvic acid (787).

When this knowledge on cellular respiration is directed particularly to the brain, some interesting special applications are observed. The Embden-Meyerhof scheme (the breakdown of glucose to pyruvic acid) was shown by a large group of workers to be applicable to the brain. It is also probable that the modified Krebs or tricarboxylic acid cycle and the presence of diphosphothiamin are necessary for the oxidation of pyruvic acid in the brain, the same as in other tissues. Since the brain practically oxidizes only carbohydrate, that organ is especially sensitive to the lack of vitamin B_1. Therefore, such conditions as peripheral neuropathy (1021, 1005), Wernicke's syndrome (1022), as well as characteristic changes in personality (354, 1007) all are prominent in a vitamin B_1 deficiency. Whether or not these diseases can be blamed on a vitamin B_1 deficiency, uncomplicated by additional factors, will be discussed in Chapter 8.

A further study of brain oxidations discloses a fact which is confirmed by the examination of some other tissues, namely, that all the phenonema of cerebral carbohydrate oxidations cannot be explained by the Embden-Meyerhof scheme (Fig. 9). Incontrovertible evidence from the author's (32) and other laboratories (31, 54) proves that glucose can be oxidized by the brain through pathways other than those initiated in the Embden-Meyerhof scheme. What these other paths of oxidation are, we cannot say for sure, but Harrison (450, 451), Warburg and Christian (971) as well as Dickens (234) have suggested that glucose may be oxidized directly, that is, without the intermediary splitting of pyruvic acid. These paths are detailed in the chemical analysis of this chapter, along with explanatory diagrams.

The role of insulin. Though it has been known for some time that insulin increases the rate of carbohydrate oxidation, until recently we had no idea at all as to how insulin achieved this catalytic effect. The evidence furnished by Colowick, Cori and Slein (178) has given us valuable information on a performance of insulin in carbohydrate metabolism. The inability of the diabetic organism to utilize ingested carbohydrate has been attributed by these investigators to the failure of glucose to enter the Embden-Meyerhof scheme in the absence of insulin. The processing of glucose occurs after that substance combines with phosphate, thus entering the metabolic mill. This phosphorylation, called the glucokinase reaction, is therefore an obligatory step for any further utilization of glucose. Anterior pituitary depresses this fundamental reaction and adrenal cortex reinforces the anterior pituitary effect while insulin on the contrary, lifts the depression (800, 801). Insulin thus augments the use of glucose indirectly by antagonizing the hormonal inhibition of the anterior pituitary and its auxiliary, the adrenal cortex. A second and direct action of insulin is exerted chiefly on hepatic carbohydrate metabolism which is speeded up in an adaptive fashion so that glycogenesis is faster when glucose is available (928). But the exception lies in the brain. We know that the brain of depancreatized dogs can *still* oxidize carbohydrate in undiminished amounts (519). Why? Because the brain has the unique ability to oxidize carbohydrate *without* the aid of insulin. It appears that the cerebral utilization of glucose is not retarded by the anterior pituitary and adrenal cortex and therefore does not require their antagonist, insulin. If the blood-brain barrier is impermeable to the anterior pituitary secretion it does not enter the cerebral cells to alter vital processes. Every diabetic individual is, therefore, protected from a grave deprivation of energy which he inevitably would suffer if his brain demanded the catalytic aid of insulin. In a word, though the brain must rely in greatest measure on carbohydrate oxidation for its energy, this limitation is compensated for by its independence from insulin.

II. Chemical analysis of oxidative paths

Preparatory to a chemical analysis of cerebral carbohydrate oxidations, it is necessary to clarify a few terms which will be used frequently. The first of these is a definition of enzymes. *Enzymes*[1] *are usually thermolabile*

[1] According to the Warburg school the definition of an enzyme does not only include the specific protein but also its active or prosthetic group, the coenzyme. By this formulation then, the colloidal protein plus the coenzyme together compose the enzyme.

Since Warburg's original work (967, 972), it has been generally agreed that the enzyme systems responsible for oxidations are associated with the insoluble parts of the cell. By the use of the differential centrifugation technic it has been found possible to separate several cellular fractions including mitochondria or cytoplasmic rod-shaped granules. Quantitative assays have revealed that various enzymatic actions are present in the mitochondria. Succinoxidase, cytochrome oxidase and the integrated reactions of the Krebs tricarboxylic acid cycle are found in this fraction thus demonstrating that the mitochondria contain the protein portions of these enzyme systems (588).

The respiratory enzymes of mitochondria are also concerned with the synthesis of ATP. These minute rod-shaped bodies therefore occupy a central position in cellular physiology for they are not only involved in respiration but also in the storage of energy in phosphate bonds. On the other hand, the mitochondria do not possess the complete enzymatic machinery for the conversion of carbohydrate to lactic acid. In contrast with the respiratory systems, which are associated with particulate matter, the glycolytic enzyme appears to be readily soluble (588).

The function of protein component of some enzyme systems has been further de-

colloidal protein substances on the surface of which interacting compounds are brought in close proximity to accelerate their rate of reaction (796, 65). One of the interacting substances is generally designated as foodstuff or substrate, the other as the coenzyme. *Coenzymes are thermostabile dialysable non-protein substances.* The coenzyme on the surface of the enzyme can accept a portion of the substrate. An example of a coenzyme is the triphosphonucleotide (Fig. 10), also called coenzyme II to which is transferred the hydrogen of glucose-monophosphate when both the latter and coenzyme II are adsorbed on the surface of the approprate enzyme—in this case, the dehydrogenase of glucose-monophosphate (Fig. 8).

The oxidation of foodstuffs begins with a dehydrogenation which involves transfer of the hydrogen atoms of the substrate to the coenzyme. The hydrogen liberated from the substrate is received by a coenzyme or hydrogen acceptor. The coenzyme, by accepting the hydrogen, is itself

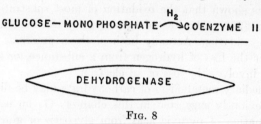

$$\text{GLUCOSE—MONO PHOSPHATE} \xrightarrow{\text{H}_2} \text{COENZYME II}$$

$$\boxed{\text{DEHYDROGENASE}}$$

FIG. 8

reduced and must be reoxidized before it can continue its activity as an hydrogen acceptor. To accomplish this the hydrogen is handed over in

fined by a study of —SH constituents (61). This study has lead Peters, Sinclair and Thompson (789) to form a theory of vesication and to explain the action of lewisite and other arsenicals by their effects to reversibly inactivate the essential —SH groups of the protein moiety in the pyruvate oxidase system. Because of this effect impairment of pyruvate oxidation is a prominent feature of vesicant action. This oxidative inhibition explains the similarity observed between some of the clinical symptoms of arsenical poisoning and of vitamin B_1 deficiency. Both diseases may have peripheral neuritis as part of their clinical manifestations. Both attack the pyruvate oxidase system but not at the same point. In the avitaminosis the coenzyme is lacking, the arsenicals on the contrary poison the collodial carrier. Such a theory of arsenical poisoning carries with it a remedy, namely the therapeutic use of dithiol groups to compete with the enzymatic proteins for arsenic and this competition has been successfully used for its antidotal action against arsenicals and other metallic poisons (914). Lacrimators in contradistinction to vesicants irreversibly inactive —SH groups of enzymes, probably in corneal nerve endings. The mustards are vesicants and interfere with many enzymes, including the phosphokinases, (enzymes which catalyze reactions involving the transfer of phosphate to or from adenylic compounds). The mustards like the arsenicals attack the colloidal protein carrier at the —SH groups. The reduction of oxygen consumption, glycolysis and other anticatalytic effects of the mustards in excised tissues are reviewed by Gilman and Philips (399).

turn to another hydrogen acceptor, a flavoprotein called cytochrome reductase. An example of this reaction may be found in Fig. 10 where the hydrogen transferred from the glucose-6-phosphate to the triphosphonucleotide is passed on from the triphosphonucleotide to cytochrome reductase. This hydrogen atom is split off from cytochrome reductase and dissociates into a hydrogen ion and an electron. The electron combines with cytochrome C to form reduced cytochrome C. The next step in this transfer is managed by cytochrome oxidase (582, 967) which reacts both with the reduced cytochrome C and oxygen in such a way that cytochrome C is oxidized as its electron is accepted by oxygen. When two electrons are taken up by oxygen in this manner (starting from the glucose-6-phosphate) the oxygen and hydrogen ions interact to form one molecule of water, and the oxidation of hydrogen is completed. Most of the energy, however, had been realized in the transfers previous to the final step.

Wieland has shown that the oxidation of most substrates involves dehydrogenation (996). The loss of hydrogen by the foodstuff may be regarded as an oxidation. Actually both of these processes are oxidations because either the loss of hydrogen from a substance, or the addition of oxygen to it, involves the loss of an electron.

The intermediary metabolism of carbohydrate may be divided into two stages, as previously suggested in this chapter: (1) an earlier anaerobic one, the formation of pyruvic acid from glycogen or glucose, and (2) a later oxidative stage whereby carbon dioxide and water are formed from pyruvic acid. The Embden-Meyerhof scheme is concerned with the first anaerobic stage, or the steps involved in the production of pyruvic acid. There may be more than one path for the formation of pyruvic acid, but the Embden-Meyerhof is the only one which is well established on experimental basis. It will therefore be described first.

A. *Embden-Meyerhof scheme*

The description of carbohydrate oxidation logically starts with glycogen since this is the relatively stable form in which carbohydrate is stored in the body. The following are the steps shown in Fig. 9: (1) glycogen in the presence of the enzyme, phosphorylase, and inorganic phosphate, is disrupted at each of its glucosidic linkages. During the reaction each of the glucose units of glycogen adds inorganic phosphate to the first carbon atom of glucose to form glucose-1-phosphate, the process of "phosphorolysis," (186). (2) Glucose-1-phosphate is transformed to glucose-6-phosphate as, with the aid of the enzyme, phosphoglucomutase,[2] the position of phos-

[2] The enzyme phosphoglucomutase is sensitive to metallic ions, zinc, copper, mercury and silver, a sensitivity which is dependent on —SH groups as it is reactivated by such reducing agents as cysteine and glutathione. This reactivation by metal-binding substances is distinct from the activation produced by glucose-1-6-phosphate (781a)(926a).

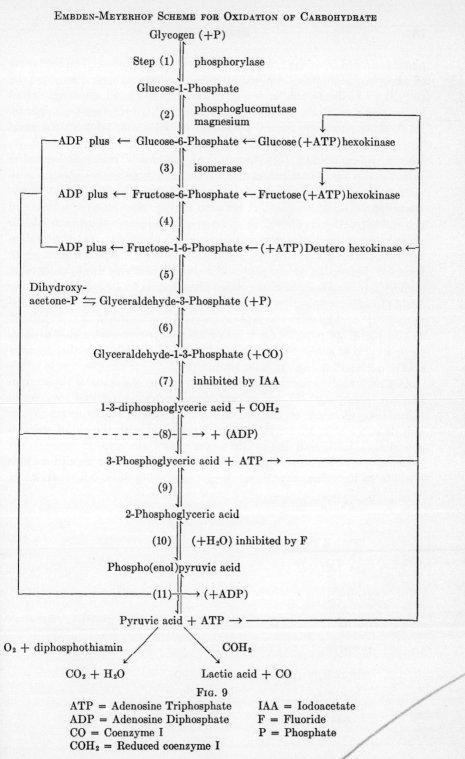

FIG. 9

ATP = Adenosine Triphosphate
ADP = Adenosine Diphosphate
CO = Coenzyme I
COH₂ = Reduced coenzyme I

IAA = Iodoacetate
F = Fluoride
P = Phosphate

phate is shifted from the first to the sixth carbon of glucose. The coenzyme of phosphoglucomutase is glucose-1-6-diphosphate. Magnesium must be present to facilitate this reaction. (3) Glucose-6-phosphate is converted in the presence of the enzyme, isomerase (679), to fructose-6-phosphate. (4) Another phosphate radical obtained from adenosine triphosphate combines with fructose-6-phosphate at the first carbon to form a diphosphate, fructose-1-6-phosphate. (5) There follows a series of reactions beginning with the slitting of each six-carbon molecule of fructose-1-6-phosphate to yield two molecules of three-carbon triosephosphate (736). This triosephosphate represents an equilibrium between dihydroxyacetone phosphate and glyceraldehyde-3-phosphate.[3] (6) The glyceraldehyde-3-phosphate adds a phosphate radical to form glyceraldehyde-1-3-phosphate. (7) Glyceraldehyde-1-3-phosphate is oxidized by coenzyme I (diphosphonucleotide) to form 1-3-diphosphoglyceric acid and reduced coenzyme I. (8) Adenosine diphosphate combines with one of the phosphates of 1-3-diphosphoglyceric acid to form 3-phosphoglyceric acid and adenosine triphosphate. (9) 3-phosphoglyceric acid gives rise to 2-phosphoglyceric acid which, (10) is changed to phospho-(enol)pyruvic acid. (11) Phosphopyruvic acid yields a phosphate radical to another molecule of adenosine diphosphate so that pyruvic acid and adenosine triphosphate appear.

At this point the aerobic phase begins. In the presence of diphosphothiamin (cocarboxylase) and oxygen, pyruvic acid is oxidized by a series of reactions discussed at the end of this section, and finally forms carbon dioxide and water. In the absence of oxygen and with the aid of reduced coenzyme I, lactic acid and oxidized coenzyme I are formed.

Starting with lactic acid and providing the appropriate conditions it is possible to have the resynthesis of glycogen (186, 927). All reactions in

[3]Formation of Triosephosphate:

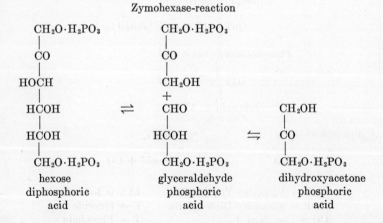

Zymohexase-reaction

the breakdown of glycogen to lactic acid are readily reversible anaerobically.[4]

By the Embden-Meyerhof scheme the oxidation of glucose can occur only after that hexose is phosphorylated in the presence of the enzyme glucokinase (191) and the coenzyme, adenosine triphosphate, yielding the phosphorylated glucose and adenosine diphosphate. Hexokinase is the name given to a group of enzymes which initiates the further metabolism of glucose, fructose and mannose. One enzyme, glucokinase aids the transformation of glucose to glucose-6-phosphate; a second, fructokinase that of fructose to fructose-1-phosphate; and a third, phosphofructokinase further catalyzes these reactions to form fructose-1-6-phosphate (928). It should be noted that brain unlike liver, muscle and yeast does not contain fructokinase (883a).[5] Ochoa (772) has demonstrated that energy obtained from the oxidation of pyruvic acid may be utilized for the phosphorylation of glucose, and Colowick, Welsh and Cori (180) have observed that the combustion of citrate, glutamate, keto-glutarate or of succinate may bring about the formation of glucose-phosphate.[6]

[4] Before the anaerobic reversal of the dephosphorylation of phosphopyruvic acid was accomplished (639), an alternative path requiring additional energy from oxidations (573, 670) was suggested. By this oxidative energy pyruvic acid combines first with carbon dioxide and then phosphate, thus temporarily forming a phosphorylated dicarboxylic acid, (phosphooxalacetate). The decarboxylation of this substance leaves phosphopyruvic acid, supposedly by the following series of reactions (957):

$$
\left.
\begin{array}{c}
\text{Pyruvate} + CO_2 \rightarrow \text{oxalacetate} \\
\updownarrow \\
\text{malate} \\
\updownarrow \\
\text{fumarate} \\
\updownarrow \\
\text{succinate}
\end{array}
\right\}
\begin{array}{c}
\rightarrow \text{phosphooxalacetate} \\
\downarrow \\
\text{phosphopyruvate} + CO_2
\end{array}
$$

Using energy obtained from oxidations, carbon dioxide is added to pyruvate to form the 4-carbon dicarboxylate, oxalacetate, which in turn is phosphorylated to form phosphooxalacetic acid. The decarboxylation of the latter results in the formation of phosphopyruvate and the liberation of carbon dioxide.

[5] For discussion of the poor ability of fructose and of succinate to support brain function see pages 20, footnote 10, 366 respectively.

[6] The formation of glucose-6-phosphate from glucose requires energy, which is afforded by an energy-rich phosphate bond from adenosine triphosphate. The importance of organic phosphate bonds as stores of energy has been emphasized by Lipmann (670) who described a phosphate cycle beginning with inorganic phosphate compounds with no readily available energy. The introduction of inorganic phosphate into ester linkage, however, absorbs about 3,000 cal./mol., energy available when the ester linkage is broken. More important are the compounds with energy-rich phosphate linkages containing about 10,000 cal./mol. Phosphocreatin and adenosine triphosphate are such structures. These linkages are built by the energy obtained either from glycolysis or from the oxidations of a variety of substances, including

The Embden-Meyerhof method for the formation of pyruvic acid on the basis of the preliminary cleavage of fructose-diphosphate has been demonstrated in skeletal muscle and heart extracts. In the liver (190), however,

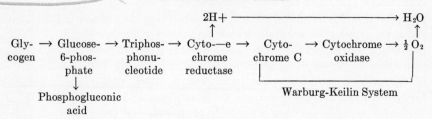

WARBURG-CHRISTIAN SCHEME

FIG. 10. The step-wise oxidation of glucose-6-phosphate includes the transfer of hydrogen atoms first to triphosphonucleotide and then to cytochrome reductase. Each hydrogen atom is then oxidized to a hydrogen ion as it loses an electron to cytochrome C. The reduced cytochrome C is next oxidized by cytochrome oxidase, which transfers the electron from cytochrome C to activated oxygen. When 2 electrons are taken up in this way, oxygen combines with 2 hydrogen ions to form one molecule of water.

this cleavage usually does not take place, to the same extent as in other organs, as the liver is rich in the enzyme, phosphatase, which splits the inorganic phosphate from the glucose-phosphate liberating free glucose.

intermediates of carbohydrate metabolism (pyruvic acid) and fat metabolism (ketone substances) as well as phospholipids (638) and the oxidative deamination of glutamate (608). Energy stored in phosphocreatin passes on to adenosine triphosphate, which in turn yields it for various biological purposes including the process of phosphorylation. In addition to the use of adenosine triphosphate in the hexokinase reactions and the oxidation of fatty acids (645), another notable example is observed in muscle function for which the breakdown of adenosine triphosphate furnishes energy. Corroborative evidence on the importance of phosphorylations in the Embden-Meyerhof scheme is the observation that insulin causes a marked increase in the turnover rates of phosphocreatin and adenosine triphosphate in resting muscle (844), and of adenosine triphosphate in the liver (576). The total concentration of adenosine triphosphate may remain the same, however, despite the more rapid turnover (525).

Another use for phosphate bond is to supply energy for acetylation as for example observed in the synthesis of acetylcholine. Nachmansohn and co-workers (763) have been able to show that choline is acetylated with the aid of the enzyme, choline acetylase (762) and at the expense of energy-rich phosphate bonds (759). The coenzyme of this system, named coenzyme A, because of its role in acetylation, is a pantothenic acid derivative (771). (See footnote 13, p. 79.) Even a brief review of the dual role played by adenosine triphosphate as a storage site for the energy produced in oxidations as well as a source of energy, a source which is depleted in proportion to the intensity of the physiological requirements, reveals that adenosine triphosphate functions as an important link between catabolism and anabolism.

This glucose is released by the liver into the blood stream to supply the carbohydrate needs of the body.

B. *Warburg-Christian-Dickens scheme*

Paths other than the Embden-Meyerhof process for the utilization of glucose have been suggested by Harrison (450, 451), and Warburg and Christian (968, 969). The data of these investigators indicate another method of the metabolism of carbohydrate in which oxygen is consumed before the formation of pyruvic acid. According to the work of Harrison, the first step in the combustion of glucose by the liver requires oxygen as glucose is oxidized to gluconic acid.[7] Two hydrogens of glucose are transferred either to coenzyme I (diphosphonucleotide) or coenzyme 2 (triphosphonucleotide) with the aid of glucose dehydrogenase and finally go to form H_2O.

The utilization of oxygen has been observed by Warburg and Christian as glucose-6-phosphate is transformed to phosphoglucconic acid. The scheme of Warburg and Christian, which was chiefly confined to the initial stage of the oxidation of glucose, was completed by the suggestion of Dickens (234, 235), that the oxidation of various intermediates is continued till pyruvic acid is produced. In the following discussion we shall first present the observations of Warburg and Christian and then complement them by those of Dickens.

The Warburg-Christian scheme is presented in its entirety in Fig. 10. In this scheme unlike the Embden-Meyerhof, a later formed anaerobic process is added to an oxygen utilization system already in function, the cytochrome-cytochrome oxidase group (see Chap. 7, pg. 155 for a discussion of the developmental order among the respiratory enzymes). The anaerobic stage starts with the dehydrogenation of glucose-6-phosphate by an enzyme, a dehydrogenase, and a coenzyme, triphosphonucleotide,

---

[7] The constitutional relationship between these compounds is as follows:

$$
\begin{array}{ccc}
CH_2 \cdot OH & & CH_2 \cdot OH \\
| & & | \\
[CH \cdot OH]_4 & \rightarrow & [CH \cdot OH]_4 \\
| & & | \\
CHO & & COOH \\
\text{Glucose} & & \text{Gluconic acid}
\end{array}
$$

The active or prothetic group of glucose oxidase obtained from *Penicillium notatum* is a flavin, alloxazine adenine dinucleotide, and the enzyme in that organism is therefore a flavoprotein (583, 584) which shows pronounced specificity for glucose. The enzyme catalyzes the oxidation of glucose to gluconic acid by molecular O_2 which is reduced to H_2O_2. This glucose oxidase may be obtained in a highly purified state from the mould and is then designated as penicillin B or notatin.

sometimes called coenzyme II (968, 969). The glucose-6-phosphate and triphosphonucleotide are both adsorbed on the surface of the dehydrogenase to facilitate the transfer of hydrogen from glucose-6-phosphate to coenzyme II. The reduced triphosphonucleotide is then dissociated from the dehydrogenase and adsorbed to the protein component of flavoprotein whereupon it gives up its recently acquired hydrogen to riboflavin, the active group of the flavoprotein complex (767). Triphosphonucleotide, thus reoxidized returns to the dehydrogenase again ready to accept hydrogen from glucose-6-phosphate (1b).

Haas, Harrer, and Hogness (432, 433) have studied the above-mentioned flavoprotein complex and named it cytochrome reductase because it not only takes on the hydrogen of reduced triphosphonucleotide, or coenzyme II, but is capable of reducing cytochrome.

Formerly it was believed that (Szent-Györgyi, 934) reduced riboflavin passes on the hydrogen to cytochrome by way of a series of four-carbon dicarboxylic acids, oxalacetic, malic, fumaric and succinic which act as hydrogen transporters.[8] Oxalacetic receives hydrogen from flavoprotein and is thus converted to malic acid under the influence of malic dehydrogenase. Malic acid, still activated by a specific dehydrogenase, may be reconverted to oxalacetic or, in the presence of fumarase, changed to fumaric acid. The latter, activated by succinic dehydrogenase, takes up hydrogen to form succinic acid. On the surface of the succinic dehydrogenase, succinic acid is reconverted to fumaric acid and two hydrogen atoms are thereby released. These hydrogens give up their electrons to the next member of the oxidative chain, cytochrome. It is obvious that the ability of cytochrome reductase to react directly with cytochrome C renders unnecessary the intermediary activity of the C_4 dicarboxylic acids in the

[8] Szent-Györgyi Cycle:

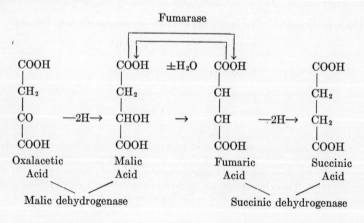

Warburg-Christian scheme, though as discussed in the next section, the Szent-Györgyi system may function as a portion of the Krebs cycle for the oxidation of pyruvic acid.

The reduced form of cytochrome reductase therefore does not release hydrogen atoms to the four-carbon dicarboxylic acids, but instead its hydrogens yield their electrons to the next member of the enzymatic chain, cytochrome C, while the hydrogen ion is dissolved in the aqueous suspending medium. Cytochrome C contains a heme with a structure consisting of a heavy metal, iron and four pyrrol nuclei.[9] It is therefore similar to the heme of hemoglobin. Hemoglobin, however, is not oxidized but forms a loose combination with oxygen while cytochrome C is oxidized or reduced as it loses or takes up electrons.[10] The enzyme to which cytochrome C yields its electron is appropriately named cytochrome oxidase (582, 972), and like cytochrome C, it contains a heme which may be oxidized or reduced. At this point the hydrogen or electron acceptor role of oxygen, comes into play, as the electrons pass from cytochrome oxidase to oxygen. When two electrons are taken up by oxygen, the latter combines with the hydrogen in aqueous solution to form water. This process of hydrogen transfers may be compared to that of a "bucket brigade." The hydrogen of the substrate is passed from one carrier to another until it combines with the oxygen activated by cytochrome oxidase. In this fashion, hydrogen atoms attached to the carbon skeleton of glucose-6-phosphate are converted to water. This long chain of oxidations and reductions liberates energy for utilization by the tissues. Most of the energy arises when hydrogen joins oxygen with the formation of water, and we remember that this is also true of the Embden-Meyerhof scheme, which is complemented by the oxidation of pyruvic acid.

We have traced the steps by which the hydrogen removed from the carbon skeleton of glucose passes on to join oxygen. Our attention next centers on the products of these dehydrogenations. The first step which deviates from the Embden-Meyerhof scheme is the combustion of glucose-6-phosphate resulting in the production of phosphogluconic acid. The phosphogluconic acid is then oxidized to 2-ketophosphogluconic acid (669, 970, 971). The latter, in turn, is oxidized to a pentosephosphate. Dickens (234, 235) using yeast has made similar observations and has extended

[9] The cytochrome system is probably more complex than indicated above and may contain copper-protein as well as iron-protein (11). In fact according to one formulation the electrons released by cytochrome reductase are taken up by cytochrome B before transfer to cytochrome C. The next intermediary is cytochrome A, which in turn transmits the electrons to cytochrome oxidase.

[10] The iron of Hb retains its Fe^{++} form unlike that of cytochrome which is reversibly oxidized $Fe^{++} \rightleftharpoons Fe^{+++} + e$.

this scheme. Beginning with glucose-6-phosphate, his studies indicate the formation first of phosphogluconic acid and then of 2-ketophosphogluconic acid. The latter substance is decarboxylated and inverted to form a pentosephosphate, d-ribose-5-phosphoric acid. Dickens suggests that

WARBURG-CHRISTIAN-DICKENS SCHEME OF CARBOHYDRATE OXIDATION

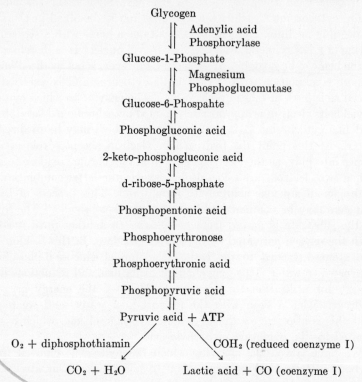

Glycogen

∥↑ Adenylic acid
∥↓ Phosphorylase

Glucose-1-Phosphate

∥↑ Magnesium
∥↓ Phosphoglucomutase

Glucose-6-Phospahte

↓↑

Phosphogluconic acid

↓↑

2-keto-phosphogluconic acid

↓↑

d-ribose-5-phosphate

↓↑

Phosphopentonic acid

↓↑

Phosphoerythronose

↓↑

Phosphoerythronic acid

↓↑

Phosphopyruvic acid

↓↑

Pyruvic acid + ATP

O_2 + diphosphothiamin COH_2 (reduced coenzyme I)

$CO_2 + H_2O$ Lactic acid + CO (coenzyme I)

FIG. 11. By this hypothetical path of carbohydrate oxidation, pyruvic acid is formed as a result of oxidations and not by the splitting of carbohydrate as has been proved for the Embden-Meyerhof path. A comparison of the two paths reveals that they diverge after glucose-6-phosphate. By the Embden-Meyerhof scheme (see Fig. 9) fructose-6-phosphate is the next step, whereas by the arrangement in this figure phosphogluconic acid is formed.

by a continuation of oxidations and decarboxylations a four-carbon sugar, phosphoerythronic acid (or phosphothreonic acid) and finally phosphopyruvic acid are formed. Coenzyme II or triphosphonucleotide may be required for these oxidations. Theoretically, by this path, pyruvic acid is manufactured in yeast as a result of the oxidation of glucose and not of its cleavage. Turning to mammalian tissues we meet the similar suggestion of Breusch (113) that liver oxidizes glucose by a scheme not involving the splitting of that substance into two 3-carbon chains. Instead, the 6-carbon compound undergoes a series of dehydrogenations via d-arabinose, d-erythrose, glyceraldehyde and glycolaldehyde. Breusch's hypothesis therefore employs the same principal as that of Warburg-Christian-Dickens. As may be seen, however, from a comparison with Figure 11 the intermediary compounds are not the same structurally nor are they phosphorylated. It must be emphasized that an enzymatic process by which pyruvic acid is produced as a result of oxidative decarboxylation of glucose has not been demonstrated. But a significant advance was made when it was shown that an enzyme, obtained from mammalian cells, converts phosphogluconic acid quantitatively to pentose phosphate and CO_2 (see Fig. 11) (540a). It is therefore important to investigate this problem further and to determine whether or not such an oxidative chain operates in the brain.

C. *Oxidation of pyruvic acid*

Because of the strategic position occupied by pyruvic acid in carbohydrate metabolism, a knowledge of its path of oxidation is important. Several paths have been suggested, but only one will be discussed at length. By that path, Krebs and co-workers (625, 627, 297), working on pigeon breast muscle, and Smyth (887) on pig heart muscle, showed that pyruvic acid combines with a four-carbon dicarboxylic acid and from this new compound three molecules of carbon dioxide are broken off in succession. The citric acid cycle of Krebs (626) includes the reaction of the four-carbon substance, oxalacetic acid, with the two-carbon chain, acetyl,[11]

[11] The intermediary metabolite which initiates the cycle has not been ascertained. An active form of acetyl phosphate has been suggested as combining with oxalacetate to form cisaconitate (771, 670) but more recently citrate rather than cisaconitate has been found to be the product of this condensation (912a).

In this scheme citric acid is found in the direct path of oxidation as originally suggested by Krebs. Because isotopic C, introduced as CO_2, together with pyruvic acid leads to the formation of a-ketoglutaric acid containing isotopic C only in the carboxyl group next to the keto group and not in the other carboxyl group, citric acid, a symmetrical compound, was ruled out as a direct intermediate (298, 910, 1018). That position was awarded to cisaconitic acid which is however in equilibrium with citric acid.

More recent work however tends to replace citric acid into the direct oxidative path. Following the suggestion of Ogston (774a) that an asymmetrical enzyme which attacks a symmetrical compound can distinguish between its identical groups, Potter and Heidelberger (797a) repeated the above work and in addition isolated the citric acid containing C-14. This citric acid was then enzymatically converted to a-ketoglutaric acid in the presence of arsenite in rat-liver homogenate. The a-ketoglutaric acid must have had all its C-14 in the carboxyl group next to the keto group produced as one molecule of carbon dioxide and two atoms of hydrogen are split off. The six-carbon substance, citric acid, is thus formed. The latter is in equilibrium with cisaconitic acid. After its rearrangement as isocitric acid, a second molecule of carbon dioxide and 2 additional atoms of hydrogen are released to form five-carbon alpha-ketoglutaric acid (713). This substance in turn yields a third molecule of carbon dioxide and 2 more hydrogen atoms to produce four-carbon succinic acid. Succinic acid then undergoes successive transformation to fumaric, malic, oxalacetic acid (Szent-Györgyi (934) system) in which form it is ready to recombine with

---

for the succinic acid formed from it was practically devoid of C-14 according to the following scheme:

$$
\begin{array}{cccccccc}
\text{COOH} & \text{COOH} & \text{COOH} & & \text{COOH} & & \text{COOH} & *\text{CO}_2 \\
| & | & | & & | & & | & + \\
\text{CO} & \text{CO} & \text{CO} & & \text{CH}_2 & & \text{CH}_2 & \text{COOH} \\
| \rightarrow & | & + | & \rightarrow \text{HOOC--C--OH} \rightarrow & | & \rightarrow & | \\
\text{CH}_3 & \text{CH}_2 & \text{CH}_3 & & \text{CH}_2 & & \text{CH}_2 & \text{CH}_2 \\
+ & | & & & | & & \text{C}{=}\text{O} & | \\
*\text{CO}_2 & *\text{COOH} & & & *\text{COOH} & & *\text{COOH} & \text{COOH}
\end{array}
$$

Pyruvic Acid + Carbon Dioxide	Oxalacetic Acid	Pyruvic Acid	Citric Acid	a-ketoglutaric Acid	Carbon Dioxide + Succinic Acid

If, unlike the formula shown in the scheme, ½ of the molecules of a-ketoglutaric acid had C-14 in the other carboxylic group, then ½ of the molecules of succinic acid would also contain C-14. But this is not the case. Thus the symmetry of citric acid is not an argument against its place in the direct line of oxidation.

Fluoroacetic acid is one of the inhibitors of the tricarboxylic acid cycle. The intraperitoneal injection of 5 mg/kg of sodium fluoroacetate into rats sacrificed one hour after the injection resulted in striking increases in the citric acid content of brain, heart and kidney (125a). It is believed that small amounts of fluorocitric acid are formed and that these interfere with the conversion of citrate to cisaconitate and the tricarboyxlic acid cycle is therefore stopped at that point (273). These observations suggest the *in vivo* existence of the tricarboxylic acid cycle. It is known that fluoroacetate interferes with the oxidation of pyruvate (548) and acetate (62) and now it appears that this interference is the indirect result of the inhibition of the tricarboxylic acid cycle.

Ammonium chloride is also effective in blocking this path. According to Potter and Recknagel (797b) ammonium chloride diverts a-ketoglutaric acid to glutamic acid. Two other inhibitors of the tricarboxylic acid cycle are aresnite which prevents the oxidation of a-ketoglutaric acid as the further progress in this cycle is prevented and malonic acid which is a competitor with succinic acid for the succinic dehydroginase.

pyruvic acid in order to re-enter the cycle.[12] Diphosphothiamin may function in each of these three decarboxylations; at least for the third one where alpha-ketoglutaric acid is decarboxylated to succinic acid, Barron and his co-workers (60) and Green and his associates (416) have found that diphosphothiamin is part of an enzymatic complex performing this transformation.[13] The dehydrogenations occurring at five different steps of this

[12] *Oxidation of fat.* Evidence is accumulating for the function of the tricarboxylic cycle in the oxidation of ketone substances, intermediates in fat metabolism (112, 122) which also react with oxalacetic acid. Thus both carbohydrate and fat utilize the same method to complete their oxidations (644).

Oxidation of alcohol. The intermediary metabolism of alcohol in some ways is like that of carbohydrate. The first step, the oxidation of alcohol to acetaldehyde, is catalyzed by a specific dehydrogenase plus a series of enzymes: diphosphonucleotide and cytochrome reductase. The mechanism is similar to that for the oxidation of glucose as suggested by Harrison (450, 451), or of glucose-6-phosphate according to the Warburg-Christian scheme with the cytochrome cytochrome-oxidase system of Keilin completing the oxidative chain (see Fig. 10) (232, 233). The oxidative steps after the production of acetaldehyde are controversial, but the formation of acetoin as an intermediary product with the aid of thiamin has been suggested (80, 922), and denied (694), while the condensation with oxalacetic acid must be considered.

Oxidation of pyruvate. Pyruvic acid may be oxidized by a pathway leading to the production of acetoacetic acid as has been demonstrated in liver homogenate. In the presence of oxalacetic acid the tricarboxylic acid cycle has a high priority but in the absence of the 4-carbon dicarboxylic acid pyruvic acid is converted to acetoacetic acid (797b).

Another method for the oxidation of pyruvic acid has been suggested by Green, Westerfeld, Vennesland, and Knox (416), who demonstrated the *in vitro* formation of acetoin as an intermediary product, a process not proved for the intact organism (694). One molecule of pyruvic acid is decarboxylated to produce acetaldehyde. The latter then reacts with another molecule of pyruvic acid to form acetoin in accordance with the following equations:

$$CH_3COCOOH \rightarrow CH_3CHO + CO_2$$
$$CH_3CHO + CH_3COCOOH \rightarrow CH_3CHOHCOCH_3 + CO_2$$

Evidently thiamin facilitates these reactions, since the brain tissue of thiamin-deficient pigeons shows a markedly lower ability to form acetoin from acetyaldehyde and pyruvate (922). Finally the direct oxidation of pyruvic acid to acetic acid and CO_2 has been discovered in mammalian tissues by Barron, Bartlett, and Kalnitsky (59).

[13] In addition to diphosphothiamin, biotin and pantothenate are somehow involved in pyruvate metabolism as demonstrated by the failure to utilize that substance in ducks that have been made deficient in either one of these two members of the vitamin B complex. In biotin deficiency cardiac tissues exhibit a depressed utilization of pyruvate, an action which may be concerned with the reversible carboxylation of pyruvate to oxalacetate (779). In the absence of pantothenate a decreased ability to use pyruvate is observed in liver slices and it is suggested by the authors (778) that pantothenate, as part of coenzyme A, (see footnote 6, p. 72) is required to aid in the formation of acetate from pyruvate.

cycle initiate hydrogen transfers which are continued by carriers until the passage is completed by the formation of water and with the aid of the cytochrome-cytochrome oxidase system as in the Warburg-Christian chain.

This tricarboxylic acid cycle with the catalytic aid of diphosphothiamin (787, 774, 35, 680) not only accounts for the CO_2 elaborated in the course of metabolism but also for most of the H_2O as the hydrogen atoms (see Figure 10) are processed in the Warburg-Christian chain. The details for the oxidation of pyruvic acid in animal tissues are in agreement with the concept of the Krebs mechanism.

In order to emphasize the continuity of the enzymatic reactions we shall take into consideration not only the tricarboxylic acid cycle but also the Embden-Meyerhof scheme. To start with the oxidation of pyruvic acid, we find that (1) $2\frac{1}{2}$ molecules of oxygen are consumed in addition to the oxygen present in the pyruvic acid molecule (2) 3 molecules of carbon dioxide are split off (Figure 12) and (3) 2 molecules of water are produced: 1 each from the hydrogen atoms removed on the formation of alpha-keto-glutaric acid and oxalacetic acid respectively.

$$C_3H_4O_3 + 2\tfrac{1}{2}\,O_2 \rightarrow 3CO_2 + 2H_2O$$

Three molecules of oxygen are used however, when we include with the $2\frac{1}{2}$ of the tricarboxylic acid cycle, the additional $\frac{1}{2}$ molecule of oxygen utilized to produce water in the cells under aerobic conditions following the dehydrogenation required for the production of 1-3-diphosphoglyceric acid in the Embden-Meyerhof process. The entire oxidation of each 3 carbon chain therefore requires 3 molecules of oxygen while yielding 3 of carbon dioxide and 3 of water. These numbers must be doubled in the consideration of the entire glucose molecule. We thus obtain an R. Q. of $\dfrac{6\ CO_2}{6\ O_2}$ and at the same time perceive the intimate reactions concerned in the manufacture of the characteristic R.Q. of unity for carbohydrate.

D. *Hormonal control of carbohydrate metabolism*

The hormonal regulation of the blood sugar level was presented in Chapter 3 but it required a description of the details of cellular carbohydrate transformations to prepare for a discussion of the processes by which the endocrine glands exert their influences. The observations of Colowick, Cori and Slein (178) reveal a significant point of hormonal attack, the phosphorylation of glucose with the formation of glucose-6-phosphate, a reaction which is driven by the energy obtained from adenosine triphosphate and catalyzed by the enzyme glucokinase in the presence of magnesium. Glucose for the most part, fails to undergo metabolic changes

THE CITRIC ACID CYCLE

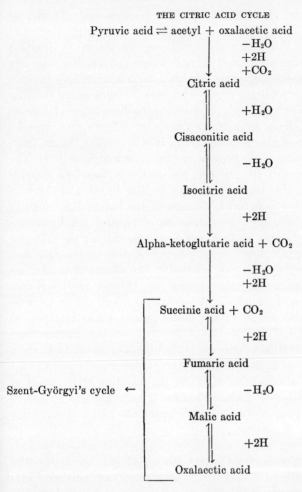

Pyruvic acid $\rightleftharpoons$ acetyl + oxalacetic acid

$-H_2O$
$+2H$
$+CO_2$

Citric acid

$+H_2O$

Cisaconitic acid

$-H_2O$

Isocitric acid

$+2H$

Alpha-ketoglutaric acid + CO_2

$-H_2O$
$+2H$

Succinic acid + CO_2

$+2H$

Fumaric acid

Szent-Györgyi's cycle ← $\qquad$ $-H_2O$

Malic acid

$+2H$

Oxalacetic acid

FIG. 12. Pyruvic acid and oxalacetic acid unite, and after splitting off 2 atoms of hydrogen and 1 molecule of carbon dioxide, form citric acid. This substance is transformed to cisaconitic acid with the elimination of water. The latter on the addition of water is changed to isocitric acid. The latter splits off two hydrogen atoms and carbon dioxide to form alpha-ketoglutaric acid, and this acid, on the addition of water and the loss of two hydrogens splits off carbon dioxide to form succinic acid. The remainder of the cycle is in accord with Szent-Györgyi as described in the footnote on page 74. The final product, oxalacetic acid again reacts with pyruvic acid to continue the cycle. In this entire process 3 carbon dioxide molecules and 10 hydrogen atoms are split off as indicated by plus (+) signs. The hydrogen transfers thus initiated are continued until water is formed with the aid of the cytochrome-cytochrome oxidase system. Five molecules of water are produced as five atoms of oxygen are utilized. But 3 molecules of water are consumed ($-4H_2O + 1H_2O$). The net exchange consists therefore, of 2 molecules of water, 5 atoms ($2\frac{1}{2}$ molecules) of oxygen and 3 molecules of carbon dioxide (see text for reaction).

until it is subjected to phosphorylation. The fundamental glucokinase reaction is retarded by the products of two glands, anterior pituitary and adrenal cortex, which thus exert their diabetogenic action to diminish glucose utilization though not that of other hexoses. The anterior pituitary influence is primary while the adrenal cortex acts in a secondary manner to intensify the anterior pituitary effect (800, 801). This hormonal retardation is curbed by insulin which tends to overcome the diabetogenic influence and permits the glucokinase reaction to proceed at a faster rate. Besides aiding the initial stage of glucose metabolism in non-nervous tissues, insulin accelerates the activity of the hepatic enzyme phosphorylase (928). The reversible reaction glycogen $\rightleftharpoons$ glucose-1-phosphate, is therefore speeded up to the left. When the level of glucose in the blood and liver is high, glycogen deposition is favored. Because of the loss of this effect of insulin in diabetic patients glycogen formation is impeded despite an excessive concentration of sugar in the blood. Strangely enough the influence of insulin on phosphorylase does not include the reaction to the right and for that reason glycogenolysis is not affected.[14] The effects of insulin are disclosed by observations in which the accumulation of lactate and pyruvate was used as an indicator of carbohydrate breakdown. Normally an increase of these two substances occurs in the blood following the intravenous injection of glucose (125). This increase fails to take place in depancreatized dogs after the administration of glucose (124, 167). The inability to form glucose-6-phosphate from glucose prevents the further metabolism of that hexose. Similarly, in patients with diabetes, the injection or ingestion of carbohydrate results either in a small increase of pyruvate and lactate or none at all depending upon the severity of the disease (604). Despite this failure to utilize injected carbohydrate it can be readily shown that the transformations occurring within the Embden-Meyerhof scheme including the formation of glucose-1-phosphate from glycogen are in no wise hindered by the absence of insulin. Both depancreatized animals (484) (526) and diabetic patients (517, 526) reveal increased blood levels of pyruvic and lactic acids as a result of exercise. It may, therefore, be concluded that even in the depancreatized individual, muscles transform glycogen to those two acids. The data on the R.Q. both in resting (510) and exercising animal (52) appear to rule out the oxidation of pyruvate in the non-nervous organs of the depancreatized animal. It is true that pyruvate injected into the diabetic organism disappears from the blood (124) but

[14] Commerical insulin preparations may contain a contaminating substance which aids glycogenolysis and raises blood sugar (929). That contaminant however does not arise in the beta cells of the islands of Langerhans and its action is not a property of endogenous insulin. Further work is necessary to determine whether the substance participates in the regulation of the blood sugar level.

this observation does not necessarily mean that the pyruvate which diffuses into the tissues is used by them. The balance of evidence for an effect of insulin on the oxidation of pyruvate via the tricarboxylic acid cycle is negative not only in experiments performed on the intact organism but also upon excised tissues (879). These results, as a group, indicate that insulin possesses at least two points of attack: one on hepatic phosphorylase and another to lift the anterior pituitary inhibition of the glucokinase reaction. But further work on the mechanism of insulin is indicated. In all non-

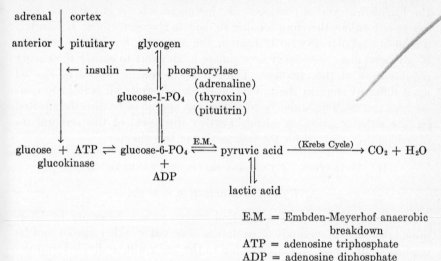

E.M. = Embden-Meyerhof anaerobic breakdown
ATP = adenosine triphosphate
ADP = adenosine diphosphate

Fig. 13. The chief stages in the path of the utilization of glucose to its ultimate products, CO_2, H_2O are presented. The sites of hormonal influences, the oxidation schemes and the direction of the energy exchanges are indicated. According to this formulation, glycogen and lactic acid lead away from the main stream of glucose utilization. The anterior pituitary does not appear to be active on brain *in situ*.

nervous tissues the progress of glucose-6-phosphate to pyruvate and subsequent oxidation is indirectly retarded by the consumption of fat. When more fat is oxidized less carbohydrate is required to maintain the caloric exchanges of the body. The processing of glucose-6-phosphate, toward glycogen, and therefore away from the direct path of utilization, is inversely related to the call for calories. The less the energy requirement is the greater storage will be; when glucose enters the Embden-Meyerhof scheme more rapidly than it is oxidized, glycogen accumulates. Each organ possesses a characteristic ceiling for this accumulation; low in brain, intermediate in muscle, and high in liver. In the liver an additional influence is the level of blood sugar for glycogen stores are spent to combat hypoglycemia just as they are stuffed to minimize hyperglycemia.

The transformations of the Embden-Meyerhof and Krebs machines are affected by other hormones; adrenaline, thyroxin, and pituitrin. Adrenaline may exert a direct action favoring the elaboration of muscle lactic acid and liver glucose at the expense of glycogen stores in the respective organs. The increased concentrations of glycogen breakdown-products stimulate carbohydrate oxidations (241) which nevertheless are inadequate to account for all of these metabolites. The levels of glucose and lactate, therefore, rise in the tissues and in the blood stream. Probably thyroxin influences the Embden-Meyerhof portion of the metabolic scheme in the same manner as adrenaline therefore tending to deplete glycogen stores. If pituitrin diminishes cellular oxygen utilization the anaerobic breakdown products of glycogen must necessarily accumulate in an effort to satisfy the energy requirements of the organism. These many hormonal influences exerted upon different steps in the utilization of carbohydrate all pertain to non-nervous tissues. The brain, *in situ*, does not appear to be directly affected by the anterior pituitary gland. Further discussion of this cerebral independence is reserved for the last section of this chapter.

III. OXIDATION OF CARBOHYDRATE BY CEREBRAL TISSUES

A. *Pyruvic acid oxidation in brain*

In an attempt to elucidate cerebral oxidation, it is necessary to determine whether the methods of oxidation observed in other tissues can be applied to the brain. The application to the brain will be divided into the same two parts, as in the previous discussion of non-nervous tissues; anaerobic and aerobic, but in this case, the oxidation of pyruvic acid will be discussed before considering the Embden-Meyerhof scheme.

The body of evidence indicates that the tricarboxylic cycle functions in the brain (60). That organ contains aconitase (566) and isocitric dehydrogenase (2), enzymes taking part in the tricarboxylic acid cycle, and we also know that citric acid synthesis occurs in the brain (111) (125a). Additional evidence in favor of the function of this cycle is afforded by the stimulating effect of four-carbon dicarboxylic acids on cerebral oxidations (35). Malonate, which is an inhibitor of succinic dehydrogenase, and therefore interferes with the Szent-Györgyi portion of the Krebs cycle, diminishes cerebral respiration (803). The significance of diphosphothiamin is firmly established in the cerebral utilization of pyruvate (787, 774, 35). Studies of brain oxidations in avitaminotic animals reveal a subnormal oxygen intake, and the addition of diphosphothiamin to these tissues restores normal oxygen consumption (787). It may be concluded that the Krebs cycle and vitamin B_1 are necessary for the oxidation of pyruvic acid in the brain.

B. *Embden-Meyerhof and other schemes*

The function of the Embden-Meyerhof scheme as applied to the brain has been established by the work of Mazza and Valeri (718), Euler *et al* (294), Meyerhof (735), Banga, Ochoa and Peters (35), Ochoa (772), Cori and co-workers (186, 190, 179), and Greville and Lehmann (422). These investigators demonstrated for the brain the various intermediary stages of carbohydrate metabolism between glycogen and pyruvic acid presented in Fig. 9. It may therefore be concluded that the Embden-Meyerhof scheme is a preparatory method for cerebral oxidation.[15] There are data, however, which indicate that this method of preparation for brain oxidation is not obligatory.

In 1929 Ashford and Holmes (23) suggested two paths for the cerebral oxidation of carbohydrate: one, starting with glycogen and involving phosphate exchanges, and the other commencing with glucose and independent of phosphate. Many observations since that time reveal that carbohydrate may be oxidized without a preliminary splitting of hexosediphosphate to two molecules of triosephosphate as occurs in the Embden-Meyerhof scheme. This evidence comes from the observation that glucose continues to be oxidized in the presence of inhibitors preventing either the formation of pyruvic acid by the Embden-Meyerhof scheme, or the oxidation of pyruvic acid. In 1935, it was first shown that despite the presence of nicotine, which prevents the oxidation of pyruvic acid, carbohydrate oxidation by the brain continues (490, 309, 32), presumably by the oxidative decarboxylation of glucose to the three carbon stage. This conception that glucose can be oxidized without previous splitting to triose is also supported by other observations made with the aid of iodoacetate (54), fluoride (309), or glyceraldehyde (31), substances which inhibit the splitting of glucose but nevertheless permit the continued, though somewhat diminished, oxidation of that substance. It is possible that paths of glucose oxidation not involving preliminary cleavage may be of greater quantitative importance than the Embden-Meyerhof scheme because the blocking of the latter path may occur with only a minor depression of cerebral oxygen consumption. The rate of cerebral oxidation of glucose may continue practically unchanged despite the action of iodoacetate inhibiting the splitting of carbohydrate from 90 to 100 per cent (54). Though this inhibition proves that there must be a route of cerebral oxidation not in-

[15] The work of Racker and Krimsky (813) shows that Theiler's F. A. virus of experimental poliomyelitis interrupts the Embden-Meyerhof pathway by preventing the phosphorylation of glucose and of fructose-6-phosphate. Pearson and Winzler (783b), also employing mouse brain but with Theiler's G.D. VII virus did not find any effect on oxygen consumption, glucose utilization and lactic acid production.

volving the Embden-Meyerhof concept, we have little knowledge of its intermediary stages. Nevertheless, some idea of the characteristics of a hypothetical path has been obtained by the use of the inhibitors, iodoacetate and nicotine. The evidence indicates that such a course is probably concerned with the formation of pyruvic acid and not its subsequent oxidation. The complete oxidation of carbohydrate, and therefore of its intermediary stage, pyruvic acid, continues in the presence of a concentration of iodoacetate strong enough to prevent the splitting of glycogen (54). But the oxidation of pyruvic acid remains unchanged irrespective of its method of manufacture. When pyruvic acid is not formed anaerobically in accordance with the Embden-Meyerhof method, it may still be produced aerobically because nicotine prevents the oxidation of pyruvic acid but does not stop the oxygen intake of cerebral tissue in the presence of glucose (32). A utilization of oxygen therefore occurs before the fabrication of pyruvic acid. In the Embden-Meyerhof plan, oxygen is used after the production of pyruvic acid. By the hypothetical scheme oxygen is required not only for the combustion of pyruvic acid but also for its formation. It is therefore necessary to seek for a design of carbohydrate oxidation in which pyruvic acid is formed as a result of oxidative processes. Suggestions for such a pattern arise in the work of Harrison on glucose (450, 451), and Warburg and Christian (968, 969) and Dickens on glucose phosphate (234, 235) as reviewed above.

With the exception of the formation of pentose phosphate from phosphogluconic acid (540a) the stages of the Warburg-Christian-Dickens path have not been demonstrated for cerebral oxidation, but brain contains materials necessary for this path: dehydrogenases (225), coenzymes containing niacin (617, 28, 933), flavoproteins containing riboflavin (156), and cytochromes (540). These substances occur in the brain and subserve various functions including the dehydrogenations of the tricarboxylic acid cycle (see Fig. 12). Further research will have to decide whether they take part in a scheme of oxidation not involving the Embden-Meyerhof path. There are some scattered bits of evidence, however, supporting the possibility of oxidative formation of pyruvic acid in cerebral tissues. For example, the first step in the Warburg-Christian path, the activation of hydrogen, is brought about by cerebral dehydrogenases (225). With the use of the dye, methylene blue, the anaerobic activity of various dehydrogenases has been demonstrated in the brain. The hydrogen of the substrate is activated on the surface of the dehydrogenase and then transferred to methylene blue which turns to methylene white as the dye is reduced. By this technic it has been possible to show that the brain contains dehydrogenases for such hexoses as glucose, fructose and galactose; for the three-carbon acids: pyruvic and lactic, as well as for the di- and tri-carboxylic acids, succinic and citric. The activities of a coenzyme of dehydrogenase in accepting this hydrogen have been shown by Quastel and Wheatley (806) who found that cozymase, or coenzyme I, markedly increases the oxidation of d-l-lactate in rat brain cortex slices.

The activity of flavoprotein, or cytochrome reductase, has been observed in the brain; for example, the oxidation of alcohol to acetaldehyde (232, 233) requires the combination of alcohol dehydrogenase, coenzyme I, flavoprotein and cytochrome-cytochrome oxidase, a mechanism similar to that for the combustion of glucose-6-phosphate as seen in the Warburg-Christian scheme (Fig. 10). The enzyme system, cytochrome-cytochrome oxidase, has been examined in brain tissue by the aid of the inhibitors, cyanide or carbon monoxide. Both cyanide and carbon monoxide may combine with the heavy metal of cytochrome oxidase, and since its affinity for the inhibitors is greater than for the oxygen, a compound is formed between the oxidase and inhibitors to the exclusion of oxygen. The oxidative chain is therefore stopped at this point. Most oxidations cease when cytochrome-cytochrome oxidase is poisoned (947).

Another way which has been used to study the Warburg-Keilin enzyme chain is the examination of the cerebral oxidation of p-phenylenediamine by the brain for this substance is oxidized directly by the cytochrome-cytochrome oxidase system of Warburg and Keilin. Holmes (535), Quastel and Wheatley (806) and Himwich *et al* (476) have studied the oxidation of p-phenylenediamine by the brain. The evidence on the application of the Warburg-Christian scheme to the brain is suggestive; the possibility of the progressive oxidative decarboxylation of glucose-6-phosphate to five-, four- and three-carbon phosphate compounds is being explored (540a). Whether the Warburg-Christian-Dickens scheme, or the Harrison, or still some other path[16] proves to be applicable, this review at least indicates that it should be profitable to investigate mechanisms of cerebral oxidation other than those starting with the Embden-Meyerhof scheme.

C. *Cerebral oxidations in the absence of insulin*

The schemes of carbohydrate metabolism just described for the brain and also for non-nervous tissues do not involve the activity of insulin. A large

[16] One of the earliest schemes for the oxidation of carbohydrate is that of Dakin and Dudley (217) and Neuberg (769) who regarded methyl glyoxal as the important product in the splitting of glucose. Ashford (21) has suggested methyl glyoxal as an intermediate for the oxidation of glucose in the brain which does not go through the Embden-Meyerhof path. Meyerhof and Lohmann (740) however have produced evidence against the importance of methyl glyoxal, and Mazza and Lenti (717) were able to exclude methyl glyoxal as a product in brain oxidations and suggest glyceraldehyde in its place. For further discussion of the position of methyl glyoxal in carbohydrate oxidations, see Needham (765) pp. 610–614.

body of evidence supports the observations of Colowick, Cori and Slein (178) that insulin is influential in initiating the metabolism of glucose as well as accelerating the formation of glycogen (928).

Briefly reviewing the action of insulin, we recall that when this hormone is administered to the normal animal or human subject, the respiratory quotient rises towards unity, and carbohydrate disappears from the body (37, 39, 86, 89, 185). By comparing the respiratory quotient with the carbohydrate content of the body, we showed (Chapter 2) that the carbohydrate which disappeared had been oxidized. Just as striking, or perhaps even more so, are the effects of the absence of insulin as seen in the depancreatized animal. In an animal so prepared the oxidation of carbohydrate is greatly depressed. Whether the diabetes is experimentally produced, or whether it is a result of pathologic processes in the diabetic patient, the diminished ability to oxidize carbohydrate is evidenced by the urinary excretion of ingested carbohydrate and a respiratory quotient of 0.7, indicating the oxidation of fat. The injection of insulin restores carbohydrate metabolism in diabetes, as indicated by the cessation of glycosuria and the rise of the respiratory quotient.

Are all the organs of the depancreatized body affected equally by this diabetic condition? A further study reveals that they are not. Muscle (821, 510) heart (210) and kidney (821, 303) have respiratory quotients of 0.7, and that of the liver (493) may be significantly below 0.7, probably because of incomplete oxidation of fat in that organ. An exception to the obligatory oxidation of fat in the absence of insulin is observed in the brain, for the cerebral respiratory quotient remains fixed at unity (519). The depancreatized animal's respiratory quotient does not represent a uniform quotient for each organ, but is the average quotient for all the organs in the body. The quotients of most the organs are close to 0.7, and the effect which the high quotient in the brain has on the respiratory quotient of the entire body is counteracted by the low quotient of the liver. These data show that the rise in quotient after the administration of insulin is due to the increased oxidation of carbohydrate by non-nervous tissues. Insulin does not exert such an effect on brain metabolism.

The first demonstration that the brain can oxidize carbohydrate in the absence of insulin was made in 1929. It was found that the brain *in situ* of the depancreatized dog possesses a respiratory quotient of unity, meaning that carbohydrate continued to be oxidized even in the absence of insulin (519). Furthermore, the cerebral arterio-venous oxygen difference remains unchanged after pancreatectomy. This observation, taken into conjunction with the fixed respiratory quotient indicates that not only is carbohydrate oxidized by the brain but that its rate of oxidation is not diminished. The respiratory quotient of cerebral tissues excised from depancreatized animals also reveals that carbohydrate oxidation was not hindered. Most of the quotients obtained from brain tissue excised from depancreatized dogs (307) and cats (32) are close to unity. Not only was carbohydrate oxidized, but the rate remained unchanged. These results are therefore in agreement with those previously described for the brain *in situ*.

Further proof of the oxidation of carbohydrate by the brain of diabetic animals is afforded by a study of the carbohydrate balance of cerebral tissues excised from depancreatized cats (32). In a typical result the utilization of glucose which could have been oxidized was *calculated*. The oxygen intake could explain the utilization of 1.2 mg. per 100 mg. dry tissue per hour of glucose; the *observed* utilization of glucose was 1.0 mg. per 100 mg. Glucose combustion therefore accounted for most of the oxygen intake, and since the respiratory quotient was close to 1.0, we know that glucose was oxidized completely. It is apparent that the absence of insulin does not decrease the ability of the brain to oxidize glucose. The consideration of insulin may therefore be omitted in any analysis of cerebral oxidation.

Observations on respiratory quotients of the brain of humans with diabetes have not been made. However, readings were taken on the cerebral arterio-venous oxygen difference of seven diabetic patients, high-grade morons whose diabetes was controlled by the administration of standard insulin.[17] On the day previous to the collection of the blood, insulin was administered before the evening meal at approximately 5 o'clock. No further dosage was given until after the observations were completed late on the morning of the next day. The average arterio-venous oxygen difference of these patients was 5.7 vol. per cent without insulin, and 5.5 vol. per cent after treatment with insulin. If no significant differences in cerebral blood flow were wrought by the treatment of insulin these preliminary results are in accord with the *in vitro* data and the human brain like that of lower mammals, does not require insulin for cerebral oxidations. The subnormal C.M.R. (cerebral metabolic rate) associated with diabetic coma is probably not due to a primary failure of cerebral carbohydrate oxidation but is rather a reflection of the pathological internal environment of the diabetic organism (see section on diabetic coma, Chapter 8).

To what are we to attribute the power of the brain to continue carbohydrate metabolism independent of insulin? This freedom from insulin is observed despite the glucokinase mechanism (773) which is present in the brain, a mechanism which requires insulin in non-nervous tissues. The anterior pituitary does not appear to depress the cerebral oxidation of carbohydrate *in vivo* and the presumption is that the cerebral capillaries

[17] Unpublished observations of the author.

or rather their surrounding glial cells occlude the passage of the anterior pituitary secretion from the blood to the brain cells.[18] In that case, the utilization of glucose would be removed from this hormonal restraint and the glucokinase reaction could proceed without the benefit of insulin.

IV. SUMMARY

A review of the methods for the cellular oxidations of carbohydrate reveals that these processes may be divided into two parts: one anaerobic, starting with glycogen and ending with the formation of pyruvic acid, and the other, aerobic, the oxidation of pyruvic acid to carbon dioxide and water. It has been demonstrated that the first part may take place by the Embden-Meyerhof path in which pyruvic acid is formed as a result of the splitting of carbohydrate. The second part requires diphosphothiamin and the Krebs cycle for the oxidation of pyruvic acid.

Upon application of these schemes to carbohydrate metabolism in the brain, it was found that the methods of pyruvic acid oxidation occuring in the brain are similar to those in other tissues, and that the Embden-Meyerhof plan also applies to the brain. Further analysis, however, reveals that in addition to the Embden-Meyerhof design, there must be another pattern of carbohydrate breakdown, because the inhibition of carbohydrate splitting or pyruvic acid oxidation does not necessarily depress cerebral oxidation of glucose. An analysis of the data indicates that this other method must involve the utilization of oxygen in the stages between glycogen and pyruvic acid. At present no such system has been uncovered in the brain, but the work of Warburg and Christian, Dickens, Harrison, Breusch, and Horecker suggests routes whereby pyruvic acid is formed as a result of oxidative decarboxylation and not from splitting carbohydrate. The oxidation of pyruvic acid to carbon dioxide and water takes place in the same manner irrespective of its method of formation.

In a consideration of the cerebral oxidations it is not necessary to include the function of insulin, since the brain, unlike non-nervous organs, does not require that hormone for the oxidation of carbohydrate. The phosphorylation of glucose, the glucokinase reaction, is the first limiting stage in cellular carbohydrate transformations. In all organs, except the brain, this reaction is depressed by the principal of the anterior pituitary which is reinforced by the product of the adrenal cortex and antagonized by insulin. The freedom of the brain from this endocrine control can be explained if that organ is impermeable to the anterior pituitary hormone. In that case, the cerebral glucokinase reaction could proceed unhindered by the secretions of the anterior pituitary and adrenal cortex and unaided by insulin.

[18] See Chapter 6, page 117 for discussion of blood-brain barrier.

ASPECTS OF CEREBRAL CIRCULATION

A book on brain metabolism would be incomplete without a description of the cerebral vasculature. Considering the latitude of the subject, we are aware that this chapter will not attempt to cover the entire framework of cerebral circulation, but will touch on only those aspects which we think are relevant to cerebral metabolism, directly or indirectly.

The brain can maintain its metabolic requirements only by receiving a continual supply of foodstuff and oxygen, and by a steady removal of the products of cellular metabolism. This work of transporting the fuel to the cells and taking away the cellular products is the specific function of the circulation. It becomes important, therefore, to examine the anatomic and physiologic characteristics of cerebral blood supply, keeping uppermost in mind the question of how they are adapted, controlled and regulated to support brain metabolism. It is essential to understand the qualitative differences in blood flow to the brain as a whole, as well as to its elemental parts. As for quantitative differences, if it were possible to determine these definitely, they would yield even more significant data. So far, the quantitative data are more limited, but even those which we now possess are of practical importance in the determination of metabolic rate of the brain *in situ*. As we have stated, two factors are involved in calculating the metabolic rate of the brain—the cerebral blood flow and the cerebral arteriovenous oxygen difference—and in this chapter we will mention only those vascular adaptations necessary to clarify the text of the following chapters.

I. SOME ANATOMIC ELEMENTS INVOLVED IN COLLECTING BLOOD SAMPLES

In its microscopic anatomy the vascular supply of the brain is not distinguished significantly from that of the other organs. In gross anatomy, however, there is a difference, for the brain is not fed from a hilum but rather from a series of vessels including the paired vertebral arteries which pour into the single basilar artery. This vessel and the two internal carotid arteries together with their respective connections form the Circle of Willis at the base of the brain. From the Circle of Willis, six large branches send out the smaller pial arteries which spread like a net over the surface of the cortex and dip into it to supply the cerebral tissues. The arterioles arising from these arteries anastomose with one another, and the capillary beds which spring from the arterioles form a continuous interlacing mesh (174, 791). Such an arrangement of the vasculature must prevent degeneration of portions of the brain if the finer arterioles should be occluded, but if a *larger* artery should be shut off, the part of the brain fed by that artery could not be sustained. In the capillaries the blood loses its oxygen to the cerebral tissues, accounting for the striking contrast in color between the arteries and veins—the bright scarlet hue of the arteries gives way to the purplish red of the veins.

The return flow from the brain is gathered in two groups of veins: one within the structure of the brain and the other on its surface. Whether within the brain or upon it, both groups empty into the intradural veins, so called because they lie within the folds of the thick dura mater which envelops the brain.

One intradural vein in particular, the superior longitudinal sinus, situated in the dural curtain between the two cerebral hemispheres, lends itself as an available site for collection of blood from an infant. This spot, commonly known as the fontanel, is an open area at the vertex of the skull and is accessible only for a limited time in the baby, until the bony borders close in to form the solid circumference of the cranium.

The superior longitudinal sinus which drains a portion of the medial surfaces of the cerebral hemispheres and most of their convex surfaces, travels posteriorly to the occipital region and there in the torcular, meets another intradural vein, the straight sinus, which also collects blood from the medial surfaces of the cerebral hemispheres, the choroid plexus, and most important, the basal ganglia. The torcular not only receives these two veins but also gives origin to the two lateral sinuses. Only rarely is the torcular a single chamber in which the venous blood mixes. Usually the superior longitudinal sinus directs most of its blood to one or the other of the lateral sinuses, while the straight sinus sends its blood to the opposite side (389, 64). Riggs (quoted in 596) examined 25 autopsy specimens and observed that most of the blood went to the right side in 15 of the specimens. In 9 instances, the superior longitudinal sinus blood in its entirety went to the right, and in one case entirely to the left lateral sinus. In an additional 100 skulls (268) a complete confluence of the superior longitudinal and straight sinuses occurred only 8 times making the percentage approximately 6 for all specimens.

To continue with the course of the venous blood, after traversing the lateral sinuses it leaves the cranial cavity chiefly by the internal jugular veins, but in part by the two vertebral veins. The same two paired exits (internal jugular and vertebral) drain the blood from the base of the brain. With two exceptions the blood collected from the internal jugular veins represents the return flow from bilaterally symmetrical portions of the brain. The midbrain, the medulla oblongata and the cerebellum are equally represented in both internal jugular veins. However, in individuals in whom the venous blood of the superior longitudinal sinus and straight sinus do

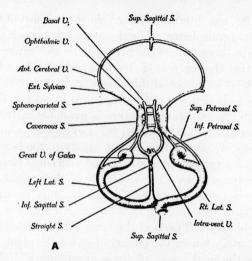

Basal U.
Ophthalmic U.
Ant. Cerebral U.
Ext. Sylvian
Spheno-parietal S.
Cavernous S.
Great U. of Galen
Left Lat. S.
Inf. Sagittal S.
Straight S.
Sup. Sagittal S.
Sup. Petrosal S.
Inf. Petrosal S.
Rt. Lat. S.
Intra-vent. U.
Sup. Sagittal S.

A

Inferior Portion of Cerebral Venous Drainage
[Hedon]

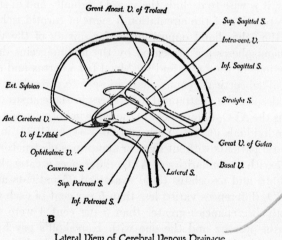

Great Anast. U. of Trolard
Sup. Sagittal S.
Intra-vent. U.
Inf. Sagittal S.
Straight S.
Ext. Sylvian
Ant. Cerebral U.
U. of L'Abbé
Ophthalmic U.
Cavernous S.
Sup. Petrosal S.
Inf. Petrosal S.
Great U. of Galen
Basal U.
Lateral S.

B

Lateral View of Cerebral Venous Drainage
[Hedon]

FIG. 14 A & B. Schematic drawings of the cerebral venous drainage which Dr. Frederic A. Gibbs had made in accordance with the description of Hedon. In these drawings the superior sagittal or longitudinal sinus sends all its blood through the right lateral sinus and to the right internal jugular vein (not labeled in the diagram). As explained in the text this arrangement of the cerebral venous drainage is only one of those which occur, however, it is here presented because it is a frequent form of the venous organization.

not mix in the torcular, one internal jugular vein carries most of the return flow from the cerebral hemispheres, while the other brings back that of the basal ganglia. Despite these differences between the two internal jugular veins, it is probable that the contents of the right and left sides are approximately the same in most instances. If this close approximation is caused by intracranial mixing of blood it can not be explained by such action on the arterial side. Though the anatomic structure is available in the Circle of Willis usually there is little mixing of blood (827) so that the contents of an internal carotid artery are distributed almost wholly to the hemisphere of the same side. Such a segregation may be expected with equal blood pressure in both internal carotid arteries. Only when one of the component tributaries of the Circle is occluded, at least partially, may its distributing potentialities be realized but even then its anastomoses may not supply an adequate volume of blood to all parts of the brain. The fact that ligation of the internal carotid artery lowers the pressure beyond the point of ligation (931a) demonstrates the inadequacy of these anastomoses. Indeed 20 to 30% of individuals may exhibit signs of anoxia after an occlusion of the artery (792a). For that reason before a carotid artery is completely ligated as a therapeutic measure, in a patient with aneurysm or arterio-venous anastomoses, it is wise to occlude the vessel gradually and in such a way as to permit restoration of the circulation if signs of carotid ischemia appear (792a). On the other hand opportunities for mixing of the venous blood from both hemispheres are presented by the midline veins draining symmetrical portions of the brain and for blood from cortex and subcortex by many cortical-subcortical venous anastomoses. As a result of this twofold mixing and despite the anatomical differences in the courses of the largest midline veins the AVO$_2$ differences are the same in both sides in the majority of normal individuals at rest. York and co-workers (1032) in 40 observations of mental patients without signs or symptoms of structural pathology found only 7 with dissimilarities of AVO$_2$ differences greater than 1 volume per cent. Gibbs and associates (399) examined 25 patients and in 17 the bilateral AVO$_2$ differences varied less than 5 per cent of each other. Of the 8 others with discrepancies greater than 5 per cent 4 were psychotics, 3 with dementia praecox and the one with Korsakoff's psychosis. The remaining 4 exhibited unilateral cerebral pathology. The lack of agreement in the patients with unilateral organic changes may be ascribed to incomplete mixing of the venous blood of the two hemispheres. Shenkin, et al (866), have found that, on the average, two-thirds of the blood coming from one internal carotid artery is returned by the internal jugular vein on the same side. But for the 4 psychotic patients of Gibbs, et al (399) and the 7 of York and co-workers (1032), it is necessary to seek some other explanation than the incomplete venous mixing across the midline to account for the dissimilar AVO_2 differences. It would seem that in this smaller group of patients, without organic pathology, the cortical-subcortical anastomoses were not adequate to make up for the anatomic differences in the distribution of the large central veins.

The normal limitations to complete cortical-subcortical venous mixing may be further restricted by thiopental anesthesia for in patients with similar AVO_2 differences on both sides under resting conditions, the imposition of light thiopental anesthesia changed the relationships so that the AVO_2 differences on both sides no longer agreed in 9 of 12 instances (Etsten, York and Himwich (293)). If light thiopental anesthesia exerts relatively greater depressant effects on cortex than subcortex, including depression of metabolic rate and blood flow, the discrepancies between cortical and subcortical blood may be magnified. This magnification makes it possible to distinguish between 2 sources; the superior longitudinal sinus and the straight sinus, in samples of blood drawn from the 2 internal jugular veins.

In 10 patients reported by Kety and Schmidt (598) the bilateral AVO_2 differences, C.B.F. and C.M.R. were in close agreement, demonstrating excellent mixing of the venous blood, probably the usual phenomenon. On the other hand, Himwich and associates (528) found dissimilar values in 4 patients. Two of these had dementia praecox and were in a deteriorated condition. The other 2 had general cerebral paresis and it is known that the degenerative processes occurring in this disease are, as a rule, more intense in the cortex than the subcortex. The bilateral differences in these 4 patients were beyond the calculated error of the method. It would be interesting to study another large series of individuals in order to determine whether the dissimilarities previously observed between the bilateral AVO_2 differences (1032, 399) would also apply to C.B.F. and C.M.R.

The blood leaving the cranial cavity whether in the internal jugular veins or in the vertebral veins may be regarded as largely of cerebral origin because there are only small communications between intracranial and extracranial vessels,[1] and few if any arterio-venous anastomoses (25). Each of these pairs of veins furnishes sources from which to draw cerebral venous blood. But, the vertebral veins, hidden as they are by the neck muscles and protected by the bony transverse processes of the cervical vertebrate can not be readily reached by a needle used for drawing blood samples. The internal jugular vein is readily accessible at or near its point of exit from the cranial cavity through the jugular foramen. It was a great technical advance

[1] Ferris and co-workers (317) have observed that with the vascular changes of hyperventilation: constriction of cerebral blood flow and increase in the extracranial circulation, the fraction of internal jugular blood coming from extracranial sources is augmented. But the contamination of internal jugular blood with extracerebral blood usually is negligible in the resting subject (866).

when Myerson, Halloran and Hirsch (756) found that this vein may be tapped by inserting a needle at a point just in front of the tip of the mastoid process, close to the lobe of the ear. On this anatomic basis, the internal jugular vein is the most logical, as well as the most convenient, place from which to draw samples of venous blood. The analysis of the venous blood tells only half the story, for without the arterial blood, we could not compare the two for oxygen, carbon dioxide, sugar, velocity of flow, or in short, for any information on the metabolic exchanges of the brain.

Fortunately, it is not necessary to puncture the deeply buried internal carotid artery to obtain a sample of blood going to the brain because the constituents of all arterial blood, no matter from what part of the body it is drawn, exhibit no demonstrable difference in content. The more superficial brachial and femoral arteries may be approached with less difficulty, and since the contents are the same regardless of the source, either of these two arteries is tapped instead of the internal carotid. The most extensively used method for studying brain metabolism is to compare the constituents of arterial and venous blood with each other. In order to support itself the brain removes sugar and oxygen from, and releases carbon dioxide into, the blood passing through it, and as a result of cerebral oxidations the arterial blood would naturally contain more oxygen and sugar, and the venous blood more carbon dioxide. Analysis of venous blood yields additional information about the brain, including the carbon dioxide and oxygen pressures within it. Investigations of Lennox and co-workers (656) and Courtice (197) have shown that one can get a better idea of the pressure of these two gases in brain tissue by examining the venous blood than from the arterial. This relationship applies to the brain in general when in a state of comparative rest, but not necessarily to any particular region which may suffer oxygen deprivation as it becomes hyperactive and its demands exceed the supply.

Work from Bronk's laboratory indicates that the oxygen pressure immediately below the surface of the cortex may be about 30 mm.; but as one goes deeper within the cortex the pressure decreases. Bronk and Brink (118) further estimated that the oxygen pressure of the internal jugular vein is approximately 10 mm. higher than that immediately below the surface of the cortex. These relationships obtain under resting conditions, but Davis, McCulloch and Roseman (227) have noted that preceding[2] a con-

---

[2] Using somewhat different methods, Davies and Rémond (226), found that the decrease in oxygen tension did not precede, but followed, the onset of electrical changes. According to these observations the metabolic rate rose in order to support the hyperactivity excited by metrazol. Though the temporal relations observed by the two groups of workers were not the same yet both groups obtained a positive correlation between activity and oxygen consumption.

vulsion caused by a stimulating drug the oxygen pressure in the brain practically disappears, while the internal jugular vein still does retain appreciable amounts of oxygen. Thus, it is seen that though the pressure difference of oxygen between the internal jugular vein and the brain itself is small during rest, it increases with cerebral activity. This greater pressure difference during activity physiologically serves to insure the passage of more oxygen from the blood to the brain at this time.

Occasionally a patient develops an arterio-venous aneurysm, in which case a portion of the arterial blood does not pass through tissue capillaries but is poured directly into the veins. In one patient of this type (541), the saturation of the hemoglobin with oxygen was 95 per cent in one internal jugular vein, approximately the same as that of arterial blood. The saturation of the other was 80 per cent. The normal is 62 per cent. The brain therefore, does not benefit from the blood passing through the aneurysm, and the cerebral AVO_2 difference is lower than the normal value of 6.7 vol. per cent (392). Hyperventilation augments still more the oxygenation of the internal jugular vein blood (678) for the fraction of blood which traverses the brain is reduced with the vasoconstriction of alkalosis. As might be expected the total cerebral blood flow is markedly accelerated with arterio-venous aneurysm and this acceleration is supported by a greater cardiac output and an enlarged heart (868).

A rapidly growing arterio-venous aneurysm may produce disastrous results and it therefore becomes necessary to tie off the internal carotid artery on the side of the aneurysm in an attempt to diminish the volume of blood within it. In one such patient of Dr. Eldridge H. Campbell,[3] the AVO_2 difference was 2.8 vol. per cent, and after a subtotal ligation it rose to an average of 5.2 vol. per cent (3 observations) demonstrating a retardation in cerebral blood flow as a result of the operative interference.

II. CONTROL OF CEREBRAL BLOOD SUPPLY

The brain is almost completely surrounded by a rigid skull which prevents any major change in the volume of the blood contained in it. At first it may seem that this inelasticity of the skull might prevent the vascular supply from adapting itself to the degree of cerebral activity. A bony encasement would indeed prove disastrous for skeletal muscle which we know runs the gamut from incomplete rest to extreme exercise. Though the brain is always active and not necessarily so at the same rate, it does not experience the wide graduations characteristic of muscle. Therefore, the encasement which encloses the brain does not interfere with the moderate vascular adaptations necessary for the acquisition of foodstuff and oxygen.

[3] Unpublished observation.

At the same time, the skull serves as a protective shield against injury. Despite the limitations imposed by the skull, there are two ways in which the cerebral blood flow may be altered.

In the first place, there may be small adjustments in the volumes of the fluid elements which go to form the cranial content and these permit minor fluctuations in the arterial blood. The quantity of arterial blood can vary if there is resorption or formation of the cerebrospinal fluid, or if the volume of blood in the intradural veins changes; or, an increase of blood in one area of the brain may be balanced by a decrease in some other area. Pathologically, edema or tumors of one type or another may decrease the arterial contents. More important however than these changes in volume is the fact that the handicap of the inelastic encasement of the brain does not prevent a greater flow of blood through the brain in a given time interval. For example, if the arterial supply is doubled and the venous return is likewise doubled, the volume of blood within the skull would not change, but each unit of blood traversing the brain would pass through at twice the speed as before. Hence, the skull barrier confines the arterial blood to small changes in volume but does not prevent variations in the rate of blood flowing through the brain per minute. The amount of blood passing through the brain at any given moment is the result of both of these factors, volume and rate, acting simultaneously, and it is this total blood flow and the mechanisms which control it which we will discuss next.

A. *Systemic blood pressure and autonomic nervous regulation*

The total blood flow through the brain is not known with certainty but from observations made on excised cerebral tissues (Chap. 8, p. 180, ft.) of an oxygen intake between 44 cc. and 32 cc. per minute and a cerebral arterio-venous oxygen difference of 6.7 vol. per cent, values between 480 cc. and 660 cc. per minute may be calculated. Schmidt, Kety and Pennes (856) using their results on simian brain *in vivo* as a basis, found the minimum of 460 cc., a mean of 660 cc., and a maximum of 1040 cc. Again Kety and Schmidt (596) observed experimentally a minimum flow of 448 cc. per minute, an average of 672 cc. per minute, a maximum of 840 cc. in 16 values ascertained on 11 men comparatively free from muscular activity. Using the same method as Kety and Schmidt, we have confirmed their results (528).[4] If we take all the above values into consideration the value may vary between 450 cc. and 850 cc. per minute. Further research will define a volume between these two extremes and using a dye to estimate

[4] In accordance with a downward revision of the partition coefficient of nitrous oxide between brain and blood these results of Kety and Schmidt as well as those of our group are reduced by 23 per cent in comparison with those previously published (594).

cerebral blood flow Gibbs and co-workers (400) report an average figure of 617 cc. per minute. The latest estimate of Kety and Schmidt (597) calculates to approximately 725 cc. for males. Whatever the exact limits of cerebral blood flow may be, the value is not a constant one but is open to fluctuations and the extent of the fluctuations is determined in part by those of the systemic blood pressure (333). This regulating mechanism works on the following principle. A sudden rise of blood pressure usually induces a faster cerebral flow, and conversely, a fall in the pressure retards the flow through the brain. Apparently, the pressure of the blood itself is a decisive factor when it comes to the amount of blood journeying through the brain.[5]

The velocity of the blood is actually influenced by the pressure difference between the cerebral arteries and the cerebral veins. The importance of systemic pressure is apparent because it is proportional to that in the cerebral arterial system. The venous pressure however is low and approaches zero in the erect position. Changes in intrathoracic pressure (440a), whether due to the respiratory process or other causes, such as lifting a heavy load or the increased venous pressure associated with cardiac decompensation are transmitted to the cerebral veins. But the cerebral venous pressure usually remains fairly constant and the rate of cerebral blood flow is therefore determined largely by the arterial blood pressure.

For this reason the vasomotor reflexes, like those of the carotid sinus, which play a significant part in limiting alterations in blood pressure, are important for the stabilization of the cerebral blood flow. The vasomotor reflexes counteract changes in arterial blood pressure by appropriate alterations in heart action and peripheral vasomotor tone which increase with the fall of blood pressure and diminish with a rise. By virtue of these reflexes, with centers in the medullary and supramedullary regions, the brain takes part in the regulation of its own blood flow. An instance, taken from the field of pathology, is the rise of blood pressure, forcing blood through the brain, against the increased intracranial pressure caused by a brain tumor (599). Thus the ability of the brain to control blood pressure subordinates the control of the systemic circulation to the maintenance of the cerebral blood supply. This phenomenon may be compared with the regulation of carbohydrate utilization in the body as a whole which is similarly subordinated to the requirement of the brain for blood sugar (see Chapter 3).

So important is systemic arterial pressure that when an individual suffers a sudden and profound fall in blood pressure he promptly faints as cerebral functions are temporarily impaired. Syncope and other signs of anoxia due either to orthostatic hypotension, Stokes-Adams syndrome, carotid sinus

[5] Schmidt and associates (856) observe that the increased blood flow during metrazol convulsions does not depend on blood pressure.

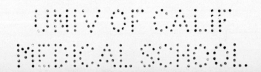

syndrome or shock may occur as consequences of the reduction in cerebral blood flow which results from a fall in blood pressure. Patients with hypertension subjected to sympathetic block as a result of differential spinal anesthesia suffer an impairment of blood pressure which may not be entirely compensated by arteriolar relaxation and for that reason signs of cerebral anoxia are observed (593a). But when the adaptive decrease in arteriolar resistance is adequate, cerebral blood flow is not reduced as for example after lumbodorsal sympathectomy (865a) or the administration of dihydroergocornine (434a). Similarly, tilting the body to an angle of 65° from the horizontal in the head-up position lowers arterial pressure and therefore slows cerebral blood flow. But because of a sufficient diminution of arterial tone, AVO_2 difference becomes larger and cerebral metabolic rate is maintained (848c).

This brings us to the second important component in the regulation of cerebral blood flow, namely cerebrovascular resistance, which according to Kety (592a) is the resultant of all factors tending to impede the flow of blood through the brain. The human brain is not altogether at the mercy of the systemic arterial pressure as the effects of the latter may be modified by the vasomotor action of the arteries and their arterioles. In fact, the contraction or dilatation of these vessels tends to counteract the otherwise monopolistic control of the systemic blood pressure. One minor element contributing to the steadying effect of the intracerebral mechanisms is observed on stimulation of the sympathetic nerves of animals. Such stimulation causes a rise of systemic blood pressure which increases the cerebral blood flow, forcing the vessels to open wider, but at the same time constricts the cerebral vessels (336, 940), diminishing somewhat their dilatation and thus acts, even though weakly, to limit the increase of cerebral blood flow. Stimulation of the parasympathetic nerves produces stronger effects and in the reverse direction (221, 336).[6] As might be expected, the responses to an injection of adrenaline (334, 331) and acetylcholine (333) are similar to those arising from a stimulation of the sympathetic and parasympathetic nerves respectively. The adrenergic neurohormone however is relatively ineffective in comparison with its extracerebral performance. But even when all buffer nerves are eliminated, the vessels shrink as blood pressure rises and enlarge when pressure falls. The vessels seem to be sensitive to the pressure within them and thus tend to maintain cerebral blood flow within normal limits.

Sympathetic constriction, weak in animals, is even more incompetent in man. Unilateral or bilateral block of the stellate ganglion usually does not augment cerebral blood flow (444a). It would therefore appear that tonic

[6] The constrictor fibers are carried to the brain in the cervical sympathetic trunk and the parasympathetic dilator branches in the great superficial petrosal nerve.

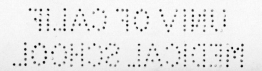

sympathetic constriction is not operative in the cerebral vessels. The benefit derived from stellate block (400a) in the relief of spasm induced by cerebral embolism or by thrombosis may be ascribed to severing a reflex pathway originating at the site of the lesion rather than to a removal of tonic sympathetic influence. The demonstration of the lack of sympathetic vasomotor constrictor tone does not however rule out the participation of the parasympathetic nerves in the regulation of the cerebral circulation. In animals stimulation of the parasympathetics yields significant results (221). Though quantitative data for man are lacking it must be remembered that acetylcholine is released not only by the parasympathetic nerves but also by the brain cells in general (803, 948, 990). This neurohormone therefore takes its place with other vasodilator products of cerebral metabolic activity. These metabolic products are acidic for the most part and include CO_2 and lactic acid. An example is afforded by a drop of systemic blood pressure, which forces the velocity of the cephalic circulation to slacken, and therefore permits the accumulation of CO_2 and also of lactic acid, if anoxia supervenes. When systemic blood pressure falls to a critical level however cerebral vasodilatation, due to the chemical changes, comes to the rescue, facilitating the flow of blood through the brain and tending to overcome the results of a fall in blood pressure. From these actions of the cerebral vessels which are sensitive to the accumulation of metabolic products we may conclude that the authority of the systemic blood pressures over cerebral circulation is checked and balanced by the vasomotor activities. But whatever the cause may be to disturb the level of blood pressure, whether it be injections of adrenaline or acetylcholine, or whether it be a rise in pressure due to asphyxia or a fall resulting from shock, the chief point is: the dangerously wide deviations of blood flow are mitigated by the cerebral vasomotor reflexes, and these, in turn, actuate a finer adjustment of the blood supply than could result without their modifying reactions.

The effect of acetylcholine to dilate the cerebral vessels is the connecting link between 3 aspects of vascular regulation: nervous control, changes wrought by deviations in the acid-base equilibrium and neuronal activity. The concentration of acetylcholine is the result not only of the amount coming from the parasympathetic fibers and the functioning brain cells, but also of that destroyed by cholinesterase. The rate of destruction however is determined by the pH of the medium, for the acidosis is not only vasodilator in its own right but also inhibits cholinesterase and stabilizes acetylcholine. Alkalosis exerts the reverse effect on cholinesterase, hastens the breakdown of the cholinergic secretion (387) thus intensifying vasoconstriction.

We have discussed the mechanisms which function within the cranial cavity in such a manner as to diminish the extent of the increases and decreases in cerebral blood flow caused by corresponding changes of blood pressures. But it must also be remembered that systemic blood pressure may act in an adaptive manner to maintain cerebral blood flow under adverse cerebral conditions. It has been previously mentioned that brain tumors may curtail the volume of blood coursing through the brain. In accordance with the Monro-Kellie Doctrine the vessels of the brain tend to collapse as a result of the heightened intracranial pressure, and this tendency is greatest in the finest vessels. The reactive rise in systemic blood pressure counteracts the influence of the intracranial pressure to diminish the calibre of the vessels and thus maintains cerebral blood flow. According to Cushing (213, 214) the mechanism depends upon cerebral ischemia with resulting stimulation of the medullary vasomotor centers and peripheral vasoconstriction. If the elevation of intracranial pressure is moderate, the corrective increment of blood pressure is adequate to prevent a measurable impairment of cerebral blood flow but when the limits of the compensatory actions are attained cerebral blood flow decreases definitely and in the observations of Kety, Shenkin and Schmidt (599) this occurred at cerebrospinal fluid pressures of 450 mm. of water or higher. The unchanged cerebral blood flow observed in essential hypertension may be regarded as an excellent example of cerebrovascular adaptation (593). The vessels close down to prevent an increased cerebral blood flow. But if the source of the hypertension lies within the skull, as in the case of brain tumor, it reveals again the preponderating role played by arterial blood pressure, which rises to maintain cerebral blood flow, a preponderance which fails when physiological adaptations can no longer cope with intracranial pathology.

Before beginning a detailed consideration of the chemical regulation of the cerebrovascular resistance it is well to mention a physical factor namely the viscosity of the blood. A slow blood flow is observed with the increase of viscosity due to the large number of the red blood cells in polycythemia vera (592a). Conversely a fast flow and diminished viscosity are associated with anemia (848c). Both in polycythemia vera and in anemia the cerebral metabolic rate of the brain may however remain normal because cerebral blood flow and AVO_2 difference vary inversely. Still another physical factor is afforded by the pressure of the cerebrospinal fluid which aids in maintaining hemodynamics during sudden and extreme pressure alterations within the cerebral vessels. Pressure changes in the veins are communicated to the cerebrospinal fluid and therefore to the cranial contents. Thus pressures both within and without the vessels may fluctuate together. With a precipitous rise of arterial and venous pressures, due to a cough or a strain of any kind, rupture of the finer vessels is prevented by a rise in pressure of the surrounding cerebrospinal fluid (440a). Similarly a protective increase of cerebrospinal fluid pressure works in favor of the flyer who is descending rapidly, for example in dive-bombing. In opposite circumstances, during the rapid ascent following the dive, arterial, venous and cerebrospinal fluid pressures all decrease together. These simultaneous changes tend to maintain cerebral blood flow as the arterio-venous pressure gradient tends to be preserved and the lower level of intracranial pressure aids in retaining the patency of the cerebral capillaries. For these reasons blood flow is continued and mental performance is carried on for a longer time than in conditions in which the fall is limited to arterial pressure, when syncope develops more rapidly (463a).

B. *Intrinsic chemical regulation*

The augmented cerebral blood flow following the rise of systemic blood pressure may act impartially to bring more blood to all parts of the brain, while the intrinsic chemical regulation is more concerned with the blood supply to the different cerebral regions. Whether the chemical control is exercised synchronously with the changes in blood pressure, or whether it acts separately, it affords in either case a more equable distribution in accordance with varied requirements of the cerebral regions, sequestering more blood for the active part than could come to it without the chemical regulation. Among the substances in this chemical control, carbon dioxide will be considered first, both in conjunction with changes in blood pressure and also independently of them in support of the localized increase of activity in a given cerebral region.

Carbon dioxide. Just as a systemic blood pressure is the strongest extracerebral factor in the regulation of cerebral circulation, so carbon dioxide is the most powerful of the intrinsic influences (653, 395, 1017). One effective operation of this gas may be traced to its synergistic action upon cerebral vasculature and systemic blood pressure to either raise or lower cerebral blood flow. As an illustration of this synergism, the inhalation of carbon dioxide forces cerebral blood vessels to dilate and, at the same time may increase systemic blood pressure by causing generalized vasoconstriction, and both of these responses to carbon dioxide accelerate cerebral blood flow (333, 557, 597). Conversely, pumping out of the carbon dioxide from the brain perhaps by overventilation sharply limits blood flow because of the localized vasoconstriction, which may be intensified by a fall in systemic blood pressure (1016, 653, 597).[7] The cerebral vasomotor reac-

---

[7] Schmidt, in a private communication, describes a decrease of cerebral blood flow during forced breathing despite a rise in blood pressure. It must be remembered, however, that such a rise occurs only infrequently, and then in part, because the direct action of alkalosis on the vasculature which diminishes the blood flow through the brain is also adequate to overcome the central depressor effect on the blood vessels in other parts of the body. For further discussion, see (90) page 250.

tions to carbon dioxide are probably direct ones exerted on the walls of the vessels, and are not mediated by nervous impulses, as are the systemic changes actuated by receptors in the carotid sinus and body and under the influence of the vasomotor centers in the medulla oblongata.

The remarkable sensitivity of the cerebral vasculature to carbon dioxide makes for an adaptive change in the circulation of any one part of the brain in accordance with the following scheme: in response to stimulation, an area of the brain goes into increased activity. The metabolism of that area must necessarily speed up to support the sudden burst of activity. The local manufacture and accumulation of carbon dioxide, which always follows any increase in metabolism, accelerates the flow of blood through the stimulated locus, thus satisfying its higher demand for oxygen (see section on *Other substances* for similar effects of other metabolites). Such an adaptive vascular response is observed when the retina is stimulated by light, and both the lateral geniculate body and the visual cortex show signs of increased blood flow (383, 846, 855). Though these nice adjustments bring a greater volume of oxygen to the active part, still the supply of this gas may be inadequate, for the oxygen tension in this region may be lower than it was in comparative rest. In fact, as described on p. 96 the hyperactive area may suffer from anoxia during a convulsive fit. In such a case, the brain reverts to an anaerobic metabolism to aid the aerobic processes in supporting activity (430, 611, 916). Lactic acid, inorganic phosphate and other metabolites accumulate so that after the fit is over, energy must be made available to reestablish the pre-convulsive biochemical pattern, and during this time the cerebral circulation is still maintained at a greater rate than before the convulsion in response to the vasodilator action of these metabolites. A dramatic instance is reported by Penfield (785) who observed the exposed brain of a patient in the aftermath of an epileptic seizure. The venous blood returning from the portion of the brain which had been active in the epileptic convulsion was of a distinctly more arterialized hue than the blood from the relatively quiescent cerebral tissue. It would seem to the writer that though each unit of blood passing through the portion which was the locus of the seizure was depleted of oxygen to a lesser extent, the oxygen absorbed was probably greater than at rest but the blood flow was so much faster that each unit volume yielded less oxygen than before the seizure. In this way the brain adjusts itself to activity by a blood flow which is not entirely capable of supporting the excessive function while it is taking place, but which remains disproportionately large after the hyperactivity subsides.

The physiologic responses to carbon dioxide detailed above not only convey more oxygen to active tissue, but also diminish the range in fluctuations of carbon dioxide pressure within the brain (656). A strong pressure of carbon dioxide hastens the cerebral blood flow, and by virtue of this acceleration, the carbon dioxide produced in the brain is washed away, tending to reduce its pressure therein. With a decrease in carbon dioxide pressure below normal, cerebral circulation is checked, which promotes an

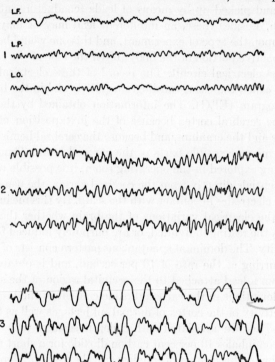

Fig. 15. Extreme overventilation in normal adult. L.F., L.P., L.O., refer to leads placed over the left frontal, the left parietal, and the left occipital portions of the scalp.

1. Before overventilation. Fairly continuous low voltage 10 per second activity in all leads, maximal in occipital.

2. After 5 minutes of overventilation. Tetany in hands. General increase in amplitude with slowing of activity to 7–9 per second.

3. After 6½ minutes of overventilation. Severe tetany. Random slow waves (2–5 per second) in all leads. Slowest and highest voltage in frontal.

accumulation of carbon dioxide, and therefore a rise of blood pressure towards normal. In a word, if there are changes in the carbon dioxide pressure in the brain, it is not *because* of the adaptive circulatory changes but *despite* them. These adaptations fail in epilepsy, as described below, and also during the depression of the nervous system and respiratory centers brought about by such extracerebral causes, as deep barbiturate narcosis (814) and profound hypoglycemia (1027).

One of the most important contributions to the study of the brain is the electroencephalograph, used most effectively by Berger in the decade beginning 1929 to establish the fundamental rhythms of the brain (81). The activity of any part of the body may be expressed in terms of electrical potentials, and picked up by means of leads (conductors) attached to the active organ. Besides these, an indifferent lead may or may not be used, depending upon the type of experiment, and this one would be fastened to a relatively inactive portion of the body (often the lobe of the ear) in order to complete the electrical circuit. The record of these electrical potentials in the heart is called the electrocardiogram (ECG) and in the brain, the electroencephalogram (EEG). The information obtained by the EEG is referable to the cerebral cortex because of the juxtaposition of the cerebral hemispheres and the cranium, and because the cerebral hemispheres are the largest and most accessible parts of the exposed brain. Though in a brain which is being explored in the operating room, it is possible to take records of these potentials directly from the cerebral cortex, the usual procedure is to bring the electrodes in contact with the scalp. By this means it is possible to observe the electrical variations of the brain whether they occur spontaneously in the resting individual, or are purposely induced for example by bodily activity. The dominant spontaneous pattern consists of regular waves usually occurring at the rate of 10 per second, and is obtained most consistently from a lead attached to the occipital region of the scalp.

Certain deviations in the carbon dioxide content of the brain modify the electrical activity of the cortex of normal subjects, as well as the pathologic potentials which are associated with epileptic seizures (655, 656). When a normal person inhales 10 per cent carbon dioxide for a short time, it speeds up the rhythm on his electroencephalogram; the usual predominant pattern gives way to a more rapid one of smaller voltage (that is, more frequent waves of smaller size). When carbon dioxide is eliminated, as by overbreathing, the normal 10 per second rhythm is replaced by waves of greater amplitude and slower activity. Figure 15 taken from the Atlas of Gibbs and Gibbs (396) shows the effect of overventilation on a normal EEG.

In addition to exerting physiologic effects, carbon dioxide may also be involved in pathologic conditions, for instance, in epilepsy. Patient T.T. was subject to petit mal epileptic seizures. The series of observations (Fig. 16) were made while he was asleep under pentobarbital (655). His EEG as seen in the top group, recorded while he was breathing pure oxygen and in the bottom group breathing room air, reveals the abnormal slow waves with intermittent sharp spikes typical of petit mal epilepsy. The middle records illustrate clearly the beneficial influence of respiring 10 per cent carbon dioxide, after which the abnormal waves are eliminated and the rhythm is stabilized. The restoration to a normal pattern is in agreement with the clinical observations that carbon dioxide mixtures inhibit petit mal seizures. On the other hand, voluntary hyperpnea which blows off carbon dioxide from the lungs, blood and brain results in slow potentials of large

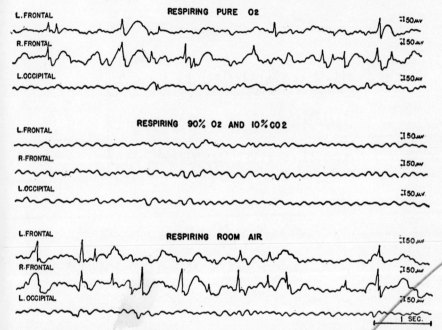

FIG. 16. Effect of the inhalation of oxygen and carbon dioxide on the electro-encephalogram of T.T. The upper trio of curves was taken while the patient was breathing pure oxygen through a mask. The middle trio is a sample of the record taken while he was breathing a mixture of 90 per cent oxygen and 10 per cent carbon dioxide. The trio at the bottom represents a control period, when he was breathing room air. Throughout the period of observation, the patient was asleep as a result of intravenous injection of pentobarbital sodium. Practically none of the abnormal sharp spikes were present during the whole period of breathing carbon dioxide.

voltage. Accordingly, overbreathing may precipitate a petit mal seizure in an epileptic.

A grand mal seizure is another thing entirely. While the three kinds of petit mal seizures include transient, but frequent lapses of consciousness, mild myoclonic jerks, and loss of posture, in grand mal the loss of contact is more prolonged and the patient bursts into a series of dramatic muscular movements. At the onset of the fit he voices a yell or "epileptic cry", then falls heavily to the floor with no regard as to what he may hit. The following stages occur in rapid succession: tonic spasms, clonic jactitations, and finally coma. Naturally we would not be surprised to find that this type of seizure

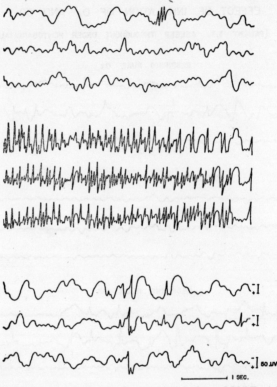

FIG. 17. Subclinical grand mal discharge during sleep. MALE, AGE 14. Deteriorated epileptic, onset of seizures at age of 6 months. Frequent grand mal, as many as 1–2 per day, average 10–16 per month, almost all nocturnal. Frontal, parietal and occipital leads, respectively.

EEG 1. Bursts of high voltage 15 per second spikes followed by slow wave in frontal lead only. Discharges occur from background of random slow activity of deep sleep.

2. No time omitted between this and preceding strip. Discharge of fast waves of increasing voltage starting with left frontal lead and spreading to left occipital. Strong 3 per second wave-and-spike component is evident. Subclinical grand mal.

3. Continuation of preceding strip. No clinical manifestations with any of these discharges.

would be expressed by tremendous hyperactivity on the EEG. A glance at Figure 17 proves this (396). Before the fit, only normal and petit mal configurations were recorded, but these gradually were replaced by outbursts of nervous electrical activity which are characteristic of grand mal seizures.

We have discussed carbon dioxide in relation to both normal and pathologic electrical activity and noted that a large amount of carbon dioxide sped up the rhythm in the brain, and conversely, a deficiency retarded it. Since petit mal is expressed on the EEG with abnormal waves, most of which are slow and of high voltage, and if we remember that an inadequate amount of carbon dioxide also decelerates the EEG, the next problem is to see whether or not these two objective measurements are interrelated. Can we say that patients with petit mal have less intrinsic carbon dioxide in their blood than non-epileptics? As for the patients with grand mal—we saw that their EEG recorded faster waves with increasing voltage and also that an excess of carbon dioxide accelerated the rhythm on the EEG. By the same reasoning applied above to petit mal, would the blood of a grand mal patient reveal a retention of carbon dioxide? To cope with both these problems, Gibbs, Lennox and Gibbs (391) examined samples of arterial and internal jugular venous blood for carbon dioxide. In 70 per cent of 94 epileptic patients (not in convulsive seizure), the carbon dioxide content of the cerebral arterial and venous blood samples was either above or below the normal range, the direction depending upon the kind of epilepsy. Though there was considerable overlapping in the values of carbon dioxide between healthy subjects and epileptics, yet, in general, they found that patients with petit mal had an abnormally low carbon dioxide content and those with grand mal, abnormally high. Patients with petit mal not only had a carbon dioxide content lower than the normal, but there was an additional fall in the content of this gas in their internal jugular venous blood immediately preceding the petit mal attack. Might there not be a causal relationship between the fall of carbon dioxide and the onset of the attack? The same investigators draw arterial blood daily from grand mal epileptics and found that the carbon dioxide of this blood climbed steadily for several days before the convulsions.[8]

Considering all these links between carbon dioxide and epilepsy, namely (1) the influence of carbon dioxide on the EEG, (2) the abnormal values for carbon dioxide in arterial and internal jugular venous blood of patients with petit and grand mal, and (3) the abnormal variations of carbon dioxide preceding grand mal and petit mal seizures in such a way as to indicate a casual relationship, we may conclude that carbon dioxide plays a significant role in the etiology of epileptic convulsion. In seeking a feasible explanation for the above reactions to carbon dioxide, we must not fail, in the first place, to recall that carbon dioxide is an acid, and that its influence both in

[8] The changes in carbon dioxide may be primary as suggested above. From another point of view the gaseous variations may be the result of excessive or deficient cortical activity and in the latter event the carbon dioxide is of intrinsic origin. In either case a correlation between carbon dioxide and the EEG rate is indicated.

health and disease may be traced in part to an unbalanced acid-base equilibrium. The next step involves Darrow's conception that cholinergic activity is at the basis of the normal EEG (221). With depletion of carbon dioxide, not only do slow waves of high potential, characteristic of petit mal, appear, but the concentration of cerebral acetylcholine is impaired. Lack of carbon dioxide is effective in this manner because alkalosis (386) enhances the activity of cholinesterase, the acetylcholine-splitting enzyme. A reduction of carbon dioxide and a decreased concentration of acetylcholine would seem to be among the events leading to a petit mal attack.

It is more difficult, however, to point to an equally direct relationship between the increase of carbon dioxide the resulting inhibition of cholinesterase and the consequent stabilization of acetylcholine to the grand mal convulsion. The inhalation of carbon dioxide only raises the frequency of the brain waves but not their amplitude, and therefore does not reproduce the EEG changes observed in grand mal epilepsy. The effect of acidosis to inhibit cholinesterase and permit the accumulation of acetylcholine is therefore not adequate to explain the grand mal picture, though these changes may be precursors to a major fit (341, 442, 742, 157, 110). It is true that the inhalation of carbon dioxide precipitates convulsions in dogs predisposed to fits by a diet containing agenized flour but the mechanism of this synergistic action is unknown (881).[9] It is possible however that the fit is a sign of subcortical release, as the cortex is depressed by excessive carbon dioxide. In accordance with the relationship between the form of epilepsy and the EEG the therapeutic agents which alleviate the petit mal seizures tend to raise the frequency toward the 10 per second rhythm while those which aid grand mal attacks depress the EEG (652).

Oxygen. The effects of oxygen (656, 597) and carbon dioxide on cerebral circulation are contradistinctive rather than similar. In the first place, the two gases on circulation in opposite directions, i.e., a surplus of carbon dioxide accelerates the blood flow through the brain, a deficiency of oxygen

[9] The toxic factor in agenized flour is a derivative of methionine to which a tentative formula has been assigned (819a):

$$
\begin{array}{c}
CH_3 \\
| \\
HN = S = O \\
| \\
CH_2 \\
| \\
CH_2 \\
| \\
H-C-NH_2 \\
| \\
COOH
\end{array}
$$

exerts the same effect. Then, an excess of oxygen and a decrease of carbon dioxide diminish the blood flow. Not only does cerebral circulation differ qualitatively in its behavior to carbon dioxide and oxygen, but quantitatively the responses are also dissimilar. The circulation of the brain is much more sensitive to small fluctuations of carbon dioxide than it is to similar changes in oxygen. But oxygen at high pressures (622a) slows cerebral blood flow to a greater extent as cerebrovascular resistance is increased (further discussion of the effects of high pressure may be found in Chapter 8). Similarly a diminution of oxygen does not greatly accelerate cerebral circulation until the anoxia becomes intense.

This conception of the relative importance of the two gases is not in accord with the observations of Dumke and Schmidt (258) who reported that the effects of anoxia were more striking than those of carbon dioxide in narcotized monkeys. In later work, however, done on healthy young men, Kety and Schmidt (597) noted the reverse relationship. Gibbs, Maxwell and Gibbs (400) suggest that the animals used by Dumke and Schmidt (258) may have suffered from varying degrees of anoxia. For that reason Gibbs and associates (400) conclude that each point of view is correct within its special milieu. When the brain is laboring under anoxia any further deprivation of oxygen serves to enhance its effect to increase cerebral blood flow and at the same time to minimize that of carbon dioxide. But when oxygen levels are within more normal limits, carbon dioxide exerts the controlling influence over the cerebral vasculature. To place each of these gases in its proper physiologic relationship to the other, and to the brain, it must be recognized that oxygen, and not carbon dioxide, is the gas required for the elaboration of cerebral energy, and that the great sensitivity of the brain and body to carbon dioxide facilitates the adaptation of the oxygen supplies to the needs of the brain. According to the tentative explanation of Gibbs and co-workers (400) however, this relationship between oxygen and carbon dioxide breaks down when the oxygen supply of the brain becomes the critical factor.

The EEG like the volume of cerebral blood flow is less susceptible to a change in pressure of oxygen than it is to that of carbon dioxide (653). Breathing pure oxygen however does affect the brain rhythm to a moderate degree, resulting in a shift towards somewhat faster frequencies (280). The lack of sensitivity to oxygen is further realized under anoxia, which must be pushed to the border of unconsciousness before it causes a significant slowing of the waves of cortical activity. Until the oxygen saturation in the internal jugular vein falls to approximately 30%, half the normal value, there is little change in cortical activity (653). Once, however, this margin is passed, notable slowing of the frequency is observed. Proof for the comparative lack of the electrical response to anoxia is the effect of inhaling 2 per cent oxygen with or without 5 per cent carbon dioxide until the subjects are rendered unconscious. In the presence of carbon dioxide there is no gross evidence of slowing; in the absence, high voltage and slow waves are a prominent feature of the record. Concurring with the work on the EEG are studies of the cerebral blood which indicate that the slow waves are largely the result of the lowered carbon dioxide tension in the brain rather than that of cerebral anoxia (397).

Two questions present themselves before we leave the subject of oxygen. The first, why does the brain permit a greater variability in its venous oxygen than in its carbon dioxide? The answer to this involves at least two points: (1) Normally, only $\frac{1}{3}$ of the oxygen content of the cerebral blood is absorbed by the brain, leaving a cushion of oxygen in the venous blood after it quits the brain. The hemoglobin of the internal jugular venous blood holds approximately 60 per cent oxygen (649). When the arterial oxygen content is reduced, such a cushion permits a further fall in the venous oxygen content and therefore impedes the diminution in the AVO_2 difference. As a result a slighter acceleration of C.B.F. is required to maintain C.M.R. For example, when the inhaled oxygen was approximately halved to 10% the AVO_2 difference was reduced only from 6.6 volumes per cent to 4.5 volumes per cent so that when cerebral blood flow was increased from 54 cc/100g./min. to 73 cc/100g./min., oxygen consumption remained statistically the same 3.4 cc/100g./min. before inhaling 10 per cent and 3.2 cc/100g./min. after the inhalation of that gas mixture (597). The brain, however, is protected only to a certain extent by this homeostatic action. Mental functions may still exhibit deterioration, a deterioration which is to be ascribed to a lower oxygen tension in the brain. These experiments show that oxygen tension may be diminished even though the utilization of oxygen is maintained. (2) As will be discussed in Chapters 7 and 10, the brain has recourse, though a slender one, to an anaerobic source of energy, but which it may carry on despite a small oxygen deficit (475, 310).

The second question concerns possible explanations for the ameliorative effect of carbon dioxide on the cerebral deterioration resulting from anoxia. It is well known that cerebral functions are impaired during anoxia, but that they may be preserved if the anoxia is accompanied by small amounts of carbon dioxide. Gellhorn reports that though the handwriting of a person (a cortically controlled function) becomes increasingly illegible in anoxia, this same person will continue to write clearly if 3 per cent carbon dioxide is added to the respiratory mixture (372). When this subject inhaled the carbon dioxide, his brain received additional supplies of oxygen. First, each unit of blood passing through his lungs was more highly arterialized because carbon dioxide is a respiratory stimulant. Not only is the volume of oxygen which hemoglobin is able to hold thus improved, but second, the amount of blood passing through his brain is expanded, resulting from a rise in systemic blood pressure and also due to cerebral vasodilatation. The enlarged oxygen supplement results in a smaller drain upon anaerobic resources: lactic acid accumulates to a lesser extent and phosphocreatin breakdown is diminished (918). Another advantage of carbon dioxide was observed in the maintenance of the acid-base equilibrium. Because of the overbreathing characteristic of anoxia, the carbon dioxide was pumped out of his body, leaving him in a state of alkalosis. But when he respired carbon dioxide, the deficiency was made up and his normal acid-base equilibrium restored. Among the benefits derived from this restoration, the oxygen combined with hemoglobin becomes more readily availalbe for the tissues and a disturbing mobilization of the sympathetic nerves is overcome (372). The reappearance of the alpha rhythm (372), mentioned above, is another indication of the improvement in cerebral function.

Other substances. The intrinsic chemical control of the cerebral vessels is not limited to carbon dioxide and oxygen, but other substances produced in cerebral metabolism become involved as the demands for energy grow more intense. The enhanced blood supply accompanying increased cerebral activity is not only a response to the more rapid formation of carbon dioxide but also to the local drop in oxygen pressure. If the enlarged supply is still not adequate to maintain cerebral oxidations, anaerobic energy sources are tapped, lactate and pyruvate accumulate and an acid shift in the pH occurs, all dilator in action and, therefore, increasing still more the oxygen supplement.[10] As emphasized by Schmidt (854) the need for increased blood is met by the production of vasodilator material, and in this category may be placed another chemical product of nervous tissue, acetylcholine (333). These vascular adaptations are largely direct responses to metabolites but are also indirect, axon reflexes mediated by perivascular nerves. These combined reactions form the nutritive reflex (465), which is sensitive to so many metabolites and makes for a nice adaptation of the blood supply to cerebral activity. Cerebral blood vessels apparently possess an inherent constrictor tone and are prevented from going into spasm by vasodilator agents. It may be concluded that the intrinsic regulation of the cephalic vasculature, whether of chemical or of nervous (parasympathetic and perivascular) origin is predominantly dilator and overcomes the constrictor influences arising within the blood vessels. But this description also reveals that the vascular reactions have their limits and cannot always assure a normal pressure of oxygen in the brain. Nevertheless, the limitations imposed upon cerebral metabolism by blood flow are not absolute but may be ameliorated, to some extent, by the anaerobic utilization of energy; for

[10] Adenosine monophosphate (253) and adenosine, breakdown products of adenosine triphosphate, are vasodilators.

example, the breakdown of cerebral glycogen stores to lactic and pyruvic acids (475, 340, 524) and the cleavage of the energy-rich phosphate bonds, especially those (430, 611) in phosphocreatin (see Chapter 5, footnote 6, page 71), while adenosine diphosphate appears at the expense of adenosine triphosphate and inorganic phosphate accumulates. The changes in the acid-base equilibrium are important determinants of the vascular reactions. The early alkaline shift (260) may limit the flow of blood to the hyperactive part while the subsequent acid shift insures the continuation of the localized hyperemia until the acid metabolites (430, 611) are finally removed and the energy-rich phosphate bonds are regenerated.

The characteristic responses to the chemicals produced within the brain may also be evoked when these substances are administered for therapeutic or other reasons. They then assume the role of pharmacologic agents, and in this classification may be included alcohol (941), ether, histamine and nitrites (333), papaverine (103), barbiturates (323) and metrazol, all dilators of pial vessels. Ergotamine tartrate (794) also dilates the arteries of the brain but constricts those of the dura. Caffeine is likewise regarded as vasoconstrictor (333), but this action is overcome by barbiturate anesthesia, and then caffeine becomes vasodilator. These conclusions, based for the main part on observations of the pia, do not necessarily hold for the parenchymal vessels nor cerebral blood flow. This objection, however, does not apply to other experiments in which cerebral blood flow was measured by the nitrous oxide technic (598). It was found that theophylline, a substance closely allied to caffeine, when administered intravenously in the form of aminophylline (theophylline ethylenediamine) causes cerebral vasoconstriction (979a). On the other hand, histamine (592a) and dihydroergocornine (434a) dilate the cerebral vessels.

An important influence of any drug on capillary activity is exerted secondarily to changes in metabolic rate. Thiopental, a barbiturate, slows cerebral blood flow (854, 538, 523, 524) when it depresses cerebral metabolic rate, while metrazol, picrotoxin and nikethamide (856) increase the volume of cerebral blood during a convulsion. The reduction in metabolic rate, induced by thiopental, is apparently accompanied by a decreased concentration of vasodilator metabolites. On the other hand, the stimulatory action of the convulsants necessarily raises cerebral metabolic rate and the concentration of metabolites, thus effecting a vasodilation. In these responses to changes in metabolic rate, physiologic and pharmacologic adaptations act on a common basis.

III. Vascularity[11] and metabolism

We have seen above that vascular reactions are the results of cerebral activity and not the cause. The physiologic adaptations whereby accelera-

[11] By vascularity we mean millimeters of capillaries per cubic millimeter of tissue.

tion of metabolism induces a larger blood supply have been discussed. We shall now present another aspect, a structural rather than functional adaptation, namely, the possibility of a positive relationship between vascularity and metabolic rate. We know that not all sections of the brain metabolize at the same rate (495). The question arises as to whether the vascularity of a certain region of the brain has anything to do with the rate at which it oxidizes foodstuff.

This problem was undertaken by Craigie (202, 203) who studied the relative vascularity in the component parts of the rat brain. He found that

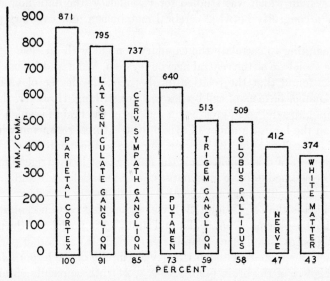

Fig. 18. Diagrammatic representation of the relative vascularity of various parts of the nervous system (cat). The average total length of blood vessels in millimeters per cubic millimeter of each tissue is indicated by columns. At the foot of the columns is expressed in per cent the approximate relative vascularity.

the grey matter is more vascular than the white, and that grey matter may be sharply divided into two groups: the motor nuclei and the nuclei with higher integrative function, the latter being most richly supplied with blood vessels. He concluded that the differences in vascularity implied a corresponding degree of metabolic activity in the regions concerned.

Wolff and his co-workers (259, 542) made similar studies on the cat and the results are presented in Figure 18. According to the graph the white matter in the brain has the lowest vascularity, and we also know that it possesses the lowest metabolic rate (535), which is in accordance with the original hypothesis of Craigie. Not only does the grey differ from the white, but in the cat as in the rat the vascularity of the various parts of grey matter differ among themselves. As can be seen from an examination of this figure, there is a diminishing richness in vascularity from the parietal cortex to the white matter. According to Wolff (259, 542) and associates this gradation probably resembles the descending order of the metabolic rates in the same cerebral areas. Along this same line is the work of Campbell (144) who found that in general there is a surprising likeness between the vascularity and the concentration of the enzyme, oxidase, in a series of regions in the cat brain, but we will not dwell on the relationship of enzymes to metabolism here since it is treated in detail in the next chapter. Though we do not know the relative metabolic rates for every portion of the central nervous system which was studied for vascularity, the data now at hand indicates a congruity between cerebral metabolism and capillary population.

In attempting to correlate the capillary content with an element in the anatomic structure of the central nervous system, Wolff and his co-workers (259, 542) found that the relationship between the degree of vascularity and the number or mass of cell bodies was not striking. However, the number of capillaries did seem greatest in regions of the brain in which the cell bodies had the largest number of synaptic structures, regions in which the axons of one cell pass on the nervous impulse to the dendrites of the next cell. In support of this conclusion is the finding that in the trigeminal ganglion, whose cell bodies have no synapses, both metabolic rate and vascularity are low (535). Then again, exceptions to this theory have been reported, one of which is that of Finley (324) who writes that certain centers in the hypothalamus—the paraventricular and supra-optic nuclei—of the monkey exhibit a greater abundance of capillaries than almost any other part of the central nervous system. Though the oxygen intake of the hypothalamus is not the highest of the brain (495, 523, 953, 244), these results obtained by two different technics are not necessarily contradictory since portions of the hypothalamus other than the supra-optic and paraventricular nuclei possess relatively poorer vascularity, and metabolic studies made on oxygen consumption of the entire hypothalamus included areas of different vascularities. Whereas Craigie's work was done on rats, and that of Dunning and Wolff on cats, Finley used monkeys for his research, and therefore his results may be distinctive of monkeys. If the rich vascular supply is not peculiar to monkeys, then it is possible that it may support other functions in addition to its oxygen requirements, functions which may be endocrine in origin. Perhaps a comparison with the blood supply of some other organ may help to make this point clear. The vascular supply of the kidney and that of the various endocrine glands is much greater than is necessary for them to maintain their requirements for energy. These organs serve important uses in the body and their activities are facilitated by a blood supply excessively large when considered only in terms of oxygen requirements.

Perhaps the hypothalamus supplies hormonal stimulation for the anterior pituitary gland (446a).

Another point favoring Craigie and Wolff in their hypothesis that metabolic rate is supported by vascularity may be adduced from Craigie's experiments on growing rats (203, 204, 206). His quantitative studies of the rat brain show that the blood supply is much lower at birth than at any other time, and that the various centers of the brain of the growing rat possess a different relationship to each other than they do in the adult. Practically all the parts studied except the cerebellar cortex show a definite rise in vascularity from the fifth to the tenth days of postnatal life when motor activity develops. Between the 10th and 21st days capillaries multiply and the characteristic differences of vascularity in the adult rat brain become established. After the 21st day the capillary supply falls off a little in most regions, and in all this growth and rearrangement the cerebral cortex tends to lag behind the other parts of the brain. This distribution of the vascular supplies appears to agree with data obtained on the development of the metabolic rates in the separate portions of the growing rat brain (953), the latter being part of the subject matter of the following chapter.

The question of metabolism versus vascularity is well on its way to a satisfactory conclusion, and though more research in this field is required, still it is safe to say that the balance of evidence today is in favor of an affirmative decision.

IV. The entrance of particles into the brain

A particle even though present in the cerebral blood stream meets various interfering membranes before entering brain cells. The cerebral capillaries are probably not very different from capillaries in other parts of the body and penetration through them depends in large measure upon the porosity of the cement lying between the cells (153). Colloidal particles suspended in the plasma go through the pores of the cement in the capillary walls chiefly by virtue of their size and then enter the adjoining perivascular spaces.[12] On the other hand between the perivascular spaces and brain tissue the pia-arachnoid glia membrane, may interpose many of the specific restraints characterized by the term blood-brain barrier. The particle in

[12] The blood vessels supplying the brain must pass through the pia-arachnoid space and carry a pial covering as they dip into the cerebral substance. In addition astrocytes surround the pia as well as the smaller arteries, capillaries and veins, the expanded ends of the astrocytes forming a supporting glial membrane for the vasculature. The larger cerebral arteries and veins are thus enfolded by perivascular spaces which are found between the vessel walls and the pia-glia membrane. The pial prolongations however come to an end on the smaller vessels and the perivascular spaces of the arterioles, capillaries and venules are separated from the parenchyma only by the glial membrane (925).

the cerebral arterial blood can however escape the cerebral capillaries and instead pass through the capillaries of the chloroid plexus as well as through the walls of the plexus. But here too specificity is not an important factor and the cerebrospinal fluid is regarded in the main as a protein-free dialysate of the blood. The pia-arachnoid glia membrane moreover not only bounds the perivascular spaces but also the subarachnoid spaces so that substances successfully permeating the cerebrospinal fluid must still traverse this membrane in order to reach brain tissue. Thus all materials entering the brain must first penetrate the glial membrane (925), epithelial in origin and possesses the specific properties of epithelial tissues, namely a relative impermeability to negatively charged ions (347).

The easy passage of oxygen into the brain and carbon dioxide outward has been mentioned at the beginning of this chapter. Water also crosses the barrier readily but other hematic contents are subjected to greater permeability restraints. Though pyruvate and lactate enter the brain relatively slowly in comparison to glucose, other organic crystalloids, like sucrose, are held back so effectively that they are used to dehydrate the brain. Two schools of thought offer different explanations for the observed phenomena. One led by Krogh (630) and Friedemann (347) is impressed by the role of the cerebral capillaries and the other represented by Chambers and Zweifach (153) relies on the function of cellular surfaces to explain permeability in general as well as that peculiar to the brain. According to Krogh (630) the barrier is relatively impermeable to ions; cations (sodium, potassium) traverse the cerebral capillaries even more slowly than anions (chloride, bromide). The chief determining factor according to this investigator is lipid solubility. This explanation is in agreement with the observation of Meyer and Overton (734) that narcotic drugs influence the brain in accordance with their solubility in lipoidal substances. Friedemann (347) emphasizes the electrical charge, for he finds that particles bearing an electronegative charge traverse the barrier slowly (neoarsphenamine, most neurotropic viruses) though others with no charge or positive ones move through the capillaries rapidly (alkaloids, sulfonamides). Either explanation accounts for the poor penetration of lactate and pyruvate, for both are ions and electronegative. In general, substances with a carboxyl group penetrate the blood-brain barrier slowly and those substances with more than one carboxyl group, i.e., glutamic acid get through even more slowly.

Chambers and Zweifach (153) on the contrary take into consideration the observations that the cells present much greater resistance to the passage of substances than do the capillaries and conclude that the latter play only a subordinate role in the regulation of permeability. Their point of view, applied to the brain, would attribute the selective permeability of that organ to the neuronal surfaces. The present trend, which appears to be entirely justified, is to ascribe greater importance to parenchymal cells and their surfaces than to capillaries. But if we add to the capillary wall that of the surrounding glial membrane we take into consideration additional factors which aid in explaining many of the observed facts.

The final analysis may find it impossible to include all the observed phenomena in a single explanation. An example of the complexity of the problem is afforded by the observations of Geiger and associates (370) who point out that the entrance of glucose into the brain is furthered by substances in the circulating blood, substances of extracerebral origin. These investigators found that the brain no longer absorbed glucose after a period of perfusion with dialysed glucose-free blood but that extracts of liver or muscle restored the normal cerebral permeability.

If loss of permeability to glucose is one of the changes occurring with protracted hypoglycemia coma, then tissue extracts, or their active principles, are suggested as a remedy in this condition, a remedy which to be entirely successful must facilitate the absorption of glucose before irreversible cerebral damage occurs. At present the members of the vitamin B complex, and especially vitamin B_1, whole blood and lyophilized serum are used therapeutically when the patient does not recover rapidly after the intravenous administration of glucose.

V. Cerebral blood flow and cerebral arterio-venous oxygen difference

We have been discussing changes in cerebral blood flow, and since these must necessarily affect AVO_2 differences, the other important factor in determining cerebral metabolic rate the relationship between the two will be briefly described. A detailed discussion is presented in Chapters 8 and 9. It should be pointed out that only recently have methods been developed which seem capable of measuring human cerebral blood flow quantitatively (400, 598). As such measurements become available, we shall speak with greater certainty on this question; but until results are obtained, it will be necessary to evaluate as carefully as possible the present data. We have noted in this chapter that vascular adaptations take place according to the requirements of the brain. An additional example is found in patients following lobotomy in whom the fall of cerebral metabolic rate can be accounted for by the decrease in cerebral blood flow (869). Though decreased activity brings on a smaller volume of blood and vice versa, the changes in blood flow are frequently not as great as those in metabolism. If the cerebral vascular changes were proportional to the requirements, the AVO_2 difference would remain unchanged. In the hypermetabolism of fever therapy, however, the AVO_2 difference rises despite a more rapid blood flow, while with the metabolic depression produced by barbiturates the oxygen difference falls even though blood flow may slow. Cerebral blood flow, then is adaptive, but not to the extent of keeping the AVO_2 difference constant.

These vascular responses to metabolic changes are characteristic but they are not the only ones. In at least one instance in which cerebral metabolism is depressed, namely anoxia, the vascular adjustment speeds the rate of cerebral blood flow. In response to the acceleration of cerebral blood flow and the curtailment of metabolic rate, the AVO_2 difference is minimized. Another kind of result is observed in cretins who received desiccated thyroid. Under the stimulation of replacement therapy the circulatory apparatus of the entire body is speeded up and cerebral blood flow increases to such an extent that cerebral AVO_2 difference falls instead of rising with brain metabolism (486).

Still another type of reaction is noted when brain metabolism is affected only indirectly as in insulin hypoglycemia, for the cerebral blood flow changes are small and AVO_2 difference decreases with brain metabolism (477, 600). The usual adaptive alterations to metabolism are therefore not observed when the respiratory enzymes are not depressed primarily but cease function only because of the lack of foodstuff (477). Vascular adaptations also fail in comas of several types (post hypoglycemia and poisoning with carbon monoxide and mercury bichloride, 478) and with acute destructive changes in the brain (as observed in a patient with acute luetic encephalopathy, 499). When the enzymes of certain portions of the brain are decreased (avitaminosis, 522 cretinism, 478), inactivated (cyanide, 304) or destroyed (499) while the remainder may be functioning normally, blood flow does not decrease to such an extent as to prevent a fall in AVO_2 difference. In fact in diabetic coma cerebral blood flow even increases somewhat and therefore intensifies the diminution in the oxygen difference produced by the fall in cerebral metabolic rate (595).

Another point of view is formulated by Schmidt, Kety and Pennes (856) who, as a result of their observations on the monkey, conclude that cerebral blood flow most frequently varies with cerebral metabolic rate so closely as to maintain the AVO_2 difference relatively unchanged. Among the three possible relationships between AVO_2 difference, blood flow and cerebral metabolism, these workers note that the correlation between the last two is the best. For example, they find that in a monkey under thiopental anesthesia, the changes in AVO_2 difference are small and variable, but blood flow always falls. Though the results have the merit of exact measurements, it must be pointed out that in man (528) and dog (538) thiopental anesthesia evokes marked reduction in cerebral AVO_2 difference. The work on human and canine subjects has revealed that the AVO_2 differences may be fairly constant under the experimental conditions employed by Schmidt and co-workers, but more generally the differences become smaller with deepening anesthesia until blood pressure falls to low levels when the AVO_2 difference increases again because cerebral blood flow is so markedly retarded. The discussion in Chapter 12 discloses that unless the control AVO_2 difference is taken in the absence of all anesthesia, and unless both right and left AVO_2 differences are obtained simultaneously, and unless the depression is not pushed beyond the limits necessary to prevent a profound fall in blood pressure, the changes observed in the deeper stages of anesthesia may not differ significantly from the lighter ones. In other observations of unanesthetized human patients, however, a constancy in the AVO_2 differences was found when slowly developing cerebral pathology had existed for some time, permitting adaptive alterations in cerebral circulation to establish themselves so that cerebral blood flow becomes slower. Accordingly, in cerebral arteriosclerosis the AVO_2 difference is unchanged and in general paresis, only slightly decreased. In hypertension too, adjustive mechanisms are successful and cerebral blood flow, AVO_2 difference and cerebral metabolic rate are not significantly changed. Not all chronic conditions, however, exhibit a comparatively steady AVO_2 difference. In cretins, for example AVO_2 difference is decreased even if blood flow is slowed. Thus, with destructive changes of the brain of long standing, blood flow gradually adapts to maintain AVO_2 difference in some instances, though not in others.

In the subject matter of this chapter not only are the effects of metabolism on cerebral blood supply emphasized but also other kinds of vascular adaptations, for example, the responses to carbon dioxide. The faster blood flow on inhalation of carbon dioxide is accompanied by a drop in AVO_2 difference while the elimination of carbon dioxide by overbeathing is associated with the slower blood flow and the larger AVO_2 difference. These results may be regarded as characteristic of agents and processes which alter the volume of blood supply to the brain, if these changes are not to be attributed to the influence of carbon dioxide on brain metabolism. Finally physical limitations imposed by disease upon cerebral blood flow may enforce metabolic restrictions. In the case of brain tumor (599) and perhaps in cerebral arteriosclerosis (141, 834) cerebral metabolic rate decreases because of the restriction in cerebral blood flow while the variations in AVO_2 difference are irregular and their average is close to normal.

From all these results some general conclusions may be drawn: the relationship between the three variables, blood flow, AVO_2 difference and C.M.R. is such that the product of the first multiplied by the second yields the third. Only when C.M.R. remains constant do blood flow and AVO_2 difference vary inversely. With alterations in C.M.R. the two other variables may change in either direction limited in extent only by the fact that their product must still conform to the rise or fall of metabolism.

Because of this latitude in cerebral blood flow and AVO_2 difference, no general rule can be drawn for their variations, but in any particular instance their changes must be established by direct observation.

VI. SUMMARY

For the purpose of simplifying subsequent terminology and setting the stage for calculating human brain metabolism, we have outlined the routes of both arterial and venous blood through the brain, and concluded that arterial blood may be drawn from any artery in the body and still be representative of cerebral arterial blood, and that the cerebral venous blood may be collected from the superior longitudinal sinus as long as the fontanel remains open, and from the internal jugular vein at all times. Because there are relatively small communications between intracephalic and extracephalic circulations, the venous blood in the internal jugular vein at the level of the mastoid process comes largely from the brain. When the subject is at rest under basal conditions, the oxygen content of the right and left internal jugular veins usually varies by less than 1 vol. per cent, probably because of intracranial mixing of the venous blood, and the values may be used interchangeably. Because of the diverse origins of the blood in the two jugulars, their oxygen contents may exhibit unequalities under certain conditions, including light thiopental anesthesia.

The AVO_2 differences are the results of cerebral exchanges, and furnish one factor necessary for the estimation of cerebral metabolism. The exact value of the other factor in the computation of cerebral metabolic rate and cerebral blood flow is still undecided and has been found to vary between wide limits, from 500 cc. to 1000 cc. per minute. Recent observations by 2 different methods disclose average values at 617 cc. per minute and at 725 cc. per min.

Despite the limiting effects of the inelastic bony skull on any variations of cerebral arterial blood volume, the blood supply of the brain may be adapted to cerebral requirements chiefly by changes in rate velocity. The most important extracranial factor governing the total cerebral blood flow is the systemic arterial pressure. The brain, however, takes part in stabilizing arterial pressure by virtue of vasomotor reflexes with centers in the medulla and to a degree subordinates systemic pressure to its own needs. The influence of systemic pressure is checked to some extent by the autonomic nervous regulation and the intrinsic vasomotor responses of the cephalic vessels. But the blood supply of any part, within limits, is largely determined by its own metabolism. The area of greatest activity is awarded the most blood in response to the localized increase in carbon dioxide, the drop in oxygen pressure, and the accumulation of lactic acid, pyruvic acid and acetylcholine. The elaboration of these and other metabolic products overcomes the inherent vasoconstrictor tone of the cerebral vasculature. Despite these adjustments, the carbon dioxide and oxygen content in the different parts of the brain may vary in accordance with their degree of activity, and with hyperactivity the region may suffer from anoxia. Carbon dioxide not only wields an influence on cerebral blood supply, but also affects the brain directly both physiologically and pathologically; studies of this gas made with the aid of the EEG have advanced the etiology of epilepsy an additional step.

The reader cannot have failed to observe that certain aspects of cerebral vascular adjustments are controversial: the effect of systemic blood pressure; the relative importance of carbon dioxide and oxygen; the relation of AVO_2 difference to C.M.R. Only by the simultaneous determination of AVO_2 difference and cerebral blood flow can these and other questions receive a final answer.

Evidence is accumulating for the conception that the capillaries of the brain are so distributed anatomically that those regions which are most active and metabolize most rapidly possess the greatest vascularity. A correlation may also exist between the aggregate sum of synapses in a given section of the brain and its vascularity. Like most biological generalizations, this one has its exceptions, but considering the evidence, this inference seems to hold for most parts of the brain.

The failure of blood glucose to enter the brain may be one cause for the production of protracted shock according to the experiments of Geiger and coworkers (370). These investigators suggested to the author, that this failure may be ascribed to the deprivation of energy and to a breakdown of energy-requiring processes such as the phosphorylation of glucose which may be essential for the passage of that foodstuff through the neuronal surface (see pages 80–84 and Fig. 13, Chapter 5). Certainly the permeability of the brain to substances other than glucose seems to be increased by hypoglycemia (1041) and by the convulsant therapies as well (1039). The transfer of some ions is notably facilitated by these treatments, a phenomenon generally observed with neuronal activity, for the cells loose their potassium and gain extracellular sodium. Such ionic shifts exert a profound influence and not only because they affect the electrolyte and water patterns of the brain cells. Potassium stimulates strongly brain oxidations while enforcing other changes on carbohydrate metabolism (22, 242, 243, 476) and these actions may be expected to fall off as cellular potassium is lost. In view of the fact that the concentration of potassium in the serum is also depressed during hypoglycemia and that the more severe hypoglycemic reactions seem to be associated with the lower levels of that ion (448, 577) it is of some interest that potassium has been used in the treatment of protracted coma (1040). This use of potassium however calls for caution because of its toxic effects exerted chiefly upon the heart.

CHAPTER 7

CEREBRAL METABOLISM DURING GROWTH OF LOWER MAMMALS

A Biochemical Basis for Neurophylogenesis

I. STATEMENT OF PROBLEM

Quantitative data on the changes of energy metabolism of the brain in lower mammals during growth will be reviewed in the present chapter. These observations and the conclusions drawn therefrom will be of aid in interpreting the results of human cerebral metabolism, which will be considered in subsequent chapters. Though the results obtained on human beings are of greater interest to us, they do not possess the same degree of quantitative exactness as the animal experiments. But if one assumes that the same general relationship which exists in the brain of infra-human mammals applies to man, then the data obtained on animals may be used as a background for evaluating the human observations.

To follow the changes in brain metabolism during growth it is necessary to know all the events from the first appearance of the anlage, or the primitive beginning, of the brain through embryonic development, and fetal life, the period of active post-natal growth, maturity and finally the senium. We still know little about cerebral metabolism during embryonic development, but our knowledge of this process during early life and maturity has been greatly amplified within recent times, so that it is now possible to compose a picture of the development of cerebral metabolism which, though still incomplete in regard to many details, is nevertheless probably correct in outline. The picture in general is that of early dependence on anaerobic processes for energy to support cerebral functions, a dependence which later shifts until at the end of the period of active growth, aerobic mechanisms are of prime importance.

In Chapter 5 we discussed the various respiratory processes by which energy is made available for the brain. The chain of events known as the Embden-Meyerhof scheme was found to function in that organ. This scheme is a basis for both anaerobic and aerobic releases of energy. It includes the breakdown of glycogen in a series of stages involving phosphorylations, and ending with the production of pyruvic acid. This process does not require oxygen, and in the continued absence of oxygen pyruvic acid is reduced to lactic acid. These reactions starting with glycogen and ending with lactic acid release energy for the brain. In the presence of oxygen and diphosphothiamin, however, pyruvic acid is oxidized to carbon dioxide and water, and if the energy releases from both processes are compared, much more energy is obtained from the oxidation of one molecule of carbohydrate than from its glycolysis.

The available evidence indicates that the rate of brain metabolism advances with growth. Both anaerobic and aerobic mechanisms become capable of greater productions of cerebral energy, but the relationship between them alters in such a way that the increase in the aerobic metabolism far exceeds that of the anaerobic. It would seem that during early embryonic development the chief release of energy occurs anaerobically, and only later do oxidations assume the role of predominant importance. This chapter is concerned chiefly with the gradual shift from anaerobic to aerobic processes, a part of the developmental phenomena of the brain. The evidence for this shift was obtained on mammals of various ages exposed to anoxia produced in several ways. The results of these experiments and an analysis of their significance form the subject matter of this chapter.

II. DURATION OF ANOXIC SURVIVAL IN RELATION TO AGE

A. Methods of producing anoxia, and their results

The most striking observation in the many experiments performed is the discovery that among all the mammalian species studied the newborn, in comparison to the adult, possesses an extraordinary resistance to anoxia. The remarkable resistance of the infant, however, is gradually lost as the animal attains maturity. In general, the effects of anoxia are the same irrespective of how it is produced. The outstanding capacity of the newborn to endure anoxia has been reemphasized in recent years, but was first reported in 1813 by Le Gallois (641). This investigator observing the respiratory movements of rabbits employed some methods used by subsequent workers: decapitation, submersion, opening the thorax, and extirpation of the heart. In 1870 Paul Bert (84) extended these observations to rats and cats and found that in these species, too, the newborn continues respiratory efforts much longer than the adult when submerged in water. More recent observations were made on mice, rats, dogs, cats, rabbits and guinea pigs (302, 27).

In mice of various ages anoxia was induced by the displacement of inspired air by one or another of a large number of gases: nitrogen, argon, hydrogen, carbon dioxide, illuminating gas, and carbon monoxide. This method of study is simple. The animal is placed in a jar so arranged that its contents of air can be rapidly replaced by that of any desired gas. Avery and Johlin (27) found that in pure concentrations of these gases the young survive exposures from 3 to 6 times as long as those which prove fatal to adults.

In the rat (302) the methods used to produce anoxia were even more extensive than in the mouse, and include not only (1) the displacement of air by some other gas, as was done with the mice, but also (2) submersion in water, and (3) injection with sodium cyanide. In the series of experiments on the rat in which the first method was employed, the air was replaced by either nitrogen, nitrous oxide, helium, carbon dioxide, or cyclopropane. The guiding criterion to indicate survival was persistence of respiratory efforts, the end-point being the time when these movements could no longer be evoked by any stimulation. Regardless of the gas used, the adult rat undergoes a short period of excitement, becomes comatose, and usually succumbs after a period of approximately 2 minutes. This short period of survival in the adult rat bereft of oxygen is in marked contrast with that of the newborn, and the one-day old, both of which in nitrogen average 60 and 50 minutes, respectively.

The duration of survival of the infant in nitrous oxide (302) is the same as that in nitrogen, and this similarity exists despite the narcotic action of nitrous oxide. Also in this category are experiments with helium (302) disclosing results corresponding to those observed with nitrogen and nitrous oxide. But, the tolerance of the newborn is not the same to all gases studied. With carbon dioxide and cyclopropane (302) the average survival periods of the 24-hour old rat are not 50 minutes as in nitrogen, but are reduced to 26 and 24 minutes respectively, periods which however far exceed those of the adult in these two gases. A probable explanation for the shorter survival periods is the depressant action of carbon dioxide and of cyclopropane on the central nervous system.

In the second method, that of submersion, the water was maintained at 37°C. In contrast to adult rats which succumbed in approximately 2 minutes, newborns continued to make respiratory movements for long periods of at least 40 minutes (302). When removed at this time, they recovered and apparently developed into normal adults. We know that water was actually drawn into their lungs because when the water contained india ink, granules of that substance could be detected in the lungs of those animals that were sacrificed. From these experiments it may be seen that at least in the newborn rats breathing movements in water for a period of 40 minutes may have no deleterious action on the continued function of the respiratory mechanisms, nor on the subsequent growth and development of the submerged infants.

The same differential effects on infants and adults produced by the first two methods can also be evoked when the third method, injection of sodium cyanide, is used. Concentrations which are lethal to adult rats in 5 minutes allow infants to make respiratory efforts for an average of 61 minutes (302). Sodium cyanide inhibits practically all tissue respiration by inactivating the heavy metal-carrying respiratory pigments, including cytochrome oxidase (see Chapter 5, page 72, figure 10). It may be expected that the responses to the injection of cyanide and to the respiration of nitrogen would be the same (60 minutes for nitrogen and 61 for cyanide) since in both instances oxidations are inhibited. Whereas the respiration of nitrogen prevents the entrance of oxygen into the body, the injection of cyanide interferes with its utilization after entrance into the body. This group of experiments on rats and mice in which anoxia was produced in many ways shows that the infant is able to live longer than the adult during anoxia, not because of a special reaction to any one of the anoxic agents used, because all the agents possess the same characteristic—that of preventing the utilization of oxygen. The difference in survival time between the infant and adult, then, must lie in their relative power to combat a lack of oxygen.

B. *Application to various species*

The difference between the adult animal and the young one in capacity to withstand anoxia has been observed not only in rats and mice but also holds true for all other species studied: dog, cat, rabbit and guinea pig (302). Because in the newborn nitrogen allows as long a period of survival as any other gas, it was used to displace air in this group of experiments. With each species the duration of survival of the adult is brief. In contrast, puppies, 1 day of age, are able to endure anoxia for an average of 23 minutes. Among the newborn of other species the following periods of survival in an atmosphere of nitrogen were observed: kittens respired on an average of 25 minutes, rabbits for about 17 minutes, and guinea pigs only 7 minutes.[1] In order to be sure that animals were really subjected to complete anoxia, analysis of samples of arterial blood from puppies were made for oxygen. After three minutes of nitrogen inhalation there was practically no oxygen in the blood, within the error of the method (302). We can safely say then that the energy for the maintenance of cerebral functions and life was obtained from anaerobic sources. These observations prove conclusively the advantage of the newborn over the adult in an atmosphere devoid of oxygen, an advantage manifest in the relatively greater resistance to anoxia, and explained by the capacity of the newborn to obtain sufficient energy for maintaining life anaerobically.

The signal ability of the newborn to withstand oxygen lack is not lost immediately after birth (Fig. 19). Rats exposed to undiluted nitrogen only gradually lose their power to withstand anoxia as they attain maturity.

[1] In all of these experiments the survival period may have been prolonged by approximately a minute since that time is required for the complete displacement of the air after the animal has been inserted in the jar.

By 17 days of age their tolerance has fallen to approximately the adult level. With the aid of a low barometric pressure chamber it can be shown that for the period from 20 to 40 days the tolerance sinks even below that of the adult (Fig. 20) and several weeks are required before the establishment of the mature performance. Except for this brief period from 20 to 40 days the adult's resistance to anoxia is always inferior to that of the neonate (116). In a similar fashion the ability of rats to resist the inhala-

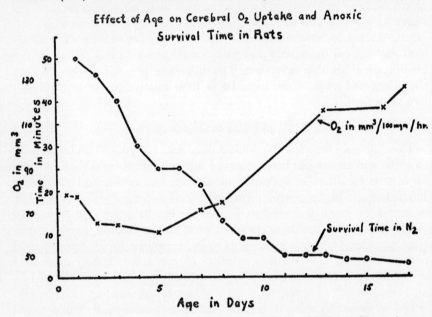

FIG. 19. The average duration of survival in nitrogen of 24 hour-old rats is seen to be 50 minutes. This duration falls, and by the 17th day reaches a value the same as that of an adult rat. Oxygen intake of minced cerebral tissues remains low until about the 8th day, after which it rises rapidly. In general, these two curves bear a reciprocal relation to each other.

tion of 100 per cent carbon dioxide diminishes with age, and at 12 days they survive for only five minutes. These results show that a loss of tolerance to anoxia occurs rather rapidly in the rat. Dogs, a species which develop more slowly than rats, retain for a longer time their infantile ability to combat anoxia. As an illustration, a puppy one month of age survives for a duration of 13 minutes in nitrogen.

Cameron (142) employed somewhat different methods in his comparative study of rodents; rats, rabbits and guinea pigs, for he exposed his animals to a mixture of 95 per cent carbon monoxide and 5 per cent air. He found that rats attained the short adult survival period in 18 days, rabbits in 13 days, while the guinea pig, an animal born in an advanced state, exhibited the adult response to carbon monoxide throughout his entire life span. Perhaps this relatively mature reaction accounts for the badly damaged brain observed in newborn pigs who were first asphyxiated and later resuscitated (1011). In the experiments of Glass, Snyder and Webster (404), who exposed their animals to the inhalation of nitrogen, newborn dogs survived 31 minutes, but when 28 days old, only for 3

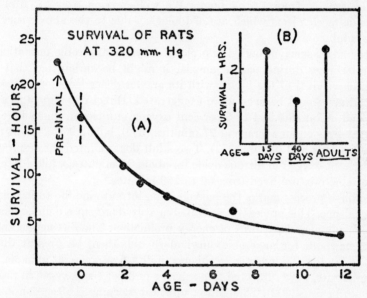

FIG. 20. The greatest tolerance to anoxia caused by reducing atmospheric pressure occurs pre-natally as seen in (a) and after birth the loss of tolerance is rapid until the third week of life when the mature level is first attained. In (b) the decrease in resistance to anoxia is observed to continue until the 40th day after which a gradual rise to the adult level occurs.

minutes, the typical adult response. Rabbits fell from 21 minutes at birth to 1½ minutes at 19 days, and guinea pigs from 6 minutes at birth to 3 minutes when 7 days old. Though the exact duration of survival varies somewhat with the methods used to produce anoxia, the different observers agree that: the intolerance to anoxia, characteristic of adult life, is gradually established though not at the same age in all species.

C. *Comparative resistance of adult, infant and fetus*

Because the mature animal is overcome so quickly under anoxic conditions, it might appear that the adult possesses no power whatsoever for enduring anoxia. But this is not the case. Under appropriate circumstances a limited ability can readily be identified even in the adult (502, 310), and is greater in the female than in the male rat (116). The experimental condition best suited for the display of the adult's anaerobic tolerance is the respiration of gas mixtures containing some oxygen, but less than the amount present in air. With this partial anoxia the energy from oxidations is not adequate, and anaerobic processes are called into activity. As a result, the adult dog in an atmosphere of 8 per cent oxygen in nitrogen can survive from 1 to 4 hours. We will examine later (p. 137) the anaerobic mechanisms which are of biologic value to the anoxic survival of the adult.

If the adult survival period is prolonged by the anaerobic formation of cerebral energy during partial anoxia, it might be anticipated that the period of survival of the infant with its greater dependence on anaerobic mechanisms should be even more exaggerated. Direct experimentation on adult and infant rats in 4 to 5 per cent oxygen in nitrogen shows that the adult rat lives on an average of 27 minutes (502), but that the infant may survive as long as 12 hours (302). Two adult dogs endured the respiration of 5 per cent oxygen in nitrous oxide for about 15 minutes, while 4 puppies in the same mixture lived from 50 to 200 minutes.

The birth process marks the passage from intrauterine life to individual independence. This process does not necessarily represent a definite change in the fundamental patterns of energy production. The distinctive ability of the newborn for anaerobic survival should, then, be present during intrauterine life. To investigate this possibility five pregnant animals, one cat and 4 rats, were subjected to a mixture of 5 per cent oxygen in nitrous oxide until exitus (302). Though the adult cat succumbed after 10 minutes, her four fetuses removed by Cesarian operation respired spontaneously in air and survived until sacrificed. Such a contrast between mother and fetus was also observed in the rats. Despite the anoxic death of the mother rats and the fact that the fetuses were permitted to remain *in utero* for five minutes thereafter, some of the rats were successfully raised by foster mothers. Indeed, in many instances the fetuses were making respiratory movements *in utero* (890).[2] The great resistance of the fetus is again noted when anoxia is produced by the injection of cyanide in the mother (302). Fetuses delivered from these mothers breathed spontaneously for a few minutes to an hour or so before the lethal effect of cyanide became evident.

These experiments show that the fetus is more resistant than the adult, but do not distinguish quantitatively between the fetal and infantile capacity to withstand anoxia. Such a study has been made by Glass, Snyder and Webster (404). They observed a series of rabbit fetuses delivered by hysterectomy at different intervals between conception and term. On the

---

[2] For discussion of fetal respiratory movements, see Windle (1010).

29th day after conception a fetus exposed to nitrogen survived as long as 44 minutes. This duration diminished for fetuses removed from the uterus at later periods and at term, 32 days after conception, the average survival was reduced to 31 minutes. The tolerance of the newborn to anoxia, extraordinary as it is, is therefore even more highly developed in the fetus, and at least within the time limits of the experiment, the younger the fetus the longer the duration of anoxic survival (compare with Figure 20). The entire series of observations made on fetuses, newborns, growing animals, and adults reveals a decreasing tolerance to anoxia which is progressive during growth, and can be explained by a shift from anaerobic to aerobic production of energy. This shift will be considered in the next section.

III. SOURCE OF ANAEROBIC ENERGY

A. *The brain as the limiting factor in anaerobic survival*

In this section we hope to show that anaerobic survival depends upon the ability of the brain to develop energy from sources other than oxidative in order to maintain cerebral functions. The evidence will be divided into two portions: first, the function of the brain in anaerobic survival, and second, the source of anaerobic energy.

A great volume of previous work has led to the suggestion that the brain is the limiting factor in tolerance to anoxia since it is the first organ to cease functioning in the absence of oxygen. The susceptibility of the brain is greater than that of other organs because of its relatively higher oxygen intake, and its inability to supply adequate energy anaerobically. This distinction between the brain and other organs is emphasized by a comparison with voluntary muscle whose continued function in anaerobiosis is well established. The heart is able to withstand anoxia less successfully than voluntary muscle. Nevertheless, the vulnerable position of the brain in comparison to that of the heart may be seen by the fact that in asphyxial death the heart may continue beating long after respiration has ceased (689, 475, 601). This is observed both in adult and infant. Once respiration has stopped and the brain has been damaged irreversibly, the maintenance of bodily function—for example, with the aid of artificial respiration—is of no avail in reviving the organism.

If the brain is the part of the body most susceptible to anoxia, then the longer survival of the infant is necessarily associated with the better ability of the infant brain to withstand anoxia. In the experiments previously described in which respiratory activities were taken as a criterion of survival, it was observed that cerebral function as evidenced by the coordination of respiratory movements are maintained for a much longer time in

the newborn than in the adult. But in these experiments the whole body
was subjected to anoxia. In Kabat's work (572) the brain was the only
organ deprived of its circulation, while that of the rest of the body was
maintained as artificial respiration was administered. Under such conditions it was possible to study the resistance of the brain uninfluenced by
the effects of anoxia on other portions of the body. When newborn and
adult animals were prepared in this manner, the newborn were able to
maintain respiratory movements 17 times as long as were the adults.

B. *Anaerobic breakdown of carbohydrate*

Effect of inhibitors. Since anoxic survival depends upon the maintenance
of cerebral functions, and these can continue only if supplied by energy
from anaerobic mechanisms, our next step is to discover the origin of this
energy. First, let us go back to Chapter 5 where we reviewed the data
showing that the Embden-Meyerhof scheme applied to excised cerebral
tissues. Starting with glycogen, among the intermediary stages in carbohydrate catabolism were glucose-phosphate → triosephosphate → phosphoglyceric acid → pyruvic acid, with the final anaerobic production of lactic
acid. We found further that this process was interrupted by iodoacetate
at triosephosphate and by fluoride at phosphoglyceric acid. If these results
can be applied to the living organism, and if it can be shown that either
iodoacetate or fluoride shortens the duration of the anoxic survival period,
this would strengthen the concept that the energy maintaining cerebral
function during anoxia is obtained from glycolysis.

As in the previous study of the duration of anoxic survival, one-day old
rats were placed in a jar in which nitrogen was substituted for air. The
controls survived 50 minutes respiring nitrogen. That this 50-minute survival was due to the anaerobic release of energy is proved by the results
of the subcutaneous injection of sodium iodoacetate, 0.18 mg. per gm. of
body weight, or of sodium fluoride, 0.5 mg. per gm. of body weight (475).
Such concentrations of iodoacetate and fluoride were not immediately
lethal, but permitted the newborn rats to live for approximately 50 minutes
when breathing air (Table 5). When other rats were injected with either
of these inhibitors of glycolysis and then exposed to nitrogen, they continued respiring on an average of only 3 minutes with iodoacetate, and 16
minutes with fluoride. Rigor set in instantaneously with death. This rigor
was of such intensity that when the animals were placed in an upright
posture they remained standing. Experiments in which lactic acid was
determined revealed no increase of this acid, showing that the rigor was
of the alactacid type (475).

Apparently concentrations of these drugs adequate to inhibit glycolysis
curtail the ability of the infants to endure anoxia (463). This curtailment

must have been brought about at least in part by suppressing the breakdown of carbohydrate in the Embden-Meyerhof scheme. In these experiments iodoacetate or fluoride affected not only the brain but all the organs of the body employing the Embden-Meyerhof process for the realization of energy. For example, following the administration of either iodoacetate or fluoride and exposure to nitrogen, the heart no longer beats after respiration has ceased, but stops practically simultaneously with respiration. In such an instance the heart rather than the brain might be the first organ to succumb to anoxia. Results obtained with the isolated head, however, would not be influenced secondarily by changes in other parts of the body.

In order to dissociate the effects on brain from those on other organs, newborn rats were decapitated after having received injections of iodoacetate or of fluoride (475). As in the experiments with the intact animal,

TABLE 5

Effect of iodoacetate and sodium fluoride on survival time and gasping reflex of newborn rats

	MG. PER GM.	AVERAGE SUR-VIVAL TIME OF INTACT ANIMAL IN AIR	AVERAGE SUR-VIVAL TIME OF INTACT ANIMAL IN NITROGEN	AVERAGE GASP-ING TIME OF ISOLATED HEAD
		minutes	*minutes*	*minutes*
Iodoacetate...................	0.18	50	3	$2\frac{1}{2}$
Sodium fluoride...............	0.5	50	16	7
Uninjected control...........		Continues to live	50	20

the persistence of respiratory movements was taken as the criterion of survival except that now only the severed head and not the entire body was observed. In a word, the duration of the gasping reflex of the isolated head was determined (862). Following decapitation, the isolated anemic head of the full grown rat gasps over a period of 10 to 20 seconds and then remains motionless. In the week-old animal the gasping time may extend over many minutes. Table 5 shows that the average gasping time of the isolated head of one-day old rats was 20 minutes and that the injection of sodium fluoride shortened this period to 7 minutes, whereas iodoacetate cut it to $2\frac{1}{2}$ minutes. These experiments on the duration of the gasping reflex of infant rats suggest that both iodoacetate and fluoride hinder the anaerobic processes in the respiratory centers, processes which produce the energy necessary for the nervous integration of gasping. Since these reagents act to stop glycolysis, we may conclude that the breakdown of carbohydrate according to the Embden-Meyerhof scheme is the anaerobic source of cerebral energy.

In the adult as well as the infant we can show that the inhibition of the anaerobic release of energy diminishes the anoxic survival period. But, in order to make such a study, the adult animals were exposed to a mixture of nitrogen containing some oxygen, in view of the fact that the mature of any species live for such a brief time in undiluted nitrogen. In these experiments (310) it was necessary first to seek a percentage of oxygen which would permit survival for a period adequate for observation; second, a concentration of iodoacetate allowing for an equally adequate period of survival for animals breathing air, but yet a dose which inhibited glycolysis markedly. By trial and error, it was found that 8 per cent oxygen in nitrogen and 32 mg. per kilo of iodoacetate were satisfactory. These concentrations were therefore used on three groups of dogs anesthetized with pentobarbital to control muscular activity (Table 6). The persistence of their respiratory movements was taken as a criterion of their survival.

TABLE 6

Survival time of adult dogs* with 8% oxygen, iodoacetate and both

CONDITION	NO. OF DOGS	AVERAGE SURVIVAL TIME
		minutes
8% oxygen in nitrogen..............	5	60–240
Iodoacetate (25–49 mg./kg.).........	17	127
8% oxygen + iodoacetate (25–49 mg./kg.).........................	10	4.3

* Pentobarbital anesthesia was employed for these adult dogs.

The first group respired 8 per cent oxygen; the second breathed air but received an injection of iodoacetate, and the third was subjected to 8 per cent oxygen after injection with iodoacetate. In contrast to the first group of animals who lived from 1 to 4 hours and the second which averaged 127 minutes, the survival period of the third group was reduced to 4.3 minutes. Since iodoacetate interferes with glycolysis, it may be concluded that the survival period of the third group of animals in partial anoxia was cut short when the anaerobic release of energy by the Embden-Meyerhof path was stopped.

The dose of iodoacetate used in these experiments, 32 mg. per kilo, inhibited glycolysis to a great extent. In support of the efficacy of this concentration of iodoacetate to depress the formation of lactic acid is the observation of Henderson and Greenberg (463) that iodoacetate in doses of 33 mg. per kilo prevented the accumulation of lactic acid in the blood despite prolonged anoxia. The chief effect of iodoacetate is therefore exerted on anaerobic rather than aerobic processes. The shortened survival of the adult animal in partial anaerobiosis following the injection of iodoacetate is presumptive evidence that the uninjected adult lived longer because cerebral energy was formed by glycolysis.

Another way to prove that the brain of these animals had to call on anaerobic resources if they were to survive, would be to establish that the oxygen supplies to the brain were not adequate. Such a proof involves the study of the oxygen content of the blood entering and leaving the brain after the animal was subjected to partial anoxia, as in the above experiment. This analysis of the blood gases revealed that the arterio-venous oxygen difference fell (310) (Table 7). We know that the fall is caused by a lack of oxygen to the brain, which in turn, excites compensatory reactions forcing the blood to flow more rapidly through the brain. The faster the flow, the greater the fall in the arterio-venous difference. Thus, such a drop in the arterio-venous oxygen difference is a sign that the brain is existing in a state of partial anoxia (198). The recovery of unanesthetized adult cats despite the depletion of their oxygen supplies resulting from

TABLE 7

Arterio-venous oxygen difference in vol. % after 8% oxygen

EXPER. NO.	CONTROL	11 MINUTES	31 MINUTES	60 MINUTES
1	11.3	7.3	5.8	
2	6.9	4.3	...	2.6
3	7.7	...	3.4	

breathing 4.5 per cent oxygen to the point of respiratory failure must be attributed in part to metabolism supported from anaerobic sources of energy (776).

Concentration of lactic acid. The inhibitory effect of iodoacetate and fluoride on the survival period is indicative of the operation of the Embden-Meyerhof scheme as an anaerobic source of energy, only if it can be shown first that the concentration of lactic acid increases with the duration of survival; and second, that the concentration of lactic acid fails to rise in those animals which do not survive following the injection of these inhibitors. Besides interrupting the process of glycolysis, iodoacetate is known to interfere with other chemical reactions probably involving the sulfhydryl group, $-SH$, and it is therefore important to prove that interference in glycolysis rather than any other reaction is the reason for the shortened survival period.

The changes in lactic acid concentration were studied both in newborns and adults. The lactic acid content of the whole newborn animal was determined before and after exposure to nitrogen (475). Some of the animals were injected with iodoacetate and others served as controls. At the end of each observation, in order to stop glycolysis, the whole body was frozen in dry ice and ether. The frozen material was then triturated in a solution of 2 per cent iodoacetate, and the lactic acid contents of the tissues and the suspending fluid were estimated by the method of Friedemann, Cotonio and Shaffer (345).

The chief point in Table 8 is the high concentration of lactic acid in those newborn rats which survived in nitrogen for 50 minutes, in contrast to the animals injected with iodoacetate and breathing nitrogen which showed no increase in lactic acid and only a brief survival. In the living

TABLE 8

Iodoacetate and anoxia in newborn rats

CONDITIONS	AVERAGE SURVIVAL TIME	AVERAGE LACTIC ACID
	minutes	*mg. %*
Iodoacetate in air....................	50	41
Iodoacetate in nitrogen..............	3	38
Nitrogen only........................	50	145*

* Determined after 40 minutes of nitrogen.

TABLE 9

Lactic acid increase in brain of newborn rats subjected to nitrogen

AGE	LACTIC ACID BEFORE ANOXIA	LACTIC ACID AFTER ANOXIA	PERIOD OF ANOXIA
days	*mg.%*	*mg.%*	*minutes*
1	63	182	40
1	55	180	40
1	50	186	40
7	29	117	20
8	26	116	20

organism, then, as in excised tissues, the cessation of glycolysis prevents anaerobic survival. It may be concluded that the anaerobic production of lactic acid and the energy released in that process maintained the life of the newborn rats in anoxia.

The increase of lactic acid in the body is the resultant of the anaerobic cleavage of carbohydrate in all of the organs of the body with the possible exception of the liver. In order to prove that the brain is involved specifically in the anaerobic manufacture of energy, it is necessary to analyze the brain for its lactic acid content (Table 9). Two groups of newborn rats were used. In the first control group the animals were decapitated and the brain examined for its lactic acid content. The second group was similarly treated except that it was exposed to nitrogen before decapitation. In every instance lactic acid increased greatly during anoxia. These experiments stress the importance of the anaerobic cleavage of carbohydrate as a source of energy for the brain. The possibility arises that the increase of lactic acid may not have been produced entirely by the anaerobic splitting of carbohydrate in the brain, but may be due in part to diffusion from the blood.

Experiments considered next will show that diffusion from the blood is only of secondary importance. In observations on adult animals, the large size of the animals permitted the chemical determinations necessary for a comparison between the lactic acid levels of the brain and of the blood, and reveal that the lactic acid was *higher* in the brain than in the blood

TABLE 10

Lactic acid mg.% in brain and blood of cats

CONDITION	MG.% LACTIC ACID IN		
	Brain		Blood
Control Breathing air	23*		21*
11% oxygen in nitrogen	24	32†	23
	35	43	19
	47	48	
8% oxygen in nitrogen	25	32‡	24
	44	44	30
	48	59	
	62	84	

* Average of 8 observations.
† Average for these 6 observations is 38 mg.%.
‡ Average for these 8 observations is 50 mg.%.

(310). Again the adult animal was exposed to an atmosphere containing some oxygen. For these experiments three groups of full-grown cats anesthetized with pentobarbital were used, the first group as controls, and the second and third being exposed to 11 per cent and 8 per cent oxygen mixtures, respectively. In the beginning of the experiment the brain was exposed through scalp and cranium, and after the gas mixtures had been respired for one hour, the experiment was terminated by a slow intravenous injection of iodoacetate, 75 mg. per kilo, in order to inhibit glycolysis. Samples of brain and blood were then removed and the lactic acid contents determined.

The respiration of 11 per cent oxygen increases the concentration of cerebral lactic acid above the normal value. With 8 per cent oxygen brain lactic acid values are still higher (475) probably because of the smaller concentration of oxygen (Table 10). The average quantity of cerebral lactic acid for the controls is 23 mg. per cent, and for blood lactic acid, 21 mg. per cent. The averages for the brain with 11 per cent and 8 per cent oxygen are 38 mg. per cent and 50 mg. per cent. As can be seen from the table, the level of blood lactic acid was not raised significantly and was lower than in the brain, which proves that the lactic acid did not diffuse from the blood to the brain, but originated there.[3]

Stone, Marshall and Nims (916) have shown that when anesthetized adult cats inhale undiluted nitrogen for a brief period, lactic acid accumulates in the cerebral cortex but promptly returns towards its normal level during recovery from the anoxia (Table 11). These authors not only observed an increase in lactic acid during anoxia, but also found that inor-

TABLE 11

Chemical pattern of cerebral cortex before, during and after a short period of breathing nitrogen

BREATHING NITROGEN	NO. OF EXPER.	(AVERAGE) LACTIC ACID MG./100 GM.	MG. P/100 GM. (AVERAGE)	
			Inorganic phosphate	Phospho-creatin
Before...................	8	17	11	13
During...................	6	55	14	8
After....................	5	25	7	14

NOTE:

(1) the advance in lactic acid production from 17 to 55 mg. % during a short period of anoxia, and the disappearance of the same after anoxia.

(2) the breakdown of phosphocreatin while breathing nitrogen, and the recovery following.

(3) the reciprocal changes in inorganic phosphate and phosphocreatin. The figures in this table were gathered from the work of Stone, Marshall and Nims (916).

ganic phosphate likewise accumulated. One source of this inorganic phosphate must have been phosphocreatin since that substance decreased in concentration during the anoxic period. Just as the excess lactic acid disappears when oxygen is again respired, so phosphocreatin is resynthesized upon introduction of oxygen. But it must be remembered that the brain may suffer from anoxia not only because the supply is inadequate but because the stepped-up demands cannot be satisfied, as for example, occurs in convulsions produced by picrotoxin or metrazol (915). Stone, Webster, and Gurdjian (917) have shown that the concentration of cerebral lactic acid increases while phosphocreatin diminishes and adenosine triphosphate is unchanged. Probably the latter is continuously rebuilt at the expense

[3] In morphinized adult dogs breathing gas mixtures low in oxygen, a correlation has been observed between the concentrations of lactic acid and electrical potentials, for a definite slowing of the brain waves and a decrease in their amplitude became evident as the lactic acid concentrations of the brain began to rise (430).

of phosphocreatin. During convulsions the brain exceeds its oxygen supply, and then like muscle, accumulates lactic acid and utilizes phosphocreatin as anaerobic sources help to sustain hyperactivity.[4]

These experiments on lactic acid lend support to the conclusion that there is some anaerobic production of energy in the brain of the adult during anoxic conditions. It is apparent that for the infant in anoxia and for the adult in partial anoxia, the anaerobic mechanisms of the Embden-Meyerhof scheme maintain the continued function of the brain.

IV. QUANTITATIVE ANALYSIS OF THE ANAEROBIC-AEROBIC SHIFT

The evidence reviewed so far shows that tolerance to anoxia is greater in the young than in the mature animal of the same species, and that the energy maintaining cerebral functions during anaerobiosis is a result of glycolysis. In the present section the changes in anaerobic and aerobic metabolism will be studied in order to compare quantiatively the two methods of energy production during growth—glycolytic and oxidative. We shall first examine quantitatively the rates of glycolysis, second, those of oxidations, and third, the shifting relationship between the two during growth.

The lactic acid production and oxygen utilization of the brain of lower animals in various age groups were determined. It was found that both processes are more rapid in the adult than in the infant. For example, comparing the formation of lactic acid in the brain of a newborn rat with a rat three weeks old, a ratio of approximately 2:1 is found in favor of the older animals[5] (475). Numerous studies of oxygen intake reveal the same

---

[4] The biochemical effects of experimental injury to the brain were studied by Gurdjian, Webster and Stone (429). The results depend largely on whether or not the cerebral tissues were contused, or torn. In apparently undamaged areas normal lactic acid levels were found most frequently, even though the animals suffered profound injury. The biochemical alterations were limited to the contused areas; lactic acid and inorganic phosphate accumulated and phosphocreatin decomposed. These changes are similar to oxygen lack, but unlike anoxia, adenosine triphosphate decreased. Following injury lactic acid and phosphocreatin were restored towards normal values. The authors attribute these reversible results both to direct injury to brain cells and to anoxia resulting from local vascular damage.

Cerebral metabolic rate and cerebral blood flow, measured from one-half to three hours after severe intracranial injury, were significantly increased (385). On the basis of the biochemical results obtained by Gurdjian and his co-workers, German et al. (385) suggested that one origin for the increased metabolism and blood flow was the payment of an oxygen debt, the additional oxidations supplying the energy to reestablish glycogen and the energy-rich phosphate bonds in the brain. A second factor was found in the rise of body temperature, the accelerated cerebral metabolism being in part a reflection of this hyperthermia.

[5] The values for lactic acid production and oxygen utilization are calculated on a basis of 100 mg. moist weight of cerebral tissue per hour. Tissue metabolism may be determined either on a basis of moist weight, which represents the original weight

phenomenon, a higher rate of metabolism in the adult than in the infant. This was first observed in infant rat brain (474), and later confirmed on the dog (495). The rates of cerebral oxygen consumption of rats at various ages are presented in Fig. 21 (953). The variations of metabolism in terms of moist weight include a rapid rise during the first four weeks of life, so that at 8 days, the oxygen intake of the rat brain has risen to approximately the adult level. Work by Tyler and van Harreveld (953) sets forth three levels of cerebral metabolism during the life-span of the rat: a low rate in the first week of life, the highest rate at approximately the fourth week, and then, a slight and slow decrease to the twentieth week.[6] These results, indicating the rapid rise of cerebral metabolism in early life, extend to rats results previously obtained on puppies that brain metabolism is lowest at birth, gradually increases to the fifth or seventh week, and then suffers a small decrease with maturity (495) (Fig. 22).[7]

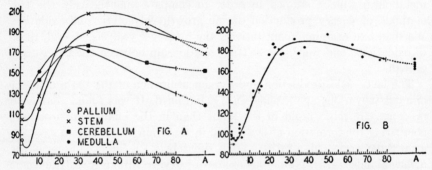

FIG. 21. Oxygen is expressed in cubic millimeters per 100 mg. of wet brain tissue per hour. Time is given in days. A stands for adult. In figure 21A the points are identification points for the curves of the various parts; they do not represent points of observation. In figure 21B each point is an observation.

of the tissues *in situ*, or by dry weight, which is the weight of tissues after water has been driven off and only solids remain. The oxygen intake of infant brain per 100 mg. dry weight of tissue approximates that of the adult. But the percentage of dry weight is greater in the older animals (248). At birth the dry weight of the brain is 12 per cent of the moist weight, 19 per cent at 22 days, and 22 per cent in the mature rat. Equal dry weights of infant and adult cerebral tissues therefore represent an original *in vivo* weight of infant brain larger than that of the adult. For that reason the rates of metabolism of the infant and adult brain appear similar on a dry weight basis. But when moist weights are compared, the metabolic rate of the adult is considerably higher. It is probable that per 100 gm. of tissue in the living animal, the infant rat brain similarly exhibits a lower metabolism than the adult, and that these results obtained from excised tissues on a moist weight basis may be applied to tissues *in situ*.

[6] Studies on the intact rat reveal that basal metabolism fluctuates within its lowest limit during the first three weeks of life and then rises rapidly to the seventh week. After that, there is a progressive fall until the 17th week (602).

[7] Reiner (819) studied the oxygen intake and the anaerobic production of lactic

Having followed glycolysis and oxidations in the brain, we are now ready to make a quantitative appraisal of the calories supplied to the brain by each of these two methods. The oxygen intake and lactic acid accumulation as measured in the Warburg manometer were calculated in terms of the calories per hour per 100 mg. of tissue. This calculation could be made because it is already known that the utilization of 100 cmm. of oxygen may produce 0.5 calories, while the anaerobic formation of 0.4 mg. of lactic

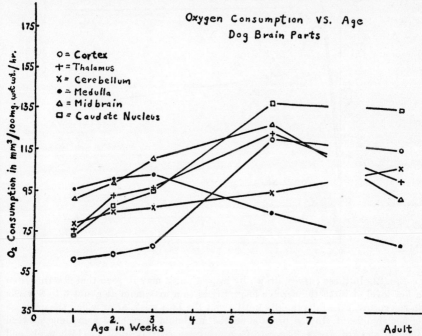

FIG. 22. The changes in oxygen consumption of the various parts of the dog brain at 1, 2, 3, and 6 weeks and in adulthood. In general, the cerebral metabolism increases during the first six weeks and then reverses slightly.

acid measured by the displacement of 100 cmm. of carbon dixoide is equivalent to 0.128 calories (132). The results for the two parts of the rat

acid on brain homogenates throughout the life span of the rat beginning in the embryo and continuing beyond the second year. He finds that the adult rate of oxygen consumption develops during the first month and continues essentially the same for two years after which time however a sharp drop is observed. Glycolysis on the other hand obtains a maximum between the second and fourth months and then exhibits a slow decline. In the early postnatal rise of cerebral metabolism and the fall with old age these results resemble those presented above. The differences in the two groups of results may be due to the methods used including the expression of the metabolic rates in terms of dry weight instead of wet weight as employed in the previous work. (See footnote 5 p. 139 for description of dry and wet weights as bases of comparison).

brain, (1) cerebral grey, and (2) the brain stem, exclusive of the corpus striatum, are arranged in Figure 23 (165). Curves A and B trace the aerobic energy production of cortex and brain stem from birth to over 500 days, and curves C and D the anaerobic energy for the same periods. If the

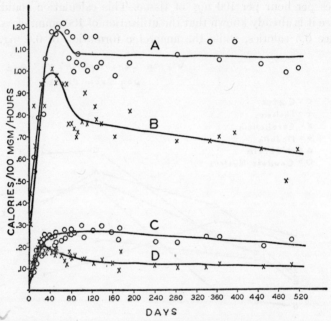

FIG. 23. In these curves, drawn by inspection, it may be seen that starting from a low level at birth the aerobic energy rises to a maximum at about 6 to 8 weeks in the cortex, then falls rapidly until about the 13th week, after which the decrease is not significant. In the brain stem the maximum is reached sometime between the 4th and 7th weeks. The rate then decreases sharply until the 15th week, and then more gradually to old age. In outline, though not in detail, the glycolysis curve matches the oxidative curve. In the cerebral cortex glycolysis accelerates greatly until about the 5th week and then more slowly for about 3 months. After this time it appears to decline slightly. The rate of glycolysis in the brain stem rises to a maximum at about 3 weeks and then decreases, precipitously at first, and then not so noticeably to old age. Each value presented in the graph is an average of a set of observations.

aerobic energy is equivalent to the caloric requirement of the excised tissues, and if the anaerobic energy represents that elaborated by these tissues during anoxia, then the difference between curves A and C for the cortex, and B and D for the stem shows the caloric deficit which would arise in these parts in the event of anoxia. The difference between the aerobic and anaerobic production, i..e the deficit, is lowest at birth. It rises rapidly thereafter and although it is already large at three weeks, the peak is reached at approximately the seventh or eighth week. An estimate of the actual rate in figures at which the deficit mounts in early life may be had by selecting three arbitrary points in the curves of Figure 23: five days, 50 days and one year. From a review of these figures (Table 12) we see that there is a decided increase in the energy debt of both the cortex and the brain stem from five to 50 days. After 50 days a noticeable fall occurs in the brain stem, but the decrease in the cortex is smaller and may not be significant. Probably for the brain as a whole the deficit becomes somewhat less with age.

The rate at which this deficit is accumulated must necessarily vary with the ability to withstand anoxia, for the magnitude of the deficit indicates the rate at which tissues suffer from increased energy debts. The changing deficit with growth, therefore, bears important physiologic significance. The infant, at five days of age, piles up its deficit at the slowest rate in its

TABLE 12

Aerobic and anaerobic energy production: calories per 100 mg. rat cerebral tissue per hour

AGE IN DAYS	OXIDATION		GLYCOLYSIS		DEFICIT	
	Cerebral Cortex A	Brain Stem B	Cerebral Cortex C	Brain Stem D	Cerebral Cortex A minus C	Brain Stem B minus D
5	0.37	0.48	0.08	0.11	0.29	0.37
50	1.18	0.99	0.26	0.18	0.92	0.81
365	1.08	0.68	0.23	0.11	0.85	0.57

life span and possesses the greatest ability to endure anoxia. By the end of the first seven weeks of life the opposite extreme is reached, the deficit grows most rapidly and this period coincides with the greatest vulnerability to oxygen lack (see Fig. 20). In the adult the accumulation of the energy debt gradually becomes slower and the ability to withstand anoxia is somewhat improved over that observed in the forty day old rat.

One other fact is of importance. Though less energy is gained by anaerobic catabolism, actually more glucose is utilized in this process. When carbohydrate is oxidized, the amount of energy released may be 12 times as great as the energy liberated in the anaerobic catabolism of the same amount of carbohydrate. The glycolysis of 12 molecules of carbohydrate would supply approximately the same amount of energy as the oxidation of one molecule. Thus, from the oxidation of 0.1 mg. of glucose, .38 calories may be obtained, and from the splitting of 1.0 mg. of glucose to lactic acid, .32 calories arise. Using these glucose equivalents, the carbohydrate utilized can be calculated from the aerobic and anaerobic production of energy presented in Table 12. These new figures for glucose catabolism are arranged in Table 13. By comparing the values for oxidation and glycolysis (col. A with C, and col. B with D) it may be seen that from 2 to 3 times as much glucose is utilized anaerobically despite the fact that the energy produced is much less. The advantage of aerobic over anaerobic metabolism in sparing carbohydrate, therefore, becomes apparent. The aerobic catabolism of glucose yields a larger amount of energy than does its glycolysis.

V. Some Factors Modifying the Requirement and Supply of Energy to the Brain

In the last section we evaluated quantitatively the aerobic and anaerobic production of energy. The aerobic production is synonymous with metabolic rate, and represents the energy *requirement* of the brain. This requirement persists irrespective of the conditions under which the brain functions, i.e. aerobic or anaerobic. Glycolysis, or the anaerobic metabolism

TABLE 13

Carbohydrate (mg.) utilized aerobically and anaerobically per 100 mg. rat cerebral tissue per hour

AGE IN DAYS	OXIDATION		GLYCOLYSIS	
	Cerebral Cortex A	Brain Stem B	Cerebral Cortex C	Brain Stem D
5	0.10	0.13	0.25	0.34
50	0.31	0.23	0.81	0.56
365	0.28	0.18	0.72	0.34

of the brain, represents the *supply* of energy which may be obtained during anaerobic conditions. Since in the absence of oxygen the requirement is greater than the supply, the difference between the two represents a deficit in the fulfillment of the caloric demands. The more rapidly the deficit accumulates, the briefer will be the anaerobic survival. Any factor which either increases or decreases this energy debt would necessarily have a corresponding effect on the anaerobic survival time. Some factors which may influence the deficit by altering the requirement (brain metabolism) are: degree of maturity, thyroxin, temperature, and at least for the rat, sex. The chief influence on the supply is the carbohydrate level of the body.

A. *Degree of maturity*

We have already shown that for the most part the ability to withstand anoxia decreases as growth proceeds. This loss of resistance is accompanied by an increasing cerebral metabolism, an increase which augments the caloric deficit. The importance of the caloric deficit is emphasized because the low tolerance of the adult occurs despite the post-natal development of reflexes which aid in the adaptive reactions to anoxia (18). A parallelism, then, may be seen between loss of tolerance to anoxia and the magnitude of the caloric deficit. Figures 19, 20, pp. 128, 129 (302) show how, in general brain metabolism increases during the period that anaerobic survival time diminishes. Thus, the greater cerebral requirement with growth limits more and more the anaerobic survival time. This holds true except for the first few post-natal days when cerebral metabolism does not increase. During the first week of life probably the poikilothermia of the newborn (302, 784), which will be discussed under "temperature", is a potent factor in lowering the cerebral requirement.

Cerebral metabolism nevertheless is an important factor in determining anoxic survival as may be seen by comparing the ages at which brain metabolism attains adult values in rats and dogs with the age at which these animals lose resistance to anoxia. The rat, which develops rapidly, first exhibits the diminished adult tolerance when it is only 18 days of age, whereas the puppy, which matures slowly, is still more resistant than the adult dog when it is 30 days old (302, 495). The distinction between the rat and dog is related to the ages at which the oxygen consumption of excised brain attains the higher values of the mature animal. In the rat at 21 days of age, the oxygen consumption of the brain is like that of the adult, while in the dog, 35 to 40 days are required for the same degree of development. These results show the correlation between the increased cerebral metabolic rate and loss of tolerance to anoxia.

Though the newborn of each species is more resistant to anoxia than the adult, there is, nevertheless, a wide divergence of the survival periods among the difference kinds of animals varying from one hour in the rat to seven minutes in the guinea pig. An analysis of this question shows, in the first place, that the neonate of various species is not equally advanced in development at the time of birth. Some species are much further along both physiologically and anatomically than are others, which accounts for the variations in the duration of survival. This, in turn, leads to the second point: that it is the physiologic and anatomic stage of the brain at birth which is a decisive factor in determining the cerebral metabolic rate. In a word, the more advanced the development, the higher the cerebral metabolism, and the less the tolerance to anoxia. The newborn rat is without hair or teeth, has unopened eyes, is totally dependent on its mother and acts like a bulbospinal animal. The newborn guinea pig, on the other hand, is a comparatively mature animal, exhibiting coordinated locomotion, righting reflexes, temperature regulation and therefore a functioning cephalad portion of the brain stem. These data suggest that the differences in the tolerance of the newborn of various species to anoxia may be attributed at least in part to cerebral metabolic rates of different intensities.

B. *Thyroxin*

One of the factors which accelerates cerebral metabolism during growth may be the secretion of the thyroid gland. Injections of thyroxin increase the basal metabolic rate, and it has been suggested that thyroxin may also increase cerebral metabolism. The data on the influence of thyroxin on metabolism of excised cerebral tissues is however controvertible since some authors have reported an increase as a result of administering thyroxin (175, 700), while others have reported no changes at all (903, 412, 305). Indirect evidence on the problem is obtained in experiments designed to study the simultaneous effects of thyroxin and anoxia on the EEG (591). Rats with or without the injection of thyroxin were subjected to the respiration of 7 per cent oxygen. Though no significant changes in the EEG were observed in the controls, the thyroxinized rats showed profound alterations: the rapid potentials were replaced by slower waves, indicating that cerebral requirements had been raised beyond the supply. These effects were reversible on readmission of air. Such an experiment emphasizes the importance of brain metabolism as a limiting factor in the ability to withstand anoxia.[8] This evidence however refers to the animal as a whole rather than specifically to the brain. Though direct measurements of cerebral metabolism in patients with hyperthyroidism do not disclose an excessive rate (848b) it is known that a normal rate fails to develop in the absence of that hormone. In cretins both brain growth and metabolism are impaired while an apparently healthy individual who becomes myxedematous suffers a reduction in brain metabolism (848b).

C. *Temperature*

Low temperature of the brain, like immaturity, or lack of thyroxin, diminishes the caloric deficit because the cerebral requirement falls. Within certain limits metabolism varies with temperature. It might therefore be expected that survival would be prolonged as the temperature is lowered (140). The newborn rat has not established temperature control but is poikilothermic and tends to assume the temperature of its environment. There are, therefore, two reasons for the unusual resistance of the newborn to anoxia: (1) at 37°C. the cerebral metabolic rate of the neonate is intrinsically less than the adult's, and (2) it is still less because the infant's body temperature is normally lower. Since metabolism varies with temperature, the cerebral requirement of the infant brain is less, the caloric deficit is diminished and the ability to survive anoxia is improved (745). For ex-

---

[8] This conclusion gains additional significance in regard to the adaptations of the organism with the observation that thyroid activity of adult rats is depressed during anoxia (954). Elimination of the thyroid secretion by thyroidectomy also affords a degree of protection (45).

ample, as temperature is diminished to 10°C., the life span is more than doubled and attains a maximum of 2 hours in rats 2 to 5 days of age (3).[9] The influence of high temperature toward shortening the anoxic survival period is substantiated by experiments in which the environmental temperature of poikilothermic newborn rats is raised from 24° to 34°C. (302). When a one-day old rat is placed in an environment of 24°C., it survives anoxia for 50 minutes. When, however, a litter mate is placed in a temperature of 34°C., life is maintained for only 21 minutes. It is true that this change from 24° to 34°C. in environmental temperature has no significant influence on the survival period of the adult because the latter has attained a more uniform regulation of its body temperature, i.e. it is homeothermic. With rise of temperature in the infant, the rate of cerebral glycolysis and the supply of energy to the brain are accelerated (242); cerebral requirements, however, are probably promoted to a greater extent than glycolysis so that the caloric deficit is increased at the higher temperature.[10] There are indications that with changes of body temperature either above normal as in fever, or below, as produced experimentally, the rate of brain metabolism is affected even in the adult, hyperpyrexia causing an increase (479) and hypothermia a diminution (308, 301a, 355). See Chapter 9 for further discussion of the role of the brain in hyperthermia.

D. *Hypoglycemia and hyperglycemia*

We have shown how the cerebral caloric deficit during anoxia is intensified as a result of augmented cerebral requirements, depending, among other factors, upon physiologic development, thyroxin, and rise of temperature. In this section we shall discuss the effect of changing the supply of carbohydrate used for the liberation of anaerobic energy. This supply originates both from the glucose brought to the brain in the blood and also from the small intrinsic cerebral glycogen stores. It would seem *a priori* that anaerobic survival should be shortened when the production of an-

[9] With a further fall of temperature however the detrimental effects of the cold become increasingly important and the survival period is shortened. This reversal which takes place at 10° in baby rats, brings into consideration a second factor namely, tolerance to cold. These two tolerances are independent of each other, ability to withstand anoxia being lost earlier in life than faculty to endure cold (3). The CNS is also involved in the kind of death which is due to freezing in the presence of air (140). The reactions of the body, making for survival at low temperatures, are coordinated by the nervous system and when body temperature falls below a certain level the CNS can function no longer, respiratory movements cease with other neural functions.

[10] Partial inanition and vitamin B_1 deficiency (155) tend to increase resistance to low barometric pressure, a phenomenon which may be attributed to diminished energy requirement. The low metabolism of inanition is well known and the diminished cerebral metabolic rate of vitamin B_1 lack is also established (790).

aerobic energy to support the brain fails. One way to change the anaerobic delivery of cerebral energy is to alter the carbohydrate stores of the body, because in anaerobic, as in aerobic metabolism, carbohydrate is the source of cerebral energy.

A series of experiments was performed on both infant and adult rats exposed to anoxia in which the carbohydrate stores and the level of blood sugar were altered. In separate experiments, hypoglycemia was induced by the injection of insulin one hour before exposure to anoxia, and hyperglycemia by the intraperitoneal or intravenous injection of glucose a few minutes before anoxia (475). When one-day old rats were subjected to hypoglycemia and anoxia, the former shortened the normal 50-minute anaerobic survival period to 20 minutes.

The decrease of tolerance resulting from hypoglycemia is observed not only in complete anoxia but also in partial anoxia (885). Infant cats breathing a mixture of 4.5 per cent oxygen in nitrogen survived for a shorter period if they had previously received a dose of insulin large enough to induce hypoglycemia. Adult rats which could withstand a gas mixture containing 4.5 per cent oxygen for 27 minutes lived only 15 minutes if they received insulin one hour before exposure to partial anoxia (502). These animals were deprived simultaneously of adequate supplies of both oxygen and carbohydrate. The anaerobic production of cerebral energy was thus limited. That the lowering of the blood sugar, and no other effect of insulin, was the cause of the curtailment of the survival period was proved in another group of adult rats who received injections of insulin one hour before being subjected to the respiration of 4.5 per cent oxygen, but in whom the hypoglycemia was overcome by intravenous injection of glucose just before being placed in the respiratory chamber. In these adult animals the average duration of survival was restored to 28 minutes.

In those experiments in which the carbohydrate stores of the body were raised by the injection of glucose, the greater resistance may be attributed to the augmentation of this anaerobic source of energy. This improved tolerance to anoxia was demonstrated on rats eight days old whose relatively brief survival period of 16 minutes was lengthened to 30 minutes after the injection of glucose (475). Similar treatment extended the duration of anoxic gasping in rats 12 to 15 days of age (861). On the other hand, it was impossible to prolong the survival period of adult rats exposed to the inhalation of undiluted nitrogen gas by raising the level of blood sugar to hyperglycemic levels, and in this way the adult is unlike the infant (475). If the injection of glucose increases the quanta of energy derived from glycolysis, which it probably does, then the greater anaerobic production of energy in the infant lessens its caloric deficit. In the adult, however, the caloric deficit is so large that this comparatively small augmentation of the anaerobic supply of energy fails to correct the caloric deficit significantly. Figure 23 illustrates the greater aceleration of the cerebral metabolic rate in the adult and the correspondingly larger difference between the anaerobic and aerobic liberations of energy. Apparently, a more rapid rate of glycolysis resulting from the higher level of blood sugar is not adequate to overcome the greater deficit in the adult. But experiments made

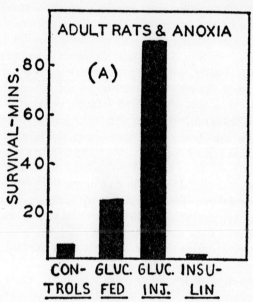

FIG. 24. The benefit derived from glucose and the disadvantage of hypoglycemia on the survival time of rats exposed to a low barometric pressure is observed in this figure. The survival time is increased manifold by glucose and significantly diminished by insulin.

at simulated high altitudes, and therefore under less taxing conditions than those of complete anoxia, do point to the advantage of a high level of blood sugar. This advantage is measured in terms of longer survival even for adult rats as presented in Figure 24 (116).

The influence of the level of the blood sugar is not necessarily confined to anoxia. In aerobic conditions hypoglycemia, by depriving the brain of foodstuff, will finally cause cessation of cerebral function and even a lethal terminus. It is possible to compare effects of anoxia and hypoglycemia since in each case the brain is deprived of one of its two necessary factors for development of energy—oxygen or glucose. Despite a parallelism in the results of anoxia and hypoglycemia, the time scale for the cerebral changes is different in the two conditions. The effects of anoxia are more rapid, and therefore anoxia cannot be withstood for as long a period as hypoglycemia.

The results of hypoglycemia on adult rats and cats breathing air will be compared with those on infant rats (502). The minimal lethal dose of insulin for adult rats and cats is approximately the same, between 10 and 15 units per kilo. There are, however, certain differences between the two species. All rats which die succumb within a period of from $1\frac{3}{4}$ to 5 hours and the cats from 8 to 16 hours. The rats which survive appear to recover completely, while the cats may receive irreversible cerebral damage during the acute episode from which they may apparently recover and yet may finally die at any time from one day to two weeks after the injection of insulin. Experiments show that rats 24 hours old are much less sensitive to hypoglycemia than are adults. The infants, even with huge doses of insulin, from 600–2000 units per kilo, survive the acute 5-hour period fatal to the adult. With equally severe hypoglycemia, the infant is able to withstand this condition for a longer time than the adult. Even the infants of course, may finally die from the delayed effects of such huge doses. The difference in susceptibility depends in part upon the lower cerebral metabolic rate of the infant. The infant rat with relatively non-functional rostral portion of the neuraxis and lower cerebral metabolism is less sensitive to hypoglycemia than the adult. The greater sensitivity of the cat to hypoglycemia in comparison to the rat may in a similar fashion be ascribed to the higher development of the rostral portion of the feline brain.

Not only the action of insulin to lower the blood sugar level but also that of other hormones to raise the level exert significant effects upon performance and survival in anoxia. The hormonal control of blood sugar has been discussed in Chapter 3. The adrenal cortex, however, deserves special mention because anoxia stimulates that gland to accelerate its characteristic effects and raise blood sugar by diminishing the utilization of sugar in non-nervous tissues and by speeding up the transformation of protein to carbohydrate. Britton and Kline (116) point out that the large size of the adrenal cortex at birth accounts in part for the astonishing resistance of the newborn to anoxia. The longer survival of the female adult rat than of the male at low barometric pressures may also be correlated with the larger adrenal gland of the female. In infant male and female rats in which adrenal weights are approximately the same, sex differences in tolerance are not observed. Probably both parts of the adrenal gland mobilize the bodily resources during anoxia, but the effects of the adrenal medulla are manifested more rapidly and those of the adrenal cortex are longer sustained. According to Van Middlesworth, Kline, and Britton (955) normal unoperated rats are apt to show hyperglycemia during the first hour or so of exposure to low barometric pressure, and hypoglycemia during the next two or more hours. The early hyperglycemia is probably an expression of sympatho-adrenaline compensatory activity. The later hypoglycemic phase does not appear in well fed or acclimatized rats. The amelioration of hypoglycemia with practice may be attributed in part to the adrenal cortex. The temporal difference in the actions of the adrenal medulla and the adrenal cortex in raising blood sugar may be imputed in part to the circuitous hormonal connections between these two organs forming the adrenal gland, a circuit which includes adrenaline, the anterior pituitary gland and ACTH (adrenocorticotrophic hormone). Adrenaline, released by the adrenal medulla stimulates the anterior pituitary to produce its various hormones including ACTH and the latter in turn arouses the adrenal cortex (see discussion of anterior pituitary in Chapter 3). The function of the anterior pituitary and the adrenocorticotrophic hormone in arousing the adrenal cortex has been stressed in Chapter 3.

As presented in detail in Chapter 5, there are at least two paths for the oxidation of carbohydrate (309): one of these, Path I, involves the preliminary splitting of hexosephosphate to triosephosphate with the formation of pyruvic acid. At this point, Path I branches: either pyruvic acid is oxidized to carbon dioxide and water, or it is reduced to lactic acid. By Path II the oxidation of hexose is accomplished without the preliminary splitting to triose. (Diagram below)

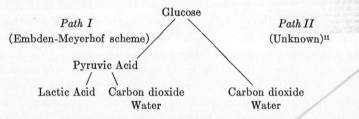

During anoxia, Path II ceases function completely, but only one of the two branches of Path I is interfered with, that of oxidation to carbon dioxide and water; the other, reduction to lactic acid is continued. This anaerobic release of energy explains the ability of the infant to sustain life in an atmosphere devoid of oxygen, and also that of the adult to remain living for some time in a mixture containing an amount of oxygen less than that in air. This difference between the infant and adult illustrates dramatically the swing from anaerobic to aerobic cerebral mechanisms as growth proceeds. This figure also explains the effect of iodoacetate or fluoride in shortening the survival period in anoxia in the infant and partial anoxia

[11] For suggestion as to what Path II may be, see Fig. 11 of Chapter 5.

in the adult, because these agents block Path I and thus inhibit the anaerobic release of energy. Though hypoglycemia and anoxia finally produce a complete block of the liberation of cerebral energy, they act at the opposite poles of the oxidative schemes. Hypoglycemia removes the substrate, while anoxia prevents its oxidation.

VI. ENZYMATIC CHANGES UNDERLYING THE ANAEROBIC-AEROBIC SHIFT

How are we going to explain the increasing rates of both anaerobic and aerobic cerebral metabolism occurring in such a fashion that the aerobic accelerates to a greater degree than the anaerobic? An analysis of this question must include a consideration of the three factors determining cerebral metabolism: oxygen, glucose and enzymes. It is probable that during most of fetal life, the supplies of glucose and oxygen to the brain are adequate.

In most mammalian species, dog, rabbit, guinea pig and rat, the level of blood sugar in the fetus is somewhat lower than that of the mother. Among the ungulates, however, including sheep, goat, and cow, the level of blood sugar in the fetus is higher than in the mother (765). But even in the ungulates according to Bacon and Bell (29a) blood glucose is lower in the fetus than in the mother and the apparently high value is due to the presence of fructose. In any case there is no deficit of blood sugar for the brain. The earliest determinations of the oxygen supply to the fetus seemed to indicate that it was inadequate, but later work in which care was taken to reproduce physiologic conditions revealed that the oxygen afforded the fetus, though necessarily less than that available to its mother since it must diffuse from the mother's blood (546, 830, 647), is nevertheless fairly adequate. For example, Barcroft and co-workers (50) observed an oxygen saturation of the blood going to the sheep fetus of more than 75 per cent until close upon term, and frequently values of 85 per cent to 95 per cent saturation during the first two-thirds of gestation. During the last week of pregnancy the saturation drops considerably. The blood going to the brain of the fetus, however, does not contain as much oxygen as that entering the fetus. The oxygenated blood leaving the placenta receives an admixture first from the liver and then from the inferior vena cava before flowing to the right auricle of the fetus. In the right auricle, moreover, there is a further small admixture with blood returning from the upper part of the body and chiefly from the superior vena cava. Most of this blood does not pass from the right auricle to the right ventricle as in extrauterine life, but instead is shunted straight across from the right auricle to the left auricle and so to the left ventricle and arch of the aorta. Because the admixtures from the liver, the inferior and superior venae cavae are small, the blood going to the brain via the carotid artery, is not much less saturated with oxygen than that leaving the placenta. During all except the last part of gestation the oxygen saturation in the carotid artery is 60 per cent, and for a time it is 65 per cent or over, though here

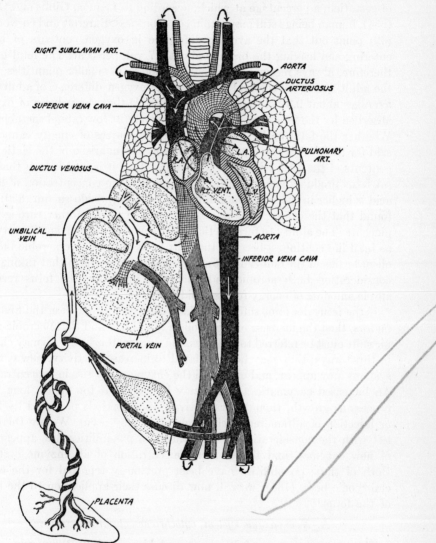

RIGHT SUBCLAVIAN ART.

AORTA

DUCTUS ARTERIOSUS

SUPERIOR VENA CAVA

PULMONARY ART.

R.A.

L.A.

DUCTUS VENOSUS

RT. VENT.

L.V.

UMBILICAL VEIN

AORTA

INFERIOR VENA CAVA

PORTAL VEIN

PLACENTA

Fig. 25. Diagram of the fetal circulation (after Gray).

again the saturation drops markedly in the last week of pregnancy. In contrast to the fetus, a saturation of 65 per cent in an adult, or approximately that at an altitude of 20,000 feet, cannot long be endured.

One can obtain some idea of the oxygen tension within the brain by a study of the venous blood in the longitudinal sinus of the sheep fetus (197). This blood may be saturated as high as 30 per cent during the middle third of gestation, a percentage at which, according to Lennox, Gibbs and Gibbs (654), human beings still may retain consciousness. Barcroft and co-workers (49) point out that the average difference in oxygen contents of blood entering and leaving the brain is about 2.7 vol. per cent. The fetal brain, therefore, always receives some oxygen though in smaller quantities than the adult brain; the cerebral arteriovenous oxygen difference of adult dogs averages about 9.3 vol. per cent. It is possible that the volume of oxygen absorbed by the fetal brain satisfies completely its low rate of metabolism. Whether the fetal brain draws on anaerobic sources of energy cannot be said for there are no results in literature on a comparison of the lactic acid contents of the fetal brain and fetal blood. But, it is well known that the rat fetus produces lactic acid rapidly, and that the concentration of lactic acid is higher in the fetus than in its mother (765). Schlossmann (850) also found that the canine fetus releases lactic acid to its mother through the placenta. The ability to form lactic acid becomes less important for survival as fetal life continues, because the shift from anaerobic to aerobic metabolism begins in the embryo (766). It would therefore seem that taking into consideration both aerobic and anaerobic processes, the fetus receives ample amounts of energy for its rapid growth.

If the fetus does not suffer from lack of oxygen or glucose, the first two factors, then the increase of metabolism after birth and the anaerobic-aerobic shift must be referred to enzymes, the third factor. Enzymes may change in three ways: they may be stimulated to increased activity, new enzyme systems may appear, and finally all the enzymes may rise in concentration. An increased enzymatic activity may be ruled out for such a long term process as growth, though for relatively short periods produced by fever or injection of adrenaline, such acceleration may occur. We are therefore left with the consideration of the other two possibilities: the appearance of new enzymes, and the greater concentration of all enzyme systems. Both of these possibilities have been previously reported for the entire embryonic body (765); we will now discuss their application to the brain of the fetus.[12]

A. *New enzyme system, cytochrome-cytochrome oxidase*

The extensive work of Warburg and his school (973) on respiratory metabolism of tissues showed that embryonic tissues possess a high rate of glycolysis in relation to oxidation. Once full growth has been attained,

[12] We do not have data for an additional possibility, namely, a change in the spacial arrangement making enzyme and substrate more available to each other during development (902).

anaerobic glycolysis declines in its importance and the aerobic source of energy takes precedence. Burrows (138) has shown the ability of cells to grow anaerobically in tissue culture declines with age. These results lead to the conclusion that the development of glycolysis preceded that of oxidations. In 1905 Pütter expressed the opinion that anaerobic metabolism was the more general or primitive scheme, and that oxidative processes developed secondarily (802). More recently Szent-Györgyi (934) made the similar suggestion that glycolysis was an earlier effort of nature to afford energy.

If this same metabolic progression applies to the brain, there should be a period when the embryo obtains its cerebral energy completely from anaerobic sources, and at some later time during intrauterine life new oxidative enzymes appear. There is some evidence that the brain does undergo such an evolution. One way of testing this suggestion is to determine whether oxidative enzymes function in the very first stages of prenatal life, or whether there may be an interval when oxidations are not significant. We may look for this evidence in the study of cytochrome-cytochrome oxidase, an enzyme system which catalyzes the greatest part of the oxygen utilized in metabolism. (This system is referred to as the Warburg-Keilin in Fig. 10 of Chapter 5). This system is formed of two components: cytochrome, usually in the form of cytochrome c which when reduced is oxidized by the second component, cytochrome oxidase. In the absence of either or both of these factors oxidations must be at a minimum.

In view of the relationship between this enzyme system and the utilization of O_2 it is significant that cytochrome c does not appear in the embryo of the chick until the fourth day of incubation (797). During this period oxidations are slight despite the presence of cytochrome oxidase as early as the 2nd day (4). If no cytochrome c can be found in the entire embryo before the fourth day, certainly it could not be expected that it would be present in the anlage of the brain which is only a portion of the embryo. In agreement with these observations on the chick are others made on the rat (920). Though small quantities of cytochrome oxidase are present in the rat embryo, there is practically no cytochrome c. At least for the chick and the rat, cytochrome c, the carrier of cytochrome oxidase seems to be lacking during earliest development, a lack which suggests a basis for the low cerebral oxygen uptake observed at the time (see pages 72–75).

Even before this cytochrome system is complete some slight oxidations do take place. That these are not caused by the cytochrome-cytochrome oxidase system is indicated by the action of sodium azide. This reagent inhibits specifically cytochrome-cytochrome oxidase activity. The work of Albaum and Worley (6) on the chick embryo shows that sodium azide does not interfere at all with the oxidations of this enzyme system on the second or third day of incubation, though respiration is checked about 70 per cent by the end of the first week. From all this work it seems that the initiation of a fast rate of oxidation is simultaneous with the appearance of this new enzyme system. Until oxidations are speeded up however, the embryo depends chiefly on anaerobic processes for the release of energy.

The next step in our analysis of this problem is to consider what substrates might be used once the cytochrome-cytochrome oxidase system begins to function. If the Embden-Meyerhof scheme is a prototype of respiration, then it might be expected that the earliest oxidations must be concerned with those substances which arise as the split products of that scheme, and that later additional substrates may also be oxidized. That this may be so can be shown in two ways: in the first place, Tyler has found that iodoacetate depresses infant respiration more than that of the adult (952). This observation can be explained if the products of the Embden-Meyerhof process of glycolysis are the chief substrates in the infant brain. Additional evidence is the observation of Himwich, Fazekas and Baker (474) that cerebral tissues excised from the rat any time during the first 11 days of life oxidize lactic acid more rapidly than glucose. The first two steps in the evolution of energy, therefore, are glycolysis and the oxidation of the products of glycolysis, probably by the Krebs cycle acting in conjunction with a hydrogen transfer chain and the cytochrome-cytochrome oxidase system. In the rat after the 11th day additional oxidative mechanisms such as those suggested by Warburg-Christian, Keilin and Dickens (Chapter 5, Figures 10 and 11) probably increase their activities: for example, a number of dehydrogenases are first observed after the presence of cytochrome oxidase is established in the chick (102, 5). These dehydrogenases act upon lactic acid, succinic acid, alphaglycerophosphate, glucose, hexosediphosphate and probably hexosemonophosphate if for no other reason than the equilibrium which exists between glucose, hexosemonophosphate and hexosediphosphate in tissues. The developmental order, therefore, seems to involve first, the Embden-Meyerhof glycolysis, second, the tricarboxylic cycle and its accompanying cytochrome oxidase mechanism, and third, a group of dehydrogenases perhaps including the one for hexosemonophosphate which also uses the Warburg-Christian oxidative chain to complete hydrogen transfer. The respiratory quotient of unity of the rat embryo in the presence of glucose is evidence for the conclusion that carbohydrate chiefly is oxidized during fetal life (239).

This review of the data indicates that during embryonic life a shift occurs from a predominantly anaerobic, glycolytic, energy mechanism to one in which the aerobic becomes more important as the cytochrome-cytochrome oxidase system develops, the entire shift of which is not completed until after birth.

B. *Increased concentration of enzymes—anaerobic and aerobic*

Anaerobic. The quantitative analysis presented diagramatically in Figure 23 shows that both aerobic and anaerobic mechanisms increase after birth. The more rapid rate of glycolysis is probably an expression of an increased concentration of enzymes. Such an increase can explain the growing capacities of two enzymes, phosphorylase and phosphoglucomutase, involved in glycolysis, as observed in the brain of young rats (864); see Chapter 5, pages 68–70, Figure 9). Phosphorylase exhibits about 60 per cent of its adult activity at birth and remains practically at the same level until the tenth day when the activity begins to rise rapidly and approximates the adult value at about 20 days. Though phosphoglucomutase appears almost inactive at birth, it also develops speedily after 10 days and attains mature performance between 20 and 30 days. A third enzyme which functions in the Embden-Meyerhof scheme, adenosine triphosphatase, is found at a low level for several days both before and after birth and then rapidly increases more than three fold by the 30th day of life (798).

Studies of anaerobic mechanisms other than glycolysis have been made on dehydrogenases (476). With the aid of methylene blue as an indicator, a substance which changes from blue to white as it is reduced by hydrogen mobilized by dehydrogenating enzymes, it can be shown that dehydrogenase activity is greater in the adult than in the infant. These observations with methylene blue reveal that the glucose dehydrogenation is slower in the young. The average decolorization time of cerebral tissues is 22.3 minutes for 22 adults, and 35.4 minutes for 25 infants, values which are significantly different. Potter examined succinic dehydrogenase of the infant rat brain and noted that it increased six-fold in content from the third through the 30th day of life (798). The evidence on the concentration of anaerobic enzymes is adequate to permit the interpretation of a concentration which enlarges with growth.

Aerobic. The greater importance of oxidations for maintaining life is evidenced by a more intense concentration and activity of the cytochrome-cytochrome oxidase system which occurs during post-natal growth (476). The average acceleration rate of the oxidation of paraphenylenediamine over a period of one hour by the infant brain is 18 per cent for the first 10 minutes, and rises gradually to 73 per cent from the 50th to the 60th minute. This result is in contrast to the effects on the respiratory metabolism of the adult brain, which is increased to 124 per cent in the first 10 minutes. The paraphenylenediamine is oxidized so rapidly by adult cerebral tissues that the substrate is soon exhausted and in the last 10 minutes of an hour the increase of metabolism over the control is only 38 per cent. The slower rise with paraphenylenediamine in the newborn indicates a smaller concentration of the cytochrome-cytochrome oxidase system. Potter has examined the cytochrome oxidase activity of the newborn rat brain and found that it was low at birth and then increased steadily during the first month of life (798). The chief point of these observations is that cytochrome-cytochrome oxidase activity, absent in an early stage of fetal development though present in the newborn, is greatly increased during the period of

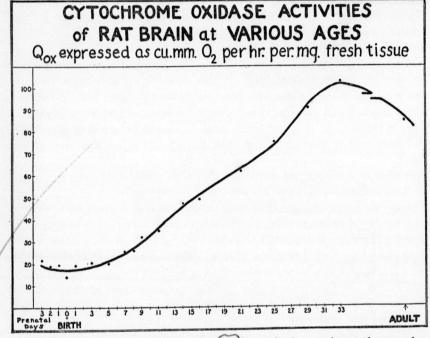

FIG. 26. Cytochrome oxidase activity Q_{ox} in rat brain remains at the same low value during the last days before birth and the first ones postpartem and then rises rapidly to a maximum at approximately the end of the first month. This graph was constructed from data kindly furnished by V. R. Potter, B. S. Schneider and G. J. Liebl (798).

active post-natal growth (Figure 26). In the pig, born in a more mature stage than the rat, a similar but earlier development occurs. The maximum rise of cytochrome oxidase takes place during the terminal quarter of gestation and at birth its value is indistinguishable from that in the adult (330).

Stimulants and inhibitors. There are many other observations which are in accord with a concentration of respiratory enzymes denser in the adult than in the infant. This increase in enzymatic population explains why the presence of potassium and of high temperature (476) has such a remarkable stimulatory effect on the grown animal. A review of Figure 27 reveals that potassium enhances liberally the aerobic metabolism of the adult rat cerebral cortex, but has only a minor effect on the infant

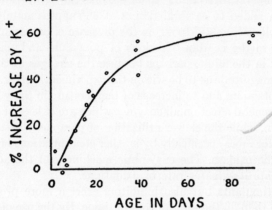

EFFECT OF AGE ON K⁺ STIMULATION

FIG. 27. The response of cerebral cortex of rats at various ages to potassium.

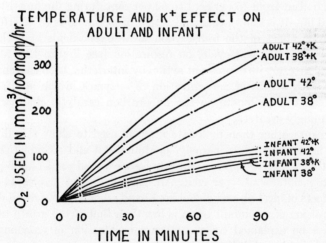

TEMPERATURE AND K⁺ EFFECT ON ADULT AND INFANT

FIG. 28. Oxygen consumption in cubic millimeters per 100 mg. wet weight of adult and infant brain.

brain. The response to potassium increases from the time of birth to 40 days of age when it is similar to that of the adult.

Rise of temperature, like potassium, increases metabolic rate. Figure 28 shows that the adult cerebral tissues exhibit a larger response than the infant. As with potassium, the infant brain has a relatively diminished reaction to elevation of the environmental temperature. It is well known that chemical processes are accelerated with increase of temperature.[13] When the elevation of temperature and increase of potassium are applied simultaneously the results are additive. The increase of metabolism due to a rise of temperature from 38° to 42°C., plus the extra stimulation from the potassium added to cerebral tissues at 38° approximately equals the rise of metabolism from 38° to 42° in the presence of potassium. The additive response to the combined actions of potassium and temperature is observed only in the adult, perhaps because the changes in the infant are of such small magnitude as to be within the experimental error. The smaller response to potassium and to increase of temperature in the young may be imputed to a general effect on all enzymes which are of lesser concentration in the newborn, while the slower utilization of paraphenylenediamine may be accounted for more specifically by smaller concentrations of cytochrome and cytochrome oxidase. The enzymatic machinery of the adult brain is able to facilitate its greater rate of oxidations.

Not only stimulants but also inhibitors exert a more profound effect on the mature than on the infant cerebral tissue. By the use of the reagent, malonate, Tyler (952) was able to show an increasing inhibition of cerebral metabolism from 15 per cent to 50 per cent during the first 10 days of post-natal life. It is known that one action of malonate is to interfere with the catalytic effect of the four-carbon dicarboxylic acids and, therefore, of the tricarboxylic acid cycle, on respiration (see Figure 12). Malonate may therefore exert its depressant action by interfering with this enzymatic activity. With a greater concentration of enzymes in the adult, the inhibitory effect of malonate on the four-carbon catalytic chain would be correspondingly greater.

Depressants other than malonate may be used to show this difference between infant and adult, namely, pentobarbital and alcohol (523). The cerebral tissues of baby and grown rats were exposed to alcohol 6 per cent and pentobarbital 0.012 per cent. An examination of Tables 14 and 16 on the effects of alcohol, and of Tables 15 and 16 on pentobarbital discloses that depression of the infant brain is less than that of the grown rat. Such results can be explained by a smaller concentration of enzymes in the infant than in the adult.[14]

[13] These results seem to be contradictory to those obtained on the intact animal in which the infant but not the adult was influenced by change of the environmental temperature from 24° to 34°C., but it must be recalled that only the intact infant rat was affected by the change in the environmental temperature since the adult had attained the ability, which the infant does not possess, to regulate its own temperature.

[14] These results obtained on excised tissues cannot be applied directly to the intact organ because of other effects in addition to those on cerebral metabolism; for

Solids and proteins. If the concentrations of cerebral enzymes, anaerobic and aerobic, become greater with the growth of the brain, then the substances which go to form enzymes must also increase. Enzyme systems are

TABLE 14

The effect of alcohol* on cerebral metabolism of various parts of the adult rat brain (cmm. O_2/100 mg. tissue/hour)

1	2	3	4	5	6
				DEPRESSION	
PART	NO. OF OBSERVATIONS	CONTROL	ALCOHOL	Absolute	Per cent
Cortex.............	19	316	195	121	38
Brain stem.........	20	251	204	47	19
Cerebellum........	20	179	111	68	38
Medulla...........	20	161	103	58	36
Total...........	79				

Column 3 presents the oxygen intake of the cerebral parts; column 4, the oxygen intake of these same cerebral parts as changed by the depressant effects of the drug; column 5, the numerical decrease from column 3 to 4; and column 6, the percentage decrease.

* 6 per cent concentration.

TABLE 15

The effect of pentobarbital* on various parts of adult rat brain (cmm. O_2/100 mg. tissue/hour)

1	2	3	4	5	6
				DEPRESSION	
PART	NO. OF OBSERVATIONS	CONTROL	PENTOBARBITAL	Absolute	Per cent
Cortex.............	40	278	170	108	38
Brain stem.........	39	226	163	63	28
Cerebellum........	40	167	106	61	37
Medulla...........	41	147	90	57	39
Total............	160				

* 0.012 per cent concentration.

composed of protein and inorganic constituents, and with growth these constituents should form a more prominent fraction of cerebral tissue when the enzyme concentration enlarges. But both protein and inorganic substances may serve other purposes than to form respiratory enzymes. For

example, infants succumb to a smaller dose of pentobarbital than adults (537, 290). To alcohol, however, infants are more resistant than the mature animal (170).

this reason, an increase of these constituents during growth does not prove that the enzymes would necessarily become more concentrated, though at least it is in accord with this conception. But it is significant that certain respiratory enzymes have been found to grow disproportionately large in comparison with the total protein (798). This increase in respiratory enzymes is, therefore, specific and occurs despite a relative diminution of other forms of protein. For this reason studies were made of the protein constituents of cerebral tissues and of their total solids during the life-span of the rat. Total solids are usually expressed as dry weight, and consist of lipids and carbohydrate in addition to protein and inorganic substances. Dry weight bears a fundamental relationship to metabolic rate. In fact, because of this relationship it is customary to measure oxygen consumption of tissues on a basis of dry weight. An examination of the table of Donaldson and Hatai (248) shows that beginning with birth there is a decreasing

TABLE 16

The effect of alcohol and pentobarbital on the infant rat brain (cmm. O_2/100 mg. tissue/hour)

1	2	3	4	5	6
				DEPRESSION	
NO. OF OBSERVATIONS	CONTROL	ALCOHOL	PENTOBAR- BITAL	Absolute	Per cent
16	102	81		21	21
44	105		83	22	22

percentage of water in the rat brain. The solids bear an inverse relationship to water and therefore increase with age. This gain is in accordance with the greater metabolism of the adult.

Koch and Koch (615) showed that significant changes occur in the constituents of the growing rat brain especially in two of the fractions which make up the total solids, specificially, protein and lipids. As a result of their findings on proteins and lipids, they divided the growth of the central nervous system into four periods: the first, during which cell division is the characteristic feature and proteins and lipids multiply, stops shortly before birth. The second period embraces the first 10 days after birth. During this time there is a rapid development of nerve fibers, and a corresponding formation of protein. During the third period from the 10th to the 20th day, the growth of the fibers attains its maximum rate, and myelinization, the laying down of the insulating lipid material around the axons, begins. These processes of growth and myelinization correspond with the increase of protein and of total lipids (963). The fourth period, after the 20th day, is that of continued myelinization. It is not likely that the higher metabolism of the adult brain can be attributed to its lipid content since white matter, formed chiefly of lipids, possesses a comparatively low metabolic rate. A more significant comparison can be made with the protein content of the brain. That a relationship exists between protein concentration and metabolism of an organism is well known (754), and may be explained by Engelhardt's suggestion that all living protein forms parts of catalytic systems (283). Since this relationship between protein and metabolism has been found to exist in the organism as a whole, it would seem logical to determine whether it applies to the brain.

Koch and Koch (615) have found that the increase of protein per mg. per day is 4.53 for one to 10 days and 5.90 from 10 to 20 days, and then falls to 0.89 from 20 to 40 days. The advance in protein concentration goes hand in hand with the accelerating rate of cerebral metabolism which is so marked during the first seven weeks of life.

VII. Phyletic order of brain changes

From the data presented in this chapter we have seen that the increase in cerebral oxidations and glycolysis occurs in such a manner that there is a swing from anaerobic towards aerobic production of energy. We will next study the pattern by which this swing takes place, and we shall be concerned first with the changes in oxidations, and then in glycolysis. It will be shown that the increase in oxidations does not occur in all parts of the brain simultaneously, but appears in the various portions at different times. The order of appearance is not a haphazard one but develops first in the caudad portions of the neuraxis and then progresses in a cephalad direction.

Such a series of changes advancing from the older to the newer parts of the brain recapitulates its phyletic development. As this process of phylogeny is carried on from one species to another, no part of the neuraxis is scrapped, but each caudad part, in turn, comes under the influence of a later developed cephalad portion, which not only possesses finer discrimination and analyzers but also exerts both reinforcing and inhibitory influences on the older parts. The evidence on the various metabolic changes of the brain appears to substantiate the conclusion that the cerebral metabolic changes occur in a phyletic fashion.

A. *Oxygen consumption*

The changes of the total cerebral metabolism throughout life, the early rapid increase and the later slight decrease, are the resultants of the distinctive metabolic rates in the discrete parts of the brain. It has been experimentally established that these metabolic rates are not equally affected by growth, but that each area possesses its own pattern of development.

In experiments on the rat (953) and the dog (495) it was found that the newer parts of the brain respire at a slower rate than the older portions at the time of birth. But as growth continues, their relative positions are reversed, and the metabolic rates of the newer parts of the brain take the lead. In Figure 21A (953) the low initial rates of the pallium and brain stem of the newborn rat can be seen. These rates rapidly rise and finally exceed those of the cerebellum and medulla after the 20th day of life. In contrast with the newborn, the adult rat exhibits the highest rate of metabolism in the phyletically newest parts of the brain. The cerebral cortex possesses the highest oxygen intake (column 3 of Tables 14 and 15); brain stem, cerebellum, and medulla follow in the order given.

A similar series of phenomena unfolds in the puppy (495) (Table 17). In the first week of life the highest rate of metabolism is found in the medulla; during the third week the most outstanding advance takes place as the midbrain changes its relative position and assumes the highest oxygen consumption. From the fifth to the seventh week, the respiratory metabolism of all parts, with the exception of the medulla, is definitely higher than the corresponding values for the first week of life. But most important, the caudate nucleus has advanced to the highest oxygen intake up to this time. In the adult the latter still retains its prime position, while the cerebral cortex ascends to second place. The cerebellum, thalamus, midbrain and medulla follow in descending order. According to Figure 22, (495) which illustrates this evolution, the relative positions of most parts of the brain are reversed during growth. Data are lacking between the seventh week and adulthood, but all parts of the brain suffer some slight decrease of metabolism as maturity is attained, though there is no further change in their order. To evaluate the significance of the differences in metabolic rates of the various parts of the brain, it must be recalled that the constituents of the brain change in concentration during growth. For example, the laying down of white matter, or myelinization, is completed only some time after birth. It is therefore probable that the fall in the metabolic rate of the older parts of the brain represents a reduction in the proportions of grey matter rather than an actual decrease in metabolic rate. On the other hand, increased rate of metabolism in the newer parts of the brain is caused by an augmentation which occurs despite a mixture of grey with white matter. The rise in metabolic rate of the newer parts of the brain represents an actual gain while the decrease in the medulla may be only apparent due to the diminished proportion of grey matter. The intrinsic oxidative rates of grey and white matter may be imputed to the concentrations of respiratory enzymes within the several parts of the brain studied. These experiments, therefore, show that grey matter in different areas possesses characteristic metabolic rates in accord with the phyletic position of the particular cerebral region.

These observations on rats and dogs reveal a metabolic progression which advances rostrally in the central nervous system. The lower parts are relatively more active than the higher ones at birth, and as development continues, the wave of metabolism presses forward so that the lower portions of the central nervous system are surpassed by the anatomically higher and phyletically more recently developed regions. The increasing rate of metabolism of the brain as a whole must therefore be attributed

TABLE 17

The oxygen intake cmm./100 mg. moist tissue/hour at different ages of dogs

PARTS OF THE BRAIN	1ST WEEK		2ND WEEK		3RD WEEK		5-7TH WEEK		ADULT	
	No.* of obs.	Averages	No. of obs.	Averages	No. of obs.	Averages	No. of obs.	Averages	No. of obs.	Averages
Cortex..................	47	61	26	64	37	68	8	121	25	116
Caudate nucleus..........	9	73	5	88	6	96	2	139	20	136
Midbrain.................	16	91	14	99	13	111	6	128	10	92
Medulla.................	14	96	15	101	19	103	6	85	16	69
Thalamus................	25	76	15	93	14	97	6	124	18	101
Cerebellum..............	14	79	19	85	25	87	9	95	22	107
Spinal cord..............	13	81	7	82	4	93			2	50

The gradual increase of the respiratory metabolism of all the parts of the brain is seen to occur from birth through the seventh week. In the adult the metabolism is slightly decreased in comparison with that observed during the 5–7th weeks. In general the order of intensity in metabolic rate observed in the adult is the reverse of that during the first week of life.

* Number of observations.

chiefly to the increasing rate in the newer parts of the brain during early life. An interesting correlation can be drawn between the rate of growth and the rate of metabolism in the rat brain. From Brody's curve (Fig. 29) it may be seen that early growth of the rat brain is rapid until the 25th day, at which time there is a rather abrupt decline in the rate. The congruity of the two rates—growth and metabolism—is apparent.

B. *Glycolysis*

In section IV of this chapter the cerebral glycolytic rates throughout the life-span of the rat were presented (165). They were found to be slowest in the newborn, increasing to a maximum in early life and declining somewhat to old age. The next point is to determine the contribution of each area in the brain making for this changing rate of glycolysis. This study necessitated the use of an animal whose brain was larger than that of a rat. Both dogs and cats were employed (168) and in several age groups: newborns to one week, three to seven weeks, three months, and adults. Samples of tissue from certain portions of the brain were inserted in the Warburg respirometer for glycolysis determination. In general, the results of the experiments on dogs and cats were similar. At birth the canine medulla oblongata revealed the highest glycolysis. From 3 to 6 weeks of age, and also at approximately 3 months, the caudate nucleus and thalamus occupied the highest positions. In the adult, however, it is the cortex that shares the most rapid metabolic rate with the caudate nucleus. In the cat,

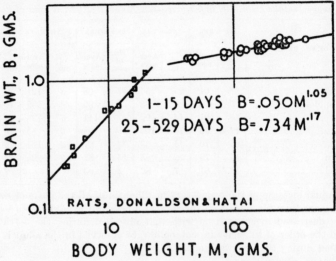

$$1-15 \text{ DAYS} \quad B=.050M^{1.05}$$
$$25-529 \text{ DAYS} \quad B=.734M^{.17}$$

RATS, DONALDSON & HATAI

BODY WEIGHT, M, GMS.

Fig. 29. Diagram of the growth curve of the rat brain. The curve advances steeply until the 15th day, and then only slightly from the 25th to the 529th day.

the medulla oblongata had the highest rate at birth, the thalamus and caudate nucleus from 3 to 7 weeks, while in the adult the caudate nucleus is above all other parts.

The results obtained in this comparative study of the glycolytic rates of the particular regions of the brain may be compared with the previous ones in which the aerobic metabolism of these same parts of the dog brain were examined (495) (see Figure 22). Qualitatively there are striking similarities, both oxidations and glycolysis moving in the same direction. Quantitatively, however, discrepancies appear because oxidations increase more than glycolysis in early life. Both the general resemblance between the two means of energy liberation, and the important divergence between them may be ascribed to the enzymatic reactions involved in oxidations and glycolysis.

Because the Embden-Meyerhof process furnished the carbohydrate split-product, pyruvic acid, which is subsequently oxidized, an increase in the concentration of enzymes responsible for glycolysis may result in the speeding up of oxidations. However, it must be recalled that other enzymes function in oxidation and are responsible for the utilization of pyruvic acid. Since different enzymes are involved in the production of carbon dioxide and water it could not be expected that glycolysis should reduplicate oxidations in all details.

The developmental progression observed in oxidations and glycolysis has also been found to exist in the distribution of cerebral glycogen, the intrinsic substrate of the brain both for oxidation and glycolysis. This glycogen distribution in the cat and dog brain has been established by quantitative determinations at three growth periods: birth, 5 to 8 weeks, and adults (164). The changing relationships of the glycogen content in seven regions of the neuraxis takes place in such a way that the concentration of glycogen in the newest parts, cerebral cortex and caudate nucleus increase with age both in the cat and dog (Fig. 30). In the intermediate areas the progress was somewhat varied for both species. The percentage of glycogen in the oldest parts, the cerebellum, medulla and cord, diminishes progressively both in the cat and in the dog, and is lowest in the adult. Not only does the glycogen content of the cerebral parts fall into a phyletic pattern, but as previously described (Chapter 4, pg. 54) the loss of glycogen provoked by hypoglycemia (166) also observes this phyletic order,[15] the medulla oblongata holding more tenaciously to its glycogen than any other part. And this, despite the fact that the medulla possesses the least glycogen to start with. The newborn presents the reverse picture, for not only do the caudad portions of the central nervous system exhibit the highest concentrations of glycogen (164) but they also suffer the greatest losses during hypoglycemia (319).

The length of time that glycogen is retained in any portion of the brain must be somewhat dependent upon the rate that it is utilized. Therefore, in the adult medulla, the glycogen is held back long after the rest of the brain has exhausted its supply, because the medullary rates of glycolysis (168) and oxidation (495) are the slowest. Such a retarded medullary metabolism is not without its biologically useful purpose, for the presence of this source of energy is needed to sustain vital activities, and does so when the rostral portions of the brain have failed. This mechanism, however, is not present in the newborn in whom the cephalad regions with their lower requirements are less susceptible to energy deprivation.

Finally, a word should be said on acetylcholine, an agent involved in nerve function. A suggested role of acetylcholine in nerve will be touched

[15] See Chapter 10, Table 34.

upon in Chapter 11, page 317. According to Welch and Hyde (990), who
studied rats, relative values for the different parts of the brain change with

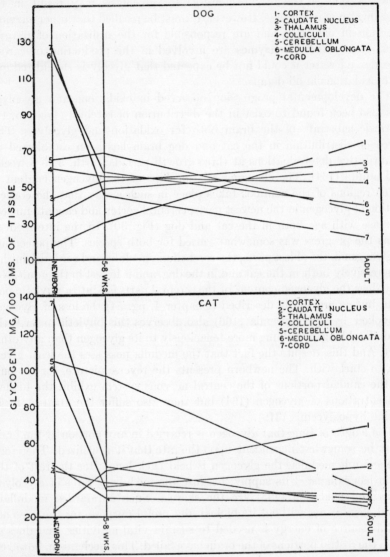

FIG. 30. Changing relationships of the glycogen content in the various parts of
the neuraxis during growth.

age: in the newborn rats the pallium is lowest in acetylcholine per unit
mass, and the medulla highest; while in adults the cerebellum is lowest and
the brain stem highest. The authors note that except for the cortex, there

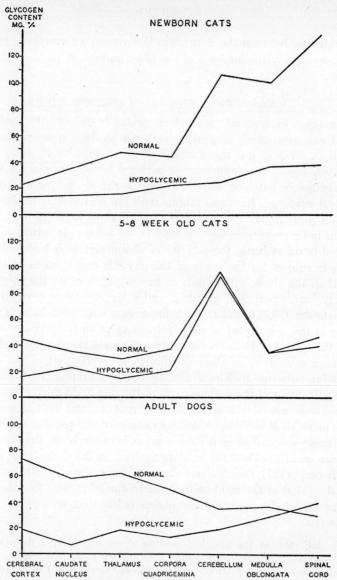

FIG. 31. These graphs show the concentrations of glycogen in the parts of the central nervous system of normal animals compared with the hypoglycemic for the three age groups. In the newborn animal, the curves for the normal and hypoglycemic animals become progressively farther separated from the cephalad to the caudad direction, while in the adult the reverse is true. In both of these age groups, those parts which have the higher concentrations of glycogen tend to show the greater fall during hypoglycemia. In the adult, these are the newer parts, while in the newborn they are the phyletically older ones. In the intermediate group, the decrease in the higher areas is of less magnitude than in the adults, and in contrast to the newborn, no significant changes occur in the lower portions (319).

is a parallelism between the changes in the oxygen consumption, glycogen content, and acetylcholine level of the older and newer parts of the brain with age.

C. *Cholinesterase, an example of enzymatic activity*

An increase in cerebral metabolism probably reflects the activity of cerebral enzymes which may also display a phyletic progression. As an illustration, we will use the enzyme cholinesterase which splits acetylcholine. In the chick cholinesterase activity accelerates during the last four days before hatching when the fetus is rapidly preparing for an independent existence. Rats and rabbits with low activities of cholinesterase at birth acquire higher values during the first three weeks of neonatal life, when the brain centers are developing.[16] In the guinea pig, with a relatively advanced brain at birth, the activity of cholinesterase is high. The sheep is a better subject for the study of the phyletic development of cholinesterase than the chick, rat, rabbit, or guinea pig, because the sheep has a relatively longer period of gestation and a larger central nervous sytem. Nachmansohn (757) found that cholinesterase is present in high concentrations in the spinal cord of sheep fetuses at an early stage of gestation; at this time it is low in the brain centers. This relationship changes as the cholinesterase activity of the cord diminishes while that of the caudate nucleus far outstrips it. The similarity between graphs (Fig. 32) on the oxygen utilization of the various parts of the dog brain during growth and the cholinesterase activities in the different regions of the embryonic sheep's neuraxis is striking. Another example of the parallel development of cholinesterase and oxygen consumption is observed in the comparison of the cerebral cortex and the caudate nucleus. In the sheep fetus, as in the adult ox brain (757), the cholinesterase activity of the cerebral hemispheres is less than that of the caudate nucleus. In the adult dog, too, the oxygen consumption of the cerebral hemispheres is less than that of the caudate nucleus (495).[17]

[16] The lethality of the anticholinesterase drug, di-isopropyl fluorophosphate (DFP) is greater in the newborn than in the adult rat (342). The brain of the newborn, with a lesser concentration of cholinesterase than that of the mature animal, possesses a smaller factor of safety against the anticholinesterase. Stated another way, an equal depression in the percentage of cholinesterase activity leaves the infant brain with a smaller absolute amount of enzyme to hydrolyze acetylcholine. Thus the neonate is rendered more susceptible to acetylcholine poisoning.

[17] This parallelism does not necessarily hold on comparing the brain with other parts of the nervous system; for example, the superior cervical ganglion, which exhibits an oxygen intake much inferior to any part of the brain, nevertheless possesses a cholinesterase activity greater than most cerebral regions, with the possible exception of the caudate nucleus (200).

Another enzyme which has been studied quantitatively both in the fetus and in the adult is carbonic anhydrase.[18] Ashby was not able to find any carbonic anhydrase in rat fetuses, but the adult rat brain was most consistent in its content of this enzyme (19). On comparing different parts of the adult rat brain, she found a greater amount of carbonic anhydrase per gram in the functionally dominant cerebral area than in the cord (20), and that this allocation was not dependent upon any anatomic distribution

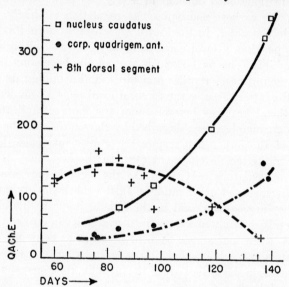

Fig. 32. Changes of acetylcholine-esterase activity in brain and spinal cord of sheep embryos during growth. This figure, revised by its author, in accordance with his conception that the esterase in conductive tissue is to be called acetyl-choline-esterase (26a). Abscissae: days of gestation. Ordinates: mg. of acetylcholine split per gm. tissue per hour.

of grey and white matter. In accordance with her suggestion, the relationship may be due to differences in the amount of enzymes contained in the neurones entering into the composition of the respective areas.[19]

[18] Carbonic anhydrase catalyzes the reaction $H_2CO_3 \rightleftarrows CO_2 + H_2O$, and is responsible for the accelerated release of carbon dioxide from the lung, though additional functions for this enzyme in the kidney, stomach and pancreas have been suggested.
[19] Davenport (223) has cast doubt on the functional importance of carbonic anhydrase because he has been able to inactivate that enzyme with thiophene-2-sulfonamide and did not observe any effect upon nervous properties. It would appear that further work is necessary in order to elucidate the role of carbonic anhydrase in the brain.

D. *Changes of cerebral function: neuromuscular control, electrical activity, and myelinization*

Neuromuscular control. If the functions of the central nervous system such as neuromuscular control and electrical activity develop in a phyletic manner, this would bring additional support for the conclusion that metabolic and enzymatic changes, which supply the biochemical basis for the neurologic functions, also develop in a phyletic plan. According to this formulation, the earliest neuromuscular regulation is chiefly spinal and bulbospinal in character. In the lowest vertebrates the midbrain occupies a prominent position, a level corresponding to the neural organization of fish and amphibia. The next stage is that of the hegemony of the basal ganglia representative of reptiles and birds, and attaining its highest expression in the latter. Finally the cerebral hemispheres commence activity as the functional patterns become more and more complicated. Such a cephalad progression has been described by Barron (57) for the respiratory mechanism of the fetus. The respiratory movements pass through four phases of intrauterine development (48). In the first, they are a part of the general musculatory movement. In the second, they are dependent upon the movements of other muscles. In the third, they occur in the absence of other movements, and in the fourth, they are inhibited by the nerve centers. By a study of the respiratory activity in fetuses with chronic brain lesions, these four stages have been shown to be dependent upon a series of centers in specific regions in the brain stem arranged serially from behind forwards, in the lower part of the medulla, the pons, and the caudad part of the midbrain.

Surgical intervention produces irreversible changes (793), but by alternate asphyxiation and revival it is possible to observe repeatedly the dissolution and reintegration of the respiratory mechanism. The relatively long period of tolerance to nitrogen in the infant dog facilitates the observation of respiratory changes in response to anoxia (302). As the metabolic depression descends from the cortex to include the pontine centers, respiration loses its rhythmicity and tends to stop in an inspiratory position. Later the predominant inspiratory character of respiration becomes biphasic as the long inspirations are divided into two by a short expiratory effort. Next the depression of all centers, except for the lowest in the medulla, becomes complete, and the respiratory act assumes a gasping character. Finally spontaneous respiration ceases though respiratory gasps may be evoked by peripheral stimulation. If at any time during this progressive depression the animals are permitted to respire air, a recapitulation of the respiratory changes is exhibited, but in reverse order and therefore similar to that of phyletic development.

Electrical activity. Another datum for the phyletic development of the central nervous system is obtained by observing the changes in the electrical activity of the cerebral cortex during growth. At birth, the medullary centers exercise their functions, but the cerebral cortex does not do so. This lack of function, as well as its gradual assumption of activity, can be followed by a study of the spontaneous electrical potentials of the cortex. Observations have been made chiefly on the cat (664) and the monkey (586). In the two- to six-day old kittens, electrical activity of the cerebral cortex is practically absent or of low amplitude. Nine-day old kittens exhibit

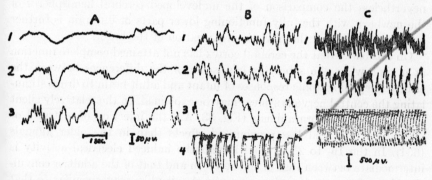

Fig. 33. Normal and metrazol activity of cerebral cortex in kitten and adult cat.
A. *Three-day old kitten.* 1. Spontaneous activity. 2. After 0.1 cc. of 10 per cent metrazol intravenously. 3. After another 0.1 cc. metrazol.
B. *Twenty-five day old kitten.* 1. Spontaneous activity. 2. After 0.1 cc. metrazol intravenously. 3. After another 0.17 cc. metrazol. 4. Another 25-day old kitten, 0.4 cc. metrazol into heart (had received 0.13 cc. metrazol into heart previously, which produced slow waves, resembling those in B2 here).
C. *Adult cat.* 1. Spontaneous activity. 2. Response after 0.2 cc. metrazol intravenously. 3. Another adult cat. 0.5 cc. metrazol intravenously.

random slow waves from the occipital and frontal regions. Kittens, 19 to 25 days of age, display considerable electrical activity in the same regions. Though the components of their EEG have a faster rhythm than in younger kittens, they are more irregular and slower than those appearing in the adult. The records obtained from a 3-day and a 25-day old kitten and an adult cat respectively are presented in Figure 33 (664). There seems to be a gradual increase with age in the frequency, regularity, and amplitude of the waves. Adult activity was not fully developed in 25-day old animals.

A similar series of changes is observed on the monkey (586) except that the period of development is longer and adult frequencies are not observed till the animals are one year of age. During the growth period the EEG becomes at once more complex and more uniform. In the infant monkey cortical potentials begin to develop at or before birth, but are not well demarcated until three or four weeks after birth. From this time until the end of the sixth month there is progressive development and elaboration of the EEG until it resembles that of the adult (Fig. 34). The more pronounced electrical activity during growth occurs on a substratum of accelerated metabolism which, in turn, is based upon the increased concentration of respiratory enzymes.

The study of the EEG reveals that at the time of birth the functional development of the cerebral cortex is not completed. Though these observations are concerned chiefly with the activities of the cerebral hemispheres, nevertheless the comparison of the undeveloped cerebral hemispheres of the newborn with the fully functioning lower parts of its brain is further evidence in favor of the phyletic organization of the brain.

On this basis, that the cerebral cortex has not attained complete function at a time when the subcortex has, some of the differences between the electroencephalographic responses of infant and adult brain to drugs stimulating the central nervous system may be explained. In the relatively silent cortex of the newborn animals (Fig. 33, A2) the injection of metrazol or strychnine produced less pronounced effects than in the older animals (664). In the 19- to 25-day old kittens the induced electrical activity is intermediate between that of the newborn and that of the adult; a convulsive dose of metrazol produces a train of spike-like waves similar to that of the adult but of lower frequency (Fig. 33, B4). The adult cortex (Fig. 33, C3) exhibits the typical rapid electrical activity of a convulsion (664).

Myelinization. We have shown that various neural functions develop in a phyletic manner. Since many nerve tracts of the central nervous sytem are myelinated, it would not be surprising to find that the process of myelinization also follows the same general phyletic pattern. Myelinization is not a prominent feature until some growth of the central nervous system has taken place. In order to account for the laying down of lipid material at this time, there must be either an appearance of new enzymes, or an increase in the concentration of enzymes already present. Chaikoff and co-workers (348, 349) studied myelinization occurring in the central nervous system by injecting radioactive phosphorus in rats of various ages and using the rate of the incorporation of the radioactive phosphorus in myelin as an indicator. They were able to do so because phosphorus is a constituent of the lecithins, the cephalins, and the sphingomyelins, substances which form myelin. These experiments revealed that the deposition of this radioactive substance is not uniform in the various divisions of the central nervous system, but maximal deposition of that substance occurred during the period of most intense myelinization. This process takes place in a phyletic order. From birth until the time the rat attains a weight of 50 gm (approximately one month) the cord is the most active part of the nervous system in deposition of lipids. During this time the medulla, cerebellum and the forebrain reveal decreasing activities and do so in that order. The cord is two or more times as active as the forebrain. The relation between the spinal and the supraspinal myelinization is reversed in the older rats; a higher concentration of radioactive substance is observed in the cerebellum, medulla, and forebrain than in the spinal cord. In summary, it may be said that myelinization reaches its peak in the spinal cord from birth to the time the rat weighs 50 gm. After this the relative activities of forebrain,

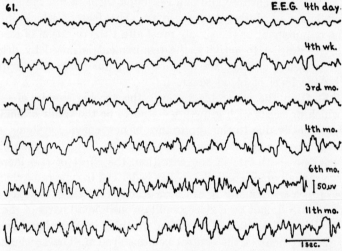

FIG. 34. EEG records at intervals during the first year of life of a *Macaca mulatta*. As the animal grows from the fourth day to the eleventh month, the amplitude, rate and complexity of pattern in his EEG are increased.

cerebellum, and medulla rise steadily, and by the time a weight of 200 or 300 gm. is attained, they are as great in those divisions as in the cord, or even greater.

VIII. SUMMARY

The newborn exhibits an extraordinary tolerance to anoxia. This tolerance was observed in many species and irrespective of the manner of producing anoxia. With the use of partial anoxia, it was shown that the adult retains sufficient resistance to be of biologic value. The first step in the analysis of this problem revealed the brain to be the limiting factor in the ability to withstand anoxia, and that the resistance of the brain depends upon the energy obtained anaerobically for that organ. Further experimentation disclosed that the anaerobic source of energy arises in the process of glycolysis. The ability to survive anoxia was found to depend upon the difference between the energy requirements of the brain, as represented by the oxygen consumption, and the energy supply produced by glycolysis. It was observed that both the anaerobic and aerobic production of energy rose as growth proceeded, but the rise was of such nature that oxygen consumption was greater than glycolysis. As a result, the difference between the caloric requirement and the anaerobic supply became more divergent in the adult, and this gradual separation is associated with poorer ability to withstand anoxia. The adult brain, however, never loses its anaerobic resources entirely and can call upon them to aid the aerobic in partial anoxia and during hyperactivity. The factors which influence either the requirement or the supply must affect the duration of anaerobic survival. In addition to activity, the requirement is raised by degree of maturity, presence of thyroxin, and rise of temperature; the supply is altered by the level of blood sugar.

The shift from the anaerobic towards the aerobic supply of cerebral energy which proceeds with growth is found to be the result of enzymatic changes, partically due to the appearance of new enzyme systems, and in part, to increased concentration of all enzymes. Though anaerobic and aerobic enzymes both rise in concentration, the effect of this increase is such that gradually more cerebral energy is derived from aerobic than from anaerobic processes. Finally it has been shown that these changes occurring with growth do not take place simultaneously in all parts of the brain but proceed in a longitudinal direction which is in accordance with the phyletic development of the central nervous system. The acceleration of metabolism, as well as the advance in glycogen concentration in various parts of the brain, both processes of which occur in a rostral direction, are paralleled by the development of cholinesterase activity. These metabolic changes form the biochemical background for the specific activities of the central nervous system, such as neuromuscular control, electrical variations and myelinization which also develop in a phyletic order within the neur axis.

CHAPTER 8

HUMAN CEREBRAL METABOLIC RATE

I. Determinants of Human Cerebral Metabolic Rate: Arterio-venous Oxygen Difference and Blood Flow

In this chapter we shall discuss normal brain metabolism in the human and the changes induced in cerebral metabolism by various pathologic conditions. It might help to clarify the meaning of the term, "cerebral metabolism" if we compare it with that of the body as a whole, usually termed "basal metabolism". Basal metabolism signifies the energy required for the maintenance of bodily functions during rest. This energy is produced by the oxidation of ingested foodstuffs and can therefore be determined by quantitative estimation of the oxygen utilized by the body. When metabolism of the body is either elevated or depressed beyond normal limits, the physician suspects a pathologic condition.

Just as the metabolism of the entire body may be measured, so the oxygen consumption of the brain alone may be determined, and this chapter presents certain preliminary efforts in that direction. The functions of the human brain, whether normal or pathologic, are performed by the energy received from cerebral metabolism. If this metabolism deviates from normal standards, as we shall see it often does, it may be a guide in diagnosing cerebral pathology, comparable to that of basal metabolism.

In the previous chapter we have shown that it is possible to measure brain metabolism by excising bits of cerebral tissues from the brain of animals and examining the oxygen intake and carbon dioxide output with the aid of the proper respirometer. It is obvious that, except for isolated instances, it would not be practical to apply this technic to the study of human brain metabolism. But, by taking two factors into consideration, it is possible to measure metabolic rate of the brain *in situ*. These two factors are: the volume of oxygen absorbed by the brain from each unit of blood traversing that organ (the arterio-venous oxygen difference), and the total volume of blood flowing through the brain per minute (cerebral blood flow). The multiplication of these two factors yields the total oxygen utilization, or the cerebral metabolic rate per minute.

This subject is still in its infancy and observations of cerebral metabolic rate (C.M.R.) are few, because methods to estimate cerebral blood flow are new but the data on cerebral arterio-venous oxygen differences (AVO_2 differences) are comparatively plentiful. In conditions in which we know only the AVO_2 differences, these data will be presented and an attempt will be made to interpret their implications in regard to cerebral metabolic

177

rate. In addition to normal subjects, studies were done on patients with a variety of diseases.

We may be able to decide from work of this kind whether the rate of cerebral metabolism can explain such nervous activities as the length of time required to respond to a given stimulus, i.e., the flashing of a light, or the ringing of a bell, or changes in personality under such conditions as high altitudes, or psychoses, and it may even help to clarify the nebulous term "consciousness". We know that alterations in basal metabolism are directly related to some pathologic condition of the body as a whole. The question at stake in this chapter is: does the cerebral metabolic rate yield any information of importance in diagnosing cerebral pathology? The answer to this question may furnish a basis for rational therapy, and also aid in the prevention of mental diseases. Some of the evidence for the solution of this broad problem is presented in this chapter and the next.

II. Cerebral metabolic rate when both determining factors are estimated

A. *Normal adults*

The first step in the evaluation of C.M.R. is to establish the normal standards, which may then be referred to as a basis of comparison with abnormal metabolism in disease. Fortunately, the largest number of data available are on normal individuals, thus assuring us a safe basis for this comparison. But even in normal subjects it has not been possible until recently to determine cerebral AVO_2 differences and blood flow simultaneously on the same individual. The technics involved in these determinations are of such a taxing nature as to render their simultaneous application difficult. We do possess, however, average results of a large number of observations of cerebral AVO_2 differences and cerebral blood flows made independently. After many years of labor it can now be quite definitely said that the average cerebral AVO_2 difference of normal[1] adults is 6.7 vol per cent (392, 391, 1025). This average is a result of 3 series of experiments comprising a total of 94 observations, and it will be used again and again throughout the book as a standard for comparing normal adults with those suffering from various diseases of the central nervous system.

[1] Normal, within the standards set by Gibbs, Lennox, Nims and Gibbs for 5 subjects in whom they determined cerebral AVO_2 differences—"intelligent, health and electroencepahlographically normal" (391). Starting from a minimum of 4. vol. per cent, which was found in only one person, there is a gradual accumulation of observations per 0.5 vol. per cent until the greatest number is found within the limits of 6.5 vol. per cent and 6.9 vol. per cent. After that, the observations again taper off to a single value at 8.5 vol. per cent. The deviation of the mean in accord with Fisher's t test is ±0.8 vol. per cent.

Unlike the cerebral AVO_2 difference, the quantitative determinations of cerebral blood flow are not in close agreement but yield results extending over a wide range. At one extreme is the value of 1 liter per minute calculated by Schneider and Schneider (858) for man on the basis of their observations on the dog, probably too high, for that figure yields an oxygen intake of 67 cc. per minute, somewhat more than $\frac{1}{4}$ of the basal energy exchanges of the entire body. At the other extreme Ferris (316) determined blood flow through the human brain experimentally and found it to be within the limits of 250 cc. and 400 cc. per minute, yielding the oxygen intakes of 16.8 cc. and 26.8 cc. per minute respectively. Ferris' estimate is somewhat low because his method depends on occlusion of the venous return from the brain, and Batson's results (64) show that Ferris' method occludes only the return from the internal jugular veins but not from the vertebrals which are protected by the bony vertebrae. While not quantitatively exact, the results of Ferris and his co-workers are reproduceable and reveal changes from the normal. With this proviso, Ferris' observations will be used in some of the following discussions.

Values between the extremes given above were obtained by three groups of investigators who determined cerebral metabolic rate by measuring simultaneously both blood flow and AVO_2 difference. Schmidt and co-workers (856, 596) applied results obtained on monkeys under light barbiturate anesthesia to man and derived a minimal oxygen consumption of 35 cc., a mean of 52 cc. and a maximal of 63 cc. per minute. In their direct observations of the human brain, in which the absorption of nitrous oxide was employed as the criterion, in 16 observations on eleven subjects a minimum of 31.2 cc., an average of 37.8 cc. and a maximum of 53.1 cc. per minute were observed assuming a brain weight of 1350 grams. Using the same method as Kety and Schmidt we obtained a somewhat lower average, 33.8 cc. per minute (528)[2]. With a brain weight of 1400 grams the averages would be 39.2 cc. per minute (596) and 35.0 per minute (528), respectively. The latter observations however were obtained on deteriorated patients, two with schizophrenia and two with general paresis and it is known that C.M.R. is reduced in general paresis (783a). Later results on other patients yielded an average of 52.0 cc. (869). Gibbs and associates (400; see Chapter 6 page 98 for cerebral blood flow in man), on the other hand, who employed a dye to measure cerebral blood flow found an average cerebral metabolic rate of 40.0 cc. per minute. Most of these determinations were made on patients with one or another type of cerebral disturbance.

Observations are available on two series of young healthy men who were studied while lying at rest. In one (598) the oxygen used by the brain, in

[2] These results (596, 528) are somewhat lower than those originally published because of the revision in the partition coefficient of nitrous oxide (594).

terms of cc/100 gm/minute, was 3.3 and in the other (848a) 3.8, astonishingly high values for C.M.R. corresponding to 46 and 53 cc/minute for the entire brain. To emphasize the magnitude of C.M.R. we shall compare the cerebral intake with the total bodily requirement at rest of approximately 250 cc. of oxygen or 1.25 calories per minute. With fractions of 46/250 and 53/250 the brain consumes a surprisingly large proportion of the total basal oxygen, approximately 18–21 per cent and its energy need is found at 0.22–0.26 calories per minute. Yet the incessantly beating heart utilizes only 10 per cent of the total basal requirement.[3]

B. *Adults in abnormal conditions*

Schizophrenia. Because of the stimulation to research given by the advent of insulin therapy, a larger number of observations have been made on patients with schizophrenia than with any other mental disease. Many investigators (481, 512, 1025) have obtained cerebral AVO₂ differences of patients with schizophrenia, not only before insulin therapy, but after therapy was completed. None of these found any variation from the normal in the arterio-venous difference. The intracranial blood flow of 16 schizophrenic patients was studied by Ferris and his collaborators (318), and according to their method the results did not differ significantly from those for the control group. In view of the fact that both cerebral AVO₂ difference and cerebral blood flow were the same as in normal subjects, we may conclude that the C.M.R. is unchanged in schizophrenia. This conclusion is supported by the work of Kety and associates (600) who measured AVO₂ difference as well as cerebral blood flow by the nitrous oxide method in a series of five patients with schizophrenia and observed C.M.R. within normal limits. In regard to our objective, the relation of C.M.R. to schizophrenia, we may call this discussion closed since this mental dis-

---

[3] Another way to make an estimate of brain metabolism is the application of *in vitro* observations. The determinations of cerebral oxygen utilization made on excised human cortex reveal values of 1.6 cc., 1.4 cc. (243) and 0.9 cc. (805) per gram of tissue per hour. These results are difficult to evaluate without knowing the relative proprotions of grey and white matter. But taking an average brain weight in the male of 1350 grams, a weight relationship of grey and white matter of 3:7, and an oxygen utilization of 3 cc. per gram of grey matter per hour and 1.5 cc. to 0.75 cc. per gram of white matter per hour, depending upon whether the oxygen intake of white matter is $\frac{1}{2}$ or $\frac{1}{4}$ that of grey (535), we may calculate the total oxygen consumption of the brain to be within the extremes of 2632 and 1924 cc. per hour. The values per minute are 44 cc. and 32 cc. Because of the lower weight of the brain in the female, averaging 1250 grams, basal C.M.R. must be slightly less between 41 and 29 cc. But both for the male and female the cerebral oxygen intake per gram per hour of mixed grey and white matter varies between 1.95 and 1.43 cc., results which are close to those obtained by direct observation of excised tissues. Finally, it should be pointed out that the higher values for the entire brain overlap the lower ones obtained *in vivo*.

ease cannot be imputed to an overall change in cerebral energy. There may, however, be an abnormal energy metabolism in an area too small to make itself felt among the other parts, and, of course, other kinds of metabolic changes are not excluded.

Insulin hypoglycemia. Because hypoglycemic coma can be produced at will during the course of the treatment of schizophrenia, we can collect blood samples for cerebral AVO_2 differences and for cerebral blood flow before, during, and after such a coma. In one series of experiments (512) the average cerebral AVO_2 difference was 6.8 vol. per cent before the injection of insulin. During profound hypoglycemia, it fell to 1.8 vol. per cent, about one fourth of the original value. After the ingestion of sugar and the re-establishment of contact with the environment, the last pair of blood samples was drawn, at which time the oxygen difference in the blood had risen to 5.1 vol. per cent. In order to estimate the change in cerebral metabolism during hypoglycemia, we must not forget to consider cerebral blood flow. The method used did not measure blood flow, but estimated accurately the percentage change from the pre-insulin value. (See Chapter 2, footnote on page 14 for discussion of the cerebral blood flow method). In one series of experiments (477) an average of 14 observations made during hypoglycemia revealed a decrease in the blood flow of 7 per cent. Considering both factors—blood flow and AVO_2 difference—the cerebral metabolic rate was decreased to 24 per cent. Another group of workers (318) observed no change or only a slight rise in cerebral blood flow during hypoglycemia. Kety and co-workers (600), using the nitrous oxide method, found that blood flow was not significantly altered by this treatment. In most cases, the difference between the values during hypoglycemia and the pre-insulin values is small enough to be disregarded.

The observations of Kety and his group (600) are of special importance because both cerebral AVO_2 differences and rates of blood flow were measured simultaneously on the same patient and C.M.R. fell to 56 per cent of its usual value before the injection of insulin. This reduction in C.M.R. is of lesser magnitude than that obtained in still another series of observations in which the patients were subjected to a more pronounced metabolic depression. As seen in the two experiments in Table 18 (477), during profound hypoglycemia, brain metabolism dropped to 22 per cent of the normal. In the second experiment it was reduced to 26 per cent before being restored to normal by the administration of carbohydrate. These results reveal the lower boundary of brain metabolism which is compatible with life (see Chapter 10 for discussion of this subject). A reduction to one-quarter of the normal metabolic rate for a limited period may not cause irreversible damage, but may still permit a rapid recovery to normal.

Effects of the inhalation of excessive and deficient carbon dioxide and oxygen. Homeostatic reactions are usually adequate to accommodate for the effects of moderate changes in carbon dioxide and oxygen so that C.M.R. is unaltered. Significant variations in the oxygen intake of the brain are not observed when the concentrations of either of these gases are increased over short periods. According to the observations of Kety and Schmidt (597) the inhalation of 5–7 per cent CO_2 accelerated C.B.F. 75 per cent

TABLE 18

Effect of insulin hypoglycemia on brain metabolism

1	2	3	4	5
		ARTERIO-VENOUS DIFFERENCE VOLUMES PER CENT		
PATIENT AND DATE	BLOOD FLOW RATIO	Observed	Corrected	BRAIN METABOLISM PER CENT
Br	1.00	6.14	6.14	100
6/21/40	0.90	4.07	3.66	60
	0.70	2.16	1.51	25
	0.90	2.33	2.09	34
	1.00	1.34	1.34	22
Br	1.00	6.57	6.57	100
7/5/40	0.70	2.45	1.72	26
	1.00	6.62	6.62	101*

The first observation on each of the two days was made before insulin was injected. In the first case, no observations of brain metabolism were made after the injection of glucose. In Br., 7/5/40 the glucose was given between the second and third recordings. Column 2 represents the ratio of blood flow after insulin to that before insulin, using 1.00 as the preinsulin value. Column 3 tabulates the oxygen removed by the brain from each 100 cc. of blood passing through it. When the values in column 3 are multiplied by those in column 2, the results are the corrected values for AVO_2 differences after considering the decrease in blood flow, and these corrected figures are enumerated in column 4. Column 5, using 100 per cent as the original observation before the injection of insulin, shows the gradual decrease in brain metabolism during coma, calculated from the corrected values in column 4.

* Observed after administration of carbohydrate.

but C.M.R. remained unchanged and AVO_2 difference decreased. Similarly the inhalation of 85 to 100 per cent oxygen slowed C.B.F. 13 per cent. Again C.M.R. was unaltered as AVO_2 difference enlarged and cerebrovascular resistance augmented.

When the inhalation of oxygen occurred for 15 minutes in an ambient pressure of $3\frac{1}{2}$ atmospheres, cerebrovascular resistance was further augmented and cerebral blood flow was reduced even more. C.M.R. however remained unchanged throughout all these observations. It must be remembered however that the individuals exposed to oxygen at high pressure for only 15 minutes were in the preconvulsant stage. It would therefore be of interest to determine whether or not a fall in C.M.R. is associated with the convulsions produced at high pressures of oxygen. The neurological alterations are the results of oxygen poisoning which will be discussed below (see pages 221–223).

A deficiency of CO_2 or O_2 may likewise fail to provoke changes in C.M.R. but nevertheless lead to significant consequences in terms of behavior. With passive hyperventilation and elimination of CO_2, the slowing of C.B.F. imposed by the alkalosis does not change C.M.R. and AVO_2 difference becomes greater. But with the fall of pH the signs and symptoms of tetany developed. Tetany is also oserved with active hyperventilation when C.M.R. rises somewhat, the fall of C.B.F. being relatively smaller then the increase of the AVO_2 difference.

Oxygen lack may also evoke serious consequences even when C.M.R. is maintained if the oxygen tension diminishes, as observed when the inhaled oxygen is reduced to 10 per cent, approximately one-half the normal value. Despite this drastic cut in the oxygen supply and consequent fall in the AVO_2 difference the acceleration of 35 per cent in C.B.F. prevents any decrease in C.M.R. But the lower oxygen tension which pervades the entire body produces the behavioral changes which are characteristic of anoxia. When greater strains are imposed, the adjustments making for a faster C.B.F. fail so that with a more profound reduction in the inhaled oxygen not only oxygen tension but also oxygen consumptoin becomes inadequate. An example may be offered by the inhalation of undiluted nitrogen continued until the AVO_2 difference falls to 1 volume per cent. With the brain weighing 1400 grams the normal C.M.R. will be approximately 46.2 cc. O_2/min., AVO_2 difference 6.1 volumes per cent and C.B.F. 756 cc/min. If the AVO_2 difference decreases to 1 volume per cent, to maintain a normal C.M.R. the C.B.F. must rise to 4620 cc/min., an improbable volume in view of the relatively fixed capacity of the cranial cavity.

In general alterations in the blood gases are surprisingly well born and C.M.R. zealously guarded. Though C.B.F. responds sensitively and more so to CO_2 than to O_2 the energy supplies of the brain are unhampered. In this manner the grave consequences of a reduction in C.M.R. are obviated or minimized. But the variations in the tensions of the two gases continue to exert potent effects. In Chapter 6 we have discussed the alterations produced by excessive oxygen and by oxygen lack. These alterations are in part responses to abnormal oxygen tensions. In this section we are content to point out that oxygen tension falls, before C.M.R. decreases, in O_2 deprivation. That is one reason why anoxia may be a more serious threat than hypoglycemia. With hypoglycemia oxygen intake is impaired but oxygen tension is well maintained.

Frontal lobotomy. Though the patient may emerge from the operation of frontal lobotomy with an immature personality, associated with loss of function of the frontal poles yet severing of the thalamic connections secures a desirable bleaching of excessive emotional tone and especially so for that of inner experience (344). Ameliorative effects are therefore observed in patients who are agitated or who respond to hallucinations with intense fear. Individuals in schizophrenic states lose their resistive and assaultive behavior. More recently this operation has been applied in the place of narcotics in the treatment of intractable pain due to organic disease. Because of the significant changes in personality it was considered worthwhile to obtain additional information on the physiologic action of this operation by a study of C.M.R.

A group (869) including Kety and using his blood flow method (596) observed 7 patients before the operation and from one to three weeks postoperatively, after full surgical recovery. On the basis of 100 grams of cerebral tissue per minute C.B.F. invariably decreased from a mean of 56 cc. to 43 cc., AVO_2 difference changed from 6.6 volumes per cent to 7.2 volumes per cent while C.M.R. fell from 3.7 cc. of oxygen to 3.1 cc. of oxygen. Thus brain metabolism is reduced 16 per cent by this operation. With a total weight of 1350 grams for the brain C.M.R. fell from 50.0 cc. to 41.9 cc. Though the results are clear their interpretation is less so. Two cerebral fractions must be taken into consideration: the lobotomized area and the remainder of the brain. With profound loss of function in the region rostral to the incision its metabolic rate falls almost to the low requirement for the maintenance of structure. This decrease must be considerable because of the high metabolism associated with the newer parts of the brain. The investigators point out however, that the impairment in C.M.R. is so great in proportion to the comparatively small amount of tissue involved that they suggest a generalized decrease in total cerebral activity reflecting a diminution in associative impulses from the lobotomized area. From this point of view the muffling of the metabolic cerebral fires is not a primary result of the operation, but secondary to retardation of function. But while the energy turnover indicates a quantitative impairment, cerebral function is not only carried on at a lower rate, but also assumes new qualities.

Diabetic coma. Studies of cerebral metabolic rate were made by Kety, Polis, Nadler, Schmidt on 14 patients with diabetes, all in severe acidosis (595). A difference was noted between those individuals still in environmental contact and others in coma. In conscious though somewhat confused patients with diabetic acidosis, cerebral metabolic rate was reduced to 82% of normal but when the metabolic depression became more profound, coma supervened and cerebral metabolic rate was found to be

52% of normal. In general a low cerebral metabolic rate correlated well with the severity of the disease for a reduction below 64% in most instances was incompatible with survival. The depression of cerebral metabolic rate was not associated with any lack of oxygen in the blood, though blood pressure was reduced. Differences were not observed between comatose and noncomatose patients in regard to the degree of acidosis, of hyperglycemia and of disturbance in the blood electrolyte pattern. It is not improbable, however, that a direct effect is exerted on cellular respiration. In this regard a suggestion comes from the demonstration of Schneider and Droll (859) that the slow intravenous infusion of acetoacetic acid produced coma in rabbits. Possibly the histotoxic phenomena observed in diabetic coma are related to the effects of ketone substances. Because they do not seem to be oxidized (407) they may exert a competitive inhibition and prevent the combustion of carbohydrate by the brain.

Brain tumors. Patients with brain tumors do not exhibit a uniform clinical picture in regard to changes in pressure whether of arterial blood or of the cerebrospinal fluid, nor do the alterations of cerebral blood flow occur in the same direction in all cases. Ask-Upmark (25) analyzed 486 of Cushing's cases between the ages of 20 and 44 years; 96 of these exhibited an abnormally low blood pressure with a systolic pressure of 100 mg. Hg or less, while 19 had an abnormally high blood pressure with a diastolic pressure of 100 mg. Hg or more. Similarly cerebrospinal fluid pressure may be low though it is more likely to be raised. Moreover the data of Kety and co-workers (599) demonstrates that cerebral blood flow may vary from patient to patient. Returning to a consideration of Ask-Upmark's analysis (25), we note that in 14 of the 19 patients with grave elevation of blood pressure the tumor was situated infratentorially. It seems that these tumors are also associated with the highest values for cerebrospinal fluid pressure and the slowest for cerebral blood flow. In general tumors, whether situated above or below the tentorium, are accompanied by an impaired cerebral metabolic rate if they are associated with an excessive cerebrospinal fluid pressure, a high blood pressure and a subnormal cerebral blood flow.

Among the factors which are involved in the impairment of the C.M.R. a reduction of C.B.F. must be considered first. If the tumor produces a significant rise in intracranial pressure it also causes a diminution in the volume of the other cranial constituents including the blood supply. At first however a reactive increase of blood pressure is able to force an adequate volume of blood through the compressed tissues. As demonstrated by Cushing (213, 214) the cerebral anemia which threatens the brain excites the vasopressor centers in the medulla and these in turn evoke a reflex peripheral vasoconstriction and a higher blood pressure. But finally systemic blood pressure does not rise any further and under the influence of the elevated intracranial pressure the vessels tend to collapse and cerebral blood flow is reduced. The brain no longer receives sufficient blood and cerebral metabolic rate decreases largely as the result of the impaired cerebral blood flow. This impairment is the important change in the causation of the low cerebral metabolic rate since either increases or decreases of the AVO$_2$ difference have been reported in different patients (1004, 195). One sign of a definite reduction in cerebral metabolic rate is the appearance of coma and in comatose patients the cerebral metabolic rate averages 76% of normal in the observations of Kety, Shenkin and Schmidt (599).

This reduction in cerebral metabolic rate is a comparatively superficial one to produce coma and therefore some suggestions are made to account for the grave clinical depression. One factor to be considered is the direct invasion of strategic areas by malignant cells with wide consequences including coma. Another factor is concerned with the method used to determine C.M.R. which is an overall measurement for all the constituents of the cranial cavity. It would seem that the estimated oxygen consumption is greater than that of the brain alone for it includes the fraction utilized by the tumor. Though the growing neoplastic cells probably respire less rapidly than the grey matter they nevertheless use oxygen that would otherwise be available to the brain. Confining our attention to that organ we must remember that the metabolic rate (oxygen per 100 grams of tissue per minute) of certain regions may be reduced far below the determined value which represents an average. Uniform pressure, equally distributed on all sides of the cell usually does not interfere with its metabolism. When however parts of the brain are forced against an unyielding ledge, whether fibrous tentorium or bony structure, the blood vessels undergo distortion and an added bar is interposed in front of the blood supply. The local metabolic rate necessarily falls and then destructive effects may be expected with functional and finally structural consequences.

Such irreversible damage may explain certain therapeutic failures; for example, ventricular drainage does not augment cerebral blood flow significantly (867). Even though the intravenous injection of a 50% glucose solution does accelerate cerebral blood flow yet the oxygen consumption of the brain is not improved in the presence of an intracranial tumor.

The cerebrospinal fluid is involved in the pathologic hemodynamics for the fluid does not give way before the greater intracranial pressure but instead maintains itself and thus becomes part of the mechanism which induces the rise in systemic blood pressure. At first the rate of formation of cerebrospinal fluid is accelerated as a result of hypertension and the rate of resorption is impeded because of the raised venous blood pressure. Thus the cerebrospinal fluid pressure increases and a vicious cycle is set up as a further compensatory rise of blood pressure is evoked. The enhanced intracranial venous pressure continues as a potent factor in this pathologic mechanism, for when the intracranial pressure is raised so high that cerebral blood flow and presumably the formation of cerebrospinal fluid are cut down, the further increase in venous pressure retards to an even greater degree the resorption of the cerebrospinal fluid. In the observations of Kety, Shenkin and Schmidt (599) blood flow was diminished significantly when cerebropsinal fluid pressures rose to values above 450 mm. of water. At such high values the walls of the capillaries tend to collapse, an effect which can be measured in terms of heightened cerebrovascular resistance (C.V.R.). C.V.R., according to Kety and Schmidt (598), is obtained by dividing C.B.F. into the mean arterial blood pressure $\left(\dfrac{\text{mean art. BP mm. Hg}}{\text{C.B.F. cc}/100 \text{ gm. brain/min.}} \right)$. In the normal individual a pressure of 1.6 mm. of mercury is required to force 1 cc. blood through 100 gm. of brain per minute (86/54). In an outstanding example of a patient with a tuberculoma situated in the posterior fossa (599) cerebrospinal fluid pressure was found to be 840 mm. Hg, C.B.F. was reduced to 31 cc/100 gm. brain/min. and with a mean arterial blood pressure of 130, C.V.R. was 4.2. Such high pressures of C.S.F. are observed more frequently with posterior fossa tumors than with tumors in other parts of the cranial cavity. In view of the role played by the intracerebral venous pressure in the resorption of the cerebrospinal fluid[4] Courtice's suggestion (195) of greater interference with venous drainage can account in part for maintaining the volume of cerebrospinal fluid and the great intracranial pressure observed in patients with posterior fossa tumors.

[4] The clear cerebrospinal fluid fills the ventricular system and the subarachnoid space. This fluid, elaborated chiefly in the choroid plexus of the lateral ventricles traverses the foramena of Munro to join that produced by the choroid plexus of the third ventricle and then goes on through the aqueduct of Sylvius to be augmented by the plexus found in the fourth ventricle. The foramena of Magendie and Luschka in the roof of the fourth ventricle, permit the fluid to pass downward to the subarachnoid space of the spinal cord as well as to the base of the brain and upwards over the cerebral hemispheres. The normal hydrostatic relations are such that pressure is greatest in the arterial bed, intermediate in the cerebrospinal fluid and least in the venous blood. Hence the cerebrospinal fluid is formed, for the most part, as a dialysate of the choroidal capillaries. Similarly, filtration is apparently adequate to account for the flow of this liquid from the subarachnoid space to the venous system. This flow occurs through the arachnoid villi and also directly into the veins. Obstruction to the passage of fluid in the foramena of Munro, the aqueduct of Sylvius or the foramena of Magendie and Luschka produces internal hydrocephalus. Interference with the resorption of this fluid by way of the arachnoid villi leads to external hydrocephalus and to an elevation of cerebrospinal fluid pressure similar to that observed with brain tumor.

To summarize this discussion, an impairment of C.M.R. is associated with some brain tumors. In accordance with Cushing's early experiments (213, 214) in those instances the brain suffers from ischemia which is the chief cause for the lower metabolism, but there may be additional pressure factors in the production of coma. The developmental steps are: (1) An increased intracranial pressure which evokes a rise of systemic blood pressure and thus maintains cerebral blood flow. (2) Intracranial pressure is elevated beyond ability of the compensatory cardiovascular mechanisms to prevent a fall of cerebral blood flow and a reduction in cerebral metabolic rate ensues. The mounting venous pressure maintains the volume of cerebrospinal fluid by retarding its resorption and thus increases still further the rise of intracranial pressure caused by the tumor. (3) It is suggested that the blood vessels supplying certain cerebral areas are occluded in those parts of the brain which partially include unyielding structures. These cerebral areas suffer a more profound fall in their blood supply than other regions and are in part responsible for bringing on the loss of environmental contact. The direct invasion of strategic areas by growing tumors must also be considered in the production of coma.

Essential hypertension. We have just discussed the alterations in brain metabolism associated with intracranial tumors and found that the metabolic consequences may be divided into stages: the first stage, that of adequate compensation, occurs when the rise of blood pressure, secondary to the greater intracranial pressure, prevents a significant fall of cerebral blood flow and thus maintains an adequate cerebral metabolic rate; the other stages, during which vascular adaptations can no longer overcome the effects of increased intracranial pressure, do not concern us here for in essential hypertension vascular adjustments seem to be adequate and maintain an unchanged cerebral metabolic rate (Kety and co-workers, 593). When the source of hypertension is of unknown cause but probably of extracranial origin, the nature of the adaptation consists largely of increased vascular tone or cerebrovascular resistance which acts in such a way as to prevent an augmentation of C.B.F. Such changes have been observed by these investigators in 13 patients with hypertension. Their average mean arterial blood pressure of 159 mm. Hg divided by their average C.B.F. of 54 cc/100 gm. brain/min. yielded a value of C.V.R. of 3.0. Normally C.B.F. is 54 and C.V.R. is 1.6. These vascular adaptations which serve to keep blood flow within normal limits are not peculiar to the brain but are shared by the entire body. But whatever the pathogenesis of essential hypertension may be C.M.R. remains unchanged. When however the hypertension is limited to the upper part of the body as occurs in coarctation of the aorta (434) preliminary results, obtained on 2 patients, indicate different conclusions. Despite an increased C.V.R., C.B.F. was accelerated. C.M.R. appeared to be raised above normal even though the arterio-venous oxygen difference remain in the normal range. It would be of interest to determine whether there is a causal relationship between the increase of C.B.F. and that of C.M.R.

C.M.R. in pregnancy, normal and toxemic. C.M.R. averaged 3.5 in normal young women between 30 to 40 weeks' gestation (McCall, 719) a value which is statistically the same as 3.3 observed in a large number of normal young women. The two determinants of C.M.R. were also the same with a C.B.F. of 56 and an AVO_2 difference of 6.5. The latter normal value was obtained despite a low arterial oxygen content due to the hydremia of pregnancy. If normal pregnancy does not alter C.M.R. then the rate is the same in men and women per 100 grams of brain. On an absolute basis however the oxygen utilized by the brain of women is less because of a lower brain weight, 1250 grams vs. 1380 grams in males. With however a lower B.M.R. in the female the percentage of the total oxygen intake utilized by her brain tends to approach that of the male.

With these normal results as a basis for comparison 29 patients with toxemia of pregnancy were studied: according to the classification proposed by the American Committee of Maternal Health in 1939, 16 with hypertensive toxemia, 8 with pre-eclampsia and 5 with acute eclamptic convulsions. Only the convulsant group exhibited a difference from the normal. C.M.R. fell to 2.8, a reduction of 20%. In the absence of knowledge on the underlying cause for the toxemia of pregnancy it is difficult to determine a reason for the impairment in oxygen consumption. McCall however furnishes a clue as he finds a consistant difference between the normal and all three groups of toxemic women, namely a greater cerebrovascular resistance. It requires a greater blood pressure to force 1 cc. of blood through the brain of the toxic woman than through that of her normal control.

In discussing the alterations responsible for the greater cerebrovascular resistance McCall (719) lists intrinsic action due to vasospasm and extrinsic pressure exerted upon the vasculature by cerebral edema or increased intracranial pressure of the cerebrospinal fluid. Because edema and increased cerebrospinal fluid pressure are inconstant findings, the investigator believes that vasospasm is the most likely cause. It would therefore seem important to study the mechanism of vasospasm and determine its relationship to the reduction in C.M.R.

Depression. Another group consisting of the depressions, is composed of individuals with retarded reactions and subjective sadness who are agitated, suffer from delusions and lose weight because they refuse to eat. Thirty-three patients were studied for their cerebral AVO_2 difference, circulation time, as well as for their general physical condition (141). The average cerebral AVO_2 difference for the whole group was 6.5 vol. per cent, not statistically different from the normal. They did not exhibit abnormalities in their circulation time nor in their physical examination to make one believe that their cerebral blood flow might be abnormal. Actual observations of the cerebral blood flow are not as numerous as those on schizophrenics but Dr. Aring[5] informs us that a few patients studied with the method used by Ferris and his group showed no difference from the normal. Even though more observations, would be welcome, the indications are that the cerebral metabolic rate (C.M.R.) is normal for patients with depression.

General paresis. Unlike the psychoses of depression or schizophrenia, it can not be expected that cerebral metabolism would remain normal in general paresis, because this disease is characterized by degenerative processes in the cerebral tissue. Actual observations revealed decreases in both the determinants of C.M.R. The average of 54 observations of the AVO_2 differences made by 3 groups of investigators (1025, 479, 687) was 6.2 vol. per cent, somewhat below the normal. These patients all suffered from the advanced stages of their disease, a condition of special aid in calculating their metabolic rate because patients in the advanced stages may possess a cerebral blood flow below the average value (834).[5] Considering the cerebral AVO_2 difference and the blood flow, we may conclude that the C.M.R. in severely demented patients with general paresis is found to be subnormal. The observations of blood flow suggest that it is reduced more than the AVO_2 difference. This slowing of the blood flow may be regarded as a result of a syphilitic inflammatory process in the vascular supply of the brain. In passing, it may be added that patients with only mild symptoms showed a cerebral blood flow and an AVO_2 difference practically the same as normal subjects. Their cerebral metabolic rate would not be affected as it is in the severely demented patients.

Observations of Patterson and co-workers (783a) using the nitrous oxide method (598) on patients with paresis and meningovascular syphilis provide quantitative information which in general is in accord with previous work and in addition throws new light upon therapeutic mechanisms. The mean blood flow of these patients was 75% of normal. The patients with paresis exhibited a mean reduction of cerebral metabolic rate to 70% of normal, a deeper reduction than observed in those with meningovascular syphilis. Again in asymptomatic syphilis both cerebral metabolic rate and cerebral blood flow were unaltered. The changes produced by treatment with penicillin and malarial fever therapy were not constant. But in paresis the cerebral metabolic rate was more apt to be restored toward normal levels while in meningovascular syphilis cerebral blood flow was usually acceler-

[5] Personal communication from Dr. Charles D. Aring.

ated. The authors conclude that syphilis not only retards cerebral blood flow but also directly affects cellular metabolism.

Cerebral arteriosclerosis. In patients with advanced cerebral arteriosclerosis, the narrowing of the vascular bed restricts the blood supply of the brain and therefore interferes with the volume of oxygen brought to that organ, which ultimately leads to the destruction of the neurones, and to a reduction in the total amount of brain tissue. There may also be primary parenchymatous degenerative changes. In this organic psychosis, like that of general paresis, a fall in C.M.R. should be expected. Averages for two series of observations of the cerebral AVO$_2$ differences were normal, 6.7 vol. per cent (1025) and 6.8 vol. per cent (141), but cerebral blood flow is retarded in this disease. Again some of the evidence for the latter was obtained by Ferris and his associates (834) who disclosed that the blood flow was impaired.[6] In that case, the reduction of the blood flow is responsible for the fall in C.M.R.

Employing the nitrous oxide technic Freyhan and co-workers (344a) report a reduction in cerebral metabolic rate dependent chiefly upon a retardation of cerebral blood flow. But such a retardation is readily compensated, in the normal individual, by a relaxation of cerebrovascular resistance and therefore a larger AVO$_2$ difference so that cerebral metabolic rate remains unaltered provided the brain cells are undamaged. Thus it would seem that parenchymal changes must have taken place in these patients. What is the mechanism of the parenchymal damage? Among the factors to be considered is the morphologic pathology of the cerebral vasculature which prevents an adequate relaxation of cerebrovascular resistance and the development of a larger AVO$_2$ difference. Thus the cells suffer injury as a consequence of an impaired oxygen supply. Such a mechanism however does not rule out a direct action on cells exerted by the toxic process that brings on the arteriosclerosis. In any event the reduction of cerebral metabolic rate would not have taken place in the absence of brain cell injury. It would be interesting to make further studies on other organic psychoses with destructive cerebral changes to discover whether or not a reduction of the metabolic rate is typical or whether these instances of neurosyphilis and arteriosclerosis are isolated cases.

Injection of aminophylline. Metabolic results (979a) are at hand on the alterations observed while aminophylline, 0.5 gram, was being administered intravenously to ten patients. Aminophylline, or theophylline ethylenediamine, had two different effects on C.M.R. In six of these patients C.M.R. decreased from a mean of 3.9 to 3.3 cc/100 gm/min. and in the four other individuals, who reacted to the drug with extreme anxiety, it rose

[6] Personal communication from Dr. Charles D. Aring.

from a mean of 3.7 to 4.6 cc/100 gm/min. In both cases the experimental means were significantly different from the control values. Cerebral blood flow was reduced in all ten patients from a mean of 59.4 to 44.4 cc/100 gm/ min. This reduction does not seem to be associated with a fall of blood pressure. Aminophylline therefore produces a marked constriction of cerebral vessels and cerebrovascular resistance is augmented, an unexpected result. In view of the relative impotence of sympathetic vasoconstriction in the brain (444a) a response emanating from the medullary vasomotor centers seems to be ruled out. Further work is needed to unravel the mechanism of the vasospasm.

As noted above with small doses of aminophylline C.M.R. may either rise or fall. With larger doses, however, it is to be anticipated that an elevation in oxygen consumption will take place as the stimulating effects of the xanthine derivative become more intense (564a). This stimulation depends in part upon a direct action on cellular metabolism. The breakdown of carbohydrate to the lactic acid is accelerated (737) and basal metabolic rate is raised (256). Experiments with larger doses of aminophylline may also determine whether the vasoconstriction will be overcome by a rise in blood pressure as well as by the vasodilatation and reduction of cerebrovascular resistance, a reduction secondary to the increased accumulation of metabolites within the brain.*

Preliminary reports. Preliminary reports are available in 2 groups of patients suffering from epilepsy and parkinsonism. In idiopathic epilepsy C.M.R. and C.B.F. were not significantly different from the normal controls

---

*Amphetamine both in man (1a) and in monkey (258, 856) seemed to yield results similar to those obtained with aminophylline. In the majority of the observations both C.B.F. and C.M.R. were reduced and this reduction occurred despite the well-known stimulating effects of that drug as shown in the depressed individual, for example in narcolepsy. Quastel (803) found that the drug increased the metabolism of excised cerebral tissues under certain conditions. Though it did not affect brain oxidation directly it nevertheless reversed the inhibitory action of some amines on oxygen intake. This toxic effect, according to Quastel, is brought on chiefly by aldehydes, products of amine oxidation. Amphetamine, like other amines, has a strong affinity for amine oxidase but is not attacked by that enzyme. The oxidizable amines are therefore displaced by amphetamine and in that way the formation of their inhibitory oxidation products is prevented. But the clinical observations of its exciting action in the normal and its analeptic effect in the anesthetized individual remain unexplained (411). If amphetamine acts like adrenaline then on the basis of Marrazzi's work (709) it may inhibit synaptic transmission and perhaps give rise to a release made manifest as apparent stimulation. Such a combined depression and release is compatible with the observed reduction in C.M.R. Xanthine derivatives on the other hand are known to stimulate the synapse directly working perhaps on the post-synaptic segment which is most sensitive to some chemical agents.

(413). The observations made on postencephalitic Parkinson's disease (870) revealed a diminished C.M.R. associated with a slowed C.B.F. in 5 of 7 patients. Contrary to the usual experience with bilateral block of the stellate ganglia (444a) bilateral stellectomy seemed to increase cerebral blood flow. C.M.R. however was not restored by the operation. The change in C.M.R. occurring with coarctation of the aorta is considered at the end of the section on hypertension.

C. *Significance of the foregoing data*

In the opening of this chapter a comparison was made between cerebral and basal metabolism, stressing the fact that basal metabolism is measured when the body is at physical rest. Rest, in this sense, implies that no physical or mental work is being done. But, we must remember that during this time the heart is beating, respiratory muscles are active, skeletal musculature is in tone, glands are secreting and nerves conducting. Basal metabolism is the energy required to maintain these activities. Total metabolism, on the other hand, connotes basal metabolism plus the energy necessary for work.

In two series of resting normal male adults cerebral metabolic rate was found to average 46 cc. and 53 cc. of oxygen/minute by the nitrous oxide method. Observations on patients, by the dye method, yielded an average of 40.0 cc/minute. The variation is small when one considers the experimental error, differences in technics and in the status of the subjects, factors which have been found to alter results obtained by the well established methods of measuring B.M.R. and which may also affect the determination of C.M.R.

C.M.R. represents the energy necessary for the maintenance of cerebral functions in a comparatively quiet and restful interlude. These functions involve the interaction of cortical and subcortical elements. For example, the regulation of respiration is an unceasing activity of the pons and medulla oblongata. It is also thought that the cerebral cortex is continually reinforcing and inhibiting subcortical mechanisms. But the brain is not working at a constant rate; any performance more intense than that supported by C.M.R. calls for a more plentiful energy supply (856). This accelerated turnover may be compared with the total metabolism of an exercising individual and becomes maximal during convulsions (226, 227). (For discussion of the cerebral energy turnover, see Chapter 2, pages 9, 10).

Cerebral energy is not only raised above the level of C.M.R. by activity greater than resting, but is depressed below it by lack of foodstuff, impaired oxygen supply, narcotic agents, and in other conditions discussed in this chapter.

The cessation of cortical and of some subcortical activities when the brain is deprived of its source of energy by insulin hypoglycemia proves that a certain minimal metabolic rate must persist if nervous performance is to continue. In hypoglycemic coma reductions in cerebral metabolic rate to 56% (600) and 40% (477) of normal were observed when contact with the environment was lost and even a greater decrease of C.M.R. in extreme clinical depression. Thus in the production of coma due to a withdrawal of foodstuff the impairment of C.M.R. is of a large order. In diabetic coma (595) the cerebral metabolic rate was 52% of normal as if it too were due chiefly to a metabolic inhibition and Kety and his associates conclude that a value 64% of normal may be the lowest at which environmental contact may be retained. On the other hand, with thiopental anesthesia (528, 293) the metabolism was diminished only to 64% and yet not only was environmental contact lost but the deep stage of surgical anesthesia was observed, indicating that in addition to a metabolic impairment other factors were operative, for example, that of specific depressant nerve effects not based on a metabolic impairment as discussed in Chapter 12. In patients with brain tumors, coma occurs with a comparatively superficial reduction to 76% of normal. It must be remembered, however the determination of cerebral metabolic rate represents the total effect of rise in intracranial pressure on the oxygen intake, while coma in this instance may be a symptomatic sign of functional loss in specific cerebral areas.

Furthermore, from these experiments it is possible to make a quantitative estimate of the proportion of cerebral energy used for the maintenance of functions which fall out during hypoglycemic coma, because brain metabolism is reduced to one-quarter of C.M.R. at that time. This minimal rate of metabolism is not sufficient if the individual is to keep in contact with the environment nor to sustain the functions of the suprabulbar portions of the brain, these being compatible only with a higher rate of metabolism, approximately 4 times this minimal. It would seem that a deprivation of three-quarters of the energy requirements of the brain could be withstood for a short period but undue prolongation or repetition of this deprivation inevitably leads to disintegration of brain tissue. The conclusion that a *short* period with a metabolic rate one-quarter of the normal is adequate to maintain the functions of the medulla oblongata and to prevent structural damage in other parts of the brain is supported by the observation that the administration of carbohydrate in such cases produces complete restoration of cerebral functions.

Schmidt, Kety and Pennes (856) have observed that a reduction to less than $\frac{1}{2}$ C.M.R. due to hemorrhage was incompatible with prompt and complete recovery in the monkey. If the greater fall in man is not due to a species difference, then it may be ascribed to the experimental conditions.

Though cerebral blood flow of the monkey, unlike that of man, was measured quantitatively, the impairment of cerebral metabolism may have been an expression of a poor general condition in an operated animal subjected to hemorrhage and was a condition shared by the brain with the entire body. In the human subject, on the contrary, we observed the direct results of depressed cerebral metabolism, while other organs were not similarly obtunded, perhaps thus accounting for recovery despite the more profound cerebral depression. Nevertheless recovery after reduction to $\frac{1}{4}$ of the normal rate is surprising and should be confirmed.

The knowledge gained by the studies of the C.M.R. during hypoglycemia is of aid in interpreting the significance of the C.M.R. in patients with psychoses of proved organic origin. Inspection of the brain of patients with cerebral arteriosclerosis reveals that two processes are occurring simultaneously: destruction of cellular tissue and narrowing of the blood vessels. From the evidence at hand it is not possible to say which of these processes is the primary one. They may be equally responsible. However, if the vascular bed is the primary cause for the deterioration of the nerve cells, then arteriosclerosis may be compared with anoxia produced for example, by the inhalation of an indifferent gas, or with hypoglycemia, but instead of either oxygen or sugar alone being withheld, supplies of both substances are impaired. Therapeutic insulin hypoglycemia or the inhalation of undiluted nitrogen is both acute and profound, while the deprivation in cerebral arteriosclerosis, though relatively mild, has an incessant action and finally succeeds in destroying cerebral tissue. The lack of cerebral energy probably interferes with normal function long before irreversible damage is produced. One would think that remedial measures to increase brain metabolism would be of value only if applied before degenerative changes have begun.

In general paresis, as in arteriosclerosis, both nerve cells and blood vessels are affected, and destruction of cerebral tissue is inevitable. It is interesting to note that histologic studies reveal abnormal contents of the iron in the brain of general paretics. In view of the fact that iron is involved in oxygen transfer, this abnormality of iron may be associated with the impaired cerebral oxidations[7]. The low cerebral metabolic rate is not the cause of the cerebral damage; on the contrary, it is produced by the infective agent. The diminished C.M.R. in general paresis is the secondary result of the loss

[7] According to Spatz (899) there are characteristic changes of the iron metabolism in patients with general paresis, causing an accumulation of iron-containing pigment in the cerebral blood vessel walls. Volland (960) reports a diminution in the iron concentration of the serum. If cerebral iron metabolism is also impaired, then such a disturbance may be associated with the low C.M.R. in general paresis because iron is involved in the process of respiration. (See Chapter 5 for the role of iron in cellular respiration).

of cerebral tissues. But long enduring diminution of C.M.R. does not necessarily indicate tissue destruction. The chief cause for the fall observed after lobotomy is not loss of tissue but reduction in function though here too the reduction is conditioned by an anatomic change. Finally, the inability to disclose any impairment in the overall energy turnover in schizophrenia and in depression, does not necessarily rule out some other kind of cerebral metabolic defect, yet it does not exclude the possibility that the clinical pictures observed may be a result of a breakdown in nerve function rather than in an insufficiency of the metabolic processes supporting them. In such a case it would seem that the abnormal behavior may be a result of one or another kind of failure in the integrated action of the brain. One type of failure has been recently emphasized by Wiener (997) namely, that the disturbance may be caused by a defect in the functioning of memory patterns.

What then, are our conclusions so far:

(1) The normal rate of cerebral metabolism was found to be 46–53 cc. of oxygen per minute. These figures indicate a surprisingly high utilization, representing 18 to 21 per cent of the total oxygen consumption in the resting individual.

(2) For the patient with schizophrenia, depression, or essential hypertension C.M.R. probably does not differ from the normal.

(3) The present evidence suggests that the two psychoses, cerebral arteriosclerosis and general paresis, may be associated with a subnormal C.M.R.

(4) When contact with environment is lost due to withdrawal of foodstuff as in insulin hypoglycemia, the diminution of C.M.R. is of a large order; 56% and 40% of normal in different observations. To maintain consciousness C.M.R. must be higher than these values and Kety and coworkers suggest a reduction to 64% of normal as a minimum. Perhaps diabetic coma with a reduction to 52% of normal may be placed in this class due to metabolic inhibition. It is true that coma occurs in the case of brain tumor with a more superficial reduction of C.M.R. to 76% of normal but in that case additional factors may enter into the production of coma.

(5) Lobotomy lowers C.M.R. significantly in observations made one to three weeks postoperatively.

(6) Because C.M.R. is unchanged in schizophrenics, it is probable that hypoglycemic coma would exert the same depressant effect on normals or on patients with diabetes as in schizophrenics.

III. AVO$_2$ DIFFERENCE KNOWN; CEREBRAL BLOOD FLOW UNKNOWN

A. *Effect of age: Normals and undifferentiated mental defectives*

Among the data in which we are equipped only with the cerebral AVO$_2$ differences, we will first discuss the effects of age. Because we already know both determinants for calculating C.M.R. in normal young adults, and in elderly arteriosclerotic individuals, we will be able to use this knowledge in evaluating the significance of the AVO_2 difference through the early growth period where we have no estimates for blood flow.

The data (Fig. 35) for the arterio-venous differences were obtained in three age groups: (1) in babies less than 2 weeks of age, (2) in children and adults from 6 to 55 years (497), and (3) in order to complete the age spectrum, the older people from 59 to 97 years previously discussed under cerebral arteriosclerosis (1025, 834, 141) were included. To facilitate this examination of the influence of age on AVO_2 differences, the second group is divided into five subdivisions: 6–9 years of age, 10–14, 15–19, 20–29, and 30–55.

To begin with, the values on the newborn babies are unexpectedly high in comparison with the cerebral AVO_2 differences of adults. Observations on 11 newborn infants in whom the cerebral venous blood was drawn from the fontanel yield an average oxygen content of 8.6 vol. per cent (497). In one other observation in which the cerebral venous blood was drawn from the internal jugular vein, the difference was 8.2 vol. per cent. These surprisingly high values do not necessarily indicate an equally high C.M.R., because as have said, there are *two* determinants in the estimation of C.M.R. *in vivo* and in human babies the blood flow is still unknown. An interpretation of these values will be given after the data on all the age groups have been presented.

The data for the second group from 6 to 55 years was furnished by individuals whose intellectual capacity is below the normal (497). It will be most profitable if we first discuss those 20 years of age and over since we have for comparison so many results covering approximately the same age brackets, but with subjects of higher intelligence. Because these results were obtained on persons with low intelligence standards, it is important to note that the volume of oxygen removed from the cerebral blood does not necessarily vary with their intellectual capacity. Even in individuals whose I.Q. is below the normal, the arterio-venous exchange may remain the same. This work was done on "undifferentiated mental defectives", patients who exhibited no other stigma except that of low intelligence. The usual line of demarcation between these individuals and normals is an I.Q. of 75 to 80. If we found this group to possess cerebral AVO_2 differences like those of adults with higher I.Q., then the data obtained on these people might be used as indicative of those on more intelligent subjects. (This is fortunate because it is difficult to obtain a sufficient number of normal volunteers to submit themselves to such an examination).

The following data shows that when these two groups are compared—normals and undifferentiated mental defectives—the oxygen removed from the cerebral blood is the same for both groups. Fourteen of these individuals with I.Q. ranging from 50 to 88 yielded an average oxygen utilization of 6.5 vol. per cent, a value not significantly different from that of the normal (6.7 vol. per cent). In a further attempt to determine whether the value for the I.Q. in undifferentiated mental defectives influences the arterio-venous difference, another group of 31 with even lower I.Q. from 8 to 49 were examined. Their average AVO_2 difference was 6.7 vol. per cent, exactly the same as the normal.

Because the level of the I.Q. had no bearing on either of these two groups, all the mental defectives within the age limits of 20 to 55 were considered together. The average cerebral AVO_2 difference (45 observations) for the entire age period was 6.6 vol. per cent, and furthermore when these patients were divided according to age from 20–29 years, and 30–55 years, each of the constituent portions had an average cerebral AVO_2 difference of 6.6 vol. per cent. It is apparent that the average cerebral oxygen utilization remains unchanged from 20 to 55 years. If the normal AVO_2 difference of these mental defectives from 20 to 55 years of age may be taken as a criterion, then the possibility arises that the AVO_2 difference of younger members of this same group will also be normal. If this is true, then an examination of the cerebral oxygen exchange of these undifferentiated mental defectives might give information not only on these individuals but also on normals. It would therefore repay us to study the lower age brackets of the undifferentiated mental defectives. The averages for all this study are: 4.7 vol. per cent for 30 observations on patients from 6 to 9 years of age; 5.1 vol. per cent on 33 others from 10 to 14 years; 5.9 vol. per cent on 22 from 15 to 19 years. These averages form a progressive increase in the five groups from 6–29 years of age. From a statistical analysis it may be concluded that these results do show a progressive biological change which comes to a maximum at the age of 20–29, and then remains un-altered to the age of 55. This analysis made with the aid of Fisher's criterion (327) proves that the differences between these averages are significant (beyond experimental error) with one exception: that between the first two groups. Since this is the only difference that is not significant, we feel it likely that with a greater number of cases this difference would also become significant.

There are no data available on infants from 1 to 5 years of age. If, how-ever, the oxygen intake during this 5-year period proceeds in the same sequence as it does during the entire period of growth, then we are tempted to conclude that it would be even lower from 1 to 5 years than it is from 6 to 9 years. This suggestion is indicated by a broken line on the graph in Fig. 35. It should be emphasized that only the values from 1 to 5 years of age are unknown; the others have been determined.

Finally we shall consider the elderly subjects. The average of one series of observations, 6.7 vol. per cent, was obtained on 15 patients with arterio-sclerosis of the brain at 59–97 years of age; the second average on 25 patients with the same disease but from 60 to 87 years of age was 6.8 vol. per cent. If these patients may be taken as examples of old age, it may be said that once the maximum value for cerebral AVO$_2$ difference is attained between the ages of 20 and 29, it tends to remain constant until the end of life.

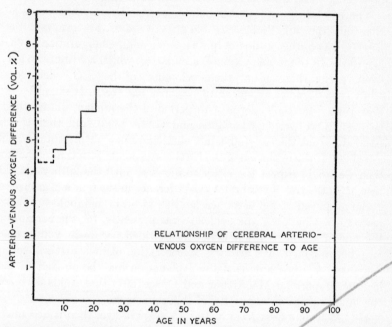

Fig. 35. Relationship of cerebral arterio-venous oxygen difference to age. The solid line represents the values between the ages of 6 and 97 years. The values from 1 to 5 years are suggestive, and filled in by the broken line.

Interpretation of the data on all age groups. The relationship of cerebral AVO$_2$ differences during the successive stages of life is presented in Fig. 35. According to this graph it is highest in the first two weeks of life, after which it falls abruptly to its lowest level, and then rises gradually in the four age periods from 6 to 29 years, remaining the same through old age.

In order to evaluate these data it is necessary to revert for a moment to Chapter 7, and the effect of age on CMR in the rat and dog. Briefly then, it was found that the metabolism of the lower animal forms a curve which rises continually until growth slows, and then tapers off gradually in later adult life (Fig. 21 of Chapter 7). Is it possible that the curve in human brain metabolism resembles that of animals? If so, would it rise from 6 to

29 years corresponding to the rise in the earlier periods of the animal's life? To answer these questions we must first decide whether C.M.R. attains its maximum during the 20–29 year period, the same time at which the cerebral AVO_2 difference first reaches its highest value. Since the oxygen consumption of the brain and the electrical potentials are related, insofar as the electrical changes subsist on an energy basis, it may be helpful in answering these questions to follow the development of the EEG.

The EEG, like cerebral AVO_2 difference, undergoes continuous modification until the time that noticeable growth ceases. For example, the waves on the EEG of the cat do not quite assume adult configuration at 25 days of age (664). In the monkey (mucaca mulatta), which continues to grow for a longer period than the cat, the development of the EEG is delayed and the adult type does not appear until 1 year of age (586). It might be expected then that with the longer growth period of the human, maturation would be even more prolonged. Gibbs and Gibbs (396) find that the human EEG does not display full adult characteristics until approximately the age of 20.[8] If the evolution of the EEG corresponds with that of metabolism, then we would expect the latter to increase until the 20th year. If this is true, then the rise of cerebral AVO_2 difference in the four age groups may be taken as an indication of an acceleration in brain metabolism during these periods. In Chapter 7 the evidence was presented for the conclusion that the amplification of brain metabolism which occurs in young mammals may be explained by a growing concentration of their cerebral respiratory enzymes. It is probable that the explanation may be applied to man. At least the report by MacArthur and Doisy (697) that solids do increase in the human being is suggestive of this conclusion.

If C.M.R. is lowest from birth to 5 years of age, then it becomes necessary to explain the anomalously high cerebral AVO_2 difference in normal infants during the first two weeks of life. According to MacArthur and Doisy, the growth curve of the human brain is steepest directly after birth. If this rapid growth requires a large complement of energy, and it seems that it should, it is possible that the high cerebral AVO_2 difference in the newborn is caused by an accelerated C.M.R. On the other hand, this possibility is rendered unlikely by direct observations on cerebral metabolism of lower mammals which reveal that metabolism is lower at birth than in any other period of extrauterine life. Similar observations on excised cerebral tissues of human origin have been made on two fetuses five and six months of age. A comparison between the fetal and adult

---

[8] With the use of the Grass Frequency Analyzer it was found that there was a general increase in component voltage in the 10 to 12 cycle band in subjects ranging in age from 71 days premature to 29 years. Higher cycles did not show any systematic increase in voltage with age but shorter cycles exhibited a decrease (398).

metabolic rates discloses a fetal rate lower than the adult[9] (812). If the cerebral metabolism is lowest at birth, then the large AVO_2 difference must be imputed to a slow blood flow through the brain. It has been observed that the rate of cerebral blood flow usually varies directly with systemic blood pressure (333). The blood pressure of 24-hour old, full-term new-born babies, averages 80/46 mm. Hg[10] (1020), and increases but slightly during the first 10 days of life. Because the infants who furnished the AVO_2 value of 8.6 vol. per cent were less than two weeks old, it is probable that their large oxygen difference may be ascribed to a slow cerebral blood flow and not to a high C.M.R. At present, however, a final decision between these two possibilities cannot be made. An interpretation of the cerebral AVO_2 difference during the senium is not necessary since the C.M.R. during this period has already been quantiatively determined, and found to be decreased (section on cerebral arteriosclerosis) though this may not apply in the normal to the same extent.

To summarize the suggestions on C.M.R.: the only values that have actually been measured are those in adults and in elderly people; others from birth until 20 years of age are merely suggested. In the beginning of this section a graph was presented showing the changes of cerebral AVO_2 differences during life. A hypothetical graph for the cerebral metabolic rate might resemble that for the AVO_2 differences with two exceptions—at both extremes of life. The entire curve of this theoretical graph, then, may build up from a low metabolism in the newborn to a maximum in adult life, and decrease somewhat during the senium.

Because of the information we have obtained from the previous chapter showing the close correlation between the rapid increases of brain metabolism (953, 495, 523, 474, 812) and brain growth (117) in the early life of the rat, it becomes pertinent to see whether any similar correlation between growth and metabolism may exist in the human brain. The answer to this question involves additional data, which are not as yet available, on the actual measurement of cerebral metabolic rate in man. When these data are obtained and a metabolic curve for the brain can be drawn, we are wondering whether it would correspond in any way with Scammon's curve (447) for the growth of the human brain (Fig. 36).

It would be interesting, however, to compare the directional changes in C.M.R., as suggested by the observations on cerebral AVO_2 difference,

[9] On a dry weight basis the oxygen intake of the cerebral cortex of two fetuses was 5.9 and 6.4 cmm/100 mg. tissue/hr., approximately the same as for the adult brain. But since a 7-month fetus has a dry weight of 9.44 per cent and a 35-year old adult of 26.80 per cent (697), as previously described in the footnote 5 of Chapter 7 p. 139, this indicates a fetal rate $\frac{1}{3}$ (or 9.44/26.80) that of the adult.

[10] 80 mm. mercury is the average systolic pressure, and 46 mm. mercury is the average diastolic pressure.

with those of basal metabolic rate (B.M.R.). According to the data of Benedict and Talbot (78), and Lewis, Kinsman and Iliff (661), basal metabolism, whether on a basis of kilos or square meter of surface area, is highest at approximately 2 years of age and then gradually falls, with a questionable secondary rise at pubescence, until the age of 20. After that there is a slight but steady regression until old age. It would seem that between the ages of 2 and 20, C.M.R. and B.M.R. are practically mirror

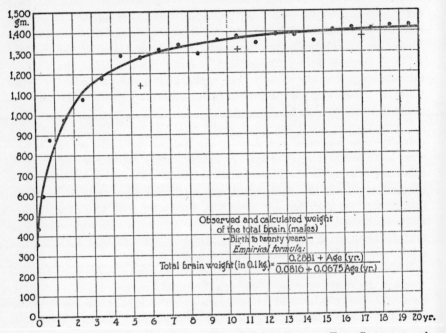

FIG. 36. Brain weight in human males from birth to 20 years. From Scammon and Dunn (105).

images of each other—changing in opposite directions. On the other hand, after maturity is reached and especially in old age the two curves bear a striking resemblance to each other as they decrease together.

B. *Avitaminosis*

Today it is not necessary to elaborate on the fact that in the absence of certain essentials in the diet, deficiency diseases or the avitaminoses, arise. In recent years diseases resulting from inadequate dietaries have been subjected to intensive study, and in this section we shall report some of the results of studies in brain metabolism on these patients. Such work was done in an attempt to find a basis for the neurologic and mental symptoms of avitaminotic persons.

Pellagra. The study of the effects of inadequate amounts of any particular vitamin is complicated by the fact that seldom is a disease caused by lack of a single vitamin; usually the patients are polyavitaminotic from a generally inadequate diet. The subjects who were examined for brain metabolism probably suffered from more than one deficiency though the effects of the lack of one or another vitamin were more prominent, and the other deficiencies were in mild or subclinical form. The work was done in co-operation with Dr. Tom D. Spies who diagnosed the patients primarily as pellagrins, suffering therefore from a niacin deficiency, among others. For example, some of the patients showed symptoms of an absence of thiamin or riboflavin, while others revealed still additional deficiencies. First, we shall present the results on 7 patients whose pellagra was apparently uncomplicated by any other deficiencies, at least not to the extent of clinical symptoms. The pellagrin symptoms displayed were: dermititis, a spotty reddening of the skin particularly pronounced on parts exposed to the sunshine, stomatitis with a fiery-red tongue, gastro-intestinal upset along with diarrhea. None of these patients were severe enough to exhibit any signs of dementia or nervous manifestations. The average cerebral AVO_2 difference of the pellagrins was 6.3 vol. per cent, which on statistical analysis proved not to be significantly different from the normal. With such a result, and no apparent acceleration or slackening in the blood flow, any deviation in the cerebral metabolic rate was not to be expected. Furthermore it must be recalled that these patients did not suffer from either neurologic or mental symptoms. In the absence of quantitative data on C.B.F. however it is impossible to conclude that C.M.R. was unchanged. Observations made on two different species yield diverse results. Cerebral tissues were excised from dogs with black tongue (617, 28), a syndrome due to lack of niacin, and therefore more or less the equivalent of pellagra in humans. The tissues of these animals did not show impairment in the oxygen utilization, nor did a study of the cerebral coenzyme I and II content (Chapter 5) disclose a decrease of these compounds, and therefore of their constituent niacin. On the other hand rats (882) on a diet deficient in nicotinic acid, exhibited subnormal levels of that substance in the brain.

The administration of niacin in the form of nicotinic acid amide to these seven pellagrins produced no significant variation in the oxygen utilization (average 6.0 vol. per cent (522)), nor did it have any effect in the velocity of the blood flow (16). The specific therapy administered to patients with niacin deficiency did not seem to change their oxygen intake. The average of the 14 observations, 7 before specific therapy and 7 after, is 6.2 vol. per cent. The difference between this and the normal value is not significant statistically.

According to Jolliffe and co-workers (567) degeneration of the brain, or encephalopathy may be caused by a niacin deficiency. These authors base their claim for this etiology upon the history of an inadequate diet and the favorable therapeutic effects following the administration of niacin. It is not improbable that encephalopathy is associated with diminished brain metabolism (see section on exogenous agents) and if the condition described by Jolliffe is due to niacin deficiency, then a rise of brain metabolism toward normal would be responsible for the favorable therapeutic effect. A possible role for niacin (a constituent of coenzymes I and II) in cellular respiration has been described in Chapter 5.

It may be of some interest to mention, before leaving our discussion of niacin deficiency, that 3 patients who showed signs of lacking both niacin and riboflavin had an average cerebral AVO_2 difference of 6.4 vol. per cent; thus, the combination of these two vitamin deficiencies produced no change in cerebral AVO_2 differences, and, as far as we know, there was no indication of a slower C.M.R.

The only pellagrins whose oxygen utilization was low were those whose disease was complicated by a vitamin B_1 deficiency, and their average value was 4.8 vol. per cent, taken from observations on 8 patients. Three hours after the intravenous administration of cocarboxylase, the diphosphoric ester of vitamin B_1 (diphosphothiamin) (35, 680), the average AVO_2 difference was 4.6 vol. per cent. Thus, 4.7 vol. per cent is obviously the mean of the complete 18 observations. It therefore becomes necessary to determine what this low value indicates in regard to C.M.R. There are three possibilities: either a decrease in brain metabolism or a quickening of cerebral blood flow, or both. Avitaminosis B_1 is characterized by increased minute volume of the heart (458, 795, 988). If such an acceleration did occur in these patients and the brain shared in the greater blood supply, cerebral blood flow would be augmented. Though a faster C.B.F. is unlikely because of the associated fall in blood pressure, yet on theoretical grounds alone it cannot be ruled out. Our next question then: was the low arteriovenous difference due to a slower metabolic rate? The first step in answering this question involves the function of vitamin B_1. A large amount of research has proved that vitamin B_1 is part of the enzyme system which oxidizes pyruvic acid (see Chapter 5) (471, 1008). Because pyruvic acid is an obligative intermediary stage in the oxidation of glucose, and the brain oxidizes glucose predominantly, cerebral tissues excised from avitaminotic B_1 animals reveal a subnormal oxidation of glucose and glucose split products, pyruvic acid and lactic acid (787, 673). Thus, both an accumulation of pyruvic acid and a depression of oxygen utilization of the central nervous system in the presence of glucose, are signs of lack of vitamin B_1. The cocarboxylase content of these avitaminotic tissues is reduced (680), and the addition of diphosphothiamin restores the normal oxygen consumption

(790), a reaction which is specific to vitamin B_1 since it is negative in tissues excised from normal or starved animals (731). The addition of thiamin does not raise oxygen intake of normal cerebral tissues because they possess adequate amounts of cocarboxylase (787). The effect of cocarboxylase on carbohydrate oxidation is exerted directly on pyruvic acid (790, 872) because the oxygen utilized by the cerebral tissues can be accounted for by the combustion of that substance. The experiments proving these conclusions were performed on the pigeon (787), chick (673), rat (362) and dog (507). These results showing the failure of carbohydrate metabolism were demonstrated on cerebral, renal (671, 873) and hepatic (671) tissues, excised from vitamin B_1 deficient animals. The human brain in patients suffering from lack of vitamin B_1 absorbed only $\frac{2}{3}$ the normal amount of glucose from each 100 cc. of blood, or 6 mg. per cent (522). In view of the observations of excised tissues one explanation for the results on patients is found in a depression of cerebral oxygen utilization.

Beriberi. Lack of diphosphothiamin is the principal cause of beriberi, a disease consisting not only of biochemical disturbances but also clinical symptoms: cardiac weakness and edema, personality changes and neurologic disturbances occurring in the part of the body controlled by the affected portions of the central nervous system. Would the nervous symptoms have any connection with the depressed brain metabolism in vitamin B_1 deficiency? If so, then a word about them might strengthen our conception that metabolism is arrested somewhat in the brain of persons suffering from vitamin B_1 inadequacy.

Though more than one part of the central nervous system may be involved as a result of lack of diphosphothiamin in the diet, the ensuing disorders are not equally profound throughout the nervous system. The symptoms may indicate that the predominant metabolic depression occurs either in the peripheral nerves and cord, the brain stem or the cerebral hemispheres. In any case, for want of vitamin B_1 to oxidize it, pyruvic acid may accumulate in the affected part and pour into the blood stream. This abnormal metabolism continues until successful therapy has been instituted, or the part has endured irreversible damage and undergone degeneration. An elevated pyruvic acid content of the blood was observed by Wortis, Bueding and Jolliffe (1021) in 45 of 48 patients with "acute" peripheral neuropathy, a result of diphosphothiamin deficiency due to alcoholism. The neurologic symptoms are in accordance with the hypothesis that both the peripheral nerves and the dorsal columns of the spinal cord were among the sources for the increase of pyruvic acid concentration in the blood. Among the early motor and sensory disturbances are: burning sensation on the soles of the feet, tenderness in the calf muscles, difficulty in walking and loss of ankle jerks. When the lesion occurs higher in the neuraxis, expecially in the periaqueductal grey containing the nuclei of the third and fourth nerves which innervate extraocular muscles, Wernicke's syndrome develops. This syndrome, which is frequently preceded by peripheral neuropathy, includes such symptoms as: ophthalmoplegia (weakness or paralysis of the extraocular muscles), clouded consciousness, and ataxia (loss of muscular co-ordination which in the lower extremities produces staggering). The therapeutic test reveals the relationship between each of this triad of symptoms and avitaminosis B_1 (1022). After the administration of diphosphothiamin, the concentration of pyruvic acid in the blood diminishes; the function of the extraocular muscles is restored in one to three days, the clouding of the mind may or may not be ameliorated, but the ataxia is not affected. These results indicate that lack of diphosphothiamin has a causal relationship to the ophthalmoplegia, and also influences the mental status but does not demonstrate a relation to the ataxia.

Both in patients with beriberi (693) and in dogs with experimentally induced B_1 avitaminosis (169), the concentrations of pyruvic and lactic acids in the blood were found to vary directly (527, 815) with the severity of the disease. Though probably many parts of the body accumulate these acids from incomplete carbohydrate oxidation, yet nervous tissues are hardest hit because they cannot fall back on the oxidation of fat. Morphologic end results indicate that among the sites for pyruvic acid production are the peripheral nerves, cord, various parts of the brain stem, cerebellum, and cerebral hemispheres. A correlation between degenerative changes of the central nervous system, clinical symptoms and abnormal physiology has been observed not only in man but also in the dog and the pigeon. Prolonged subminimal intake of vitamin B_1 by dogs (924) on an otherwise adequate diet leads to degenerative changes both in the peripheral nerves and the posterior columns of the spinal cord. The leg weakness of pigeons produced by thiamin deficiency is due to degeneration of peripheral nerve fibers in the sciatic nerve (930). Only in the pig, so far, has vitamin B_1 deficiency been unattended by nervous deterioration. Though this may be a species difference, Wintrobe and co-workers (1013) suggest that nerve degeneration heretofore attributed to thiamin deficiency may be due to lack of other vitamins. If this is so, then it is possible that vitamin B_1 deficiency causes either the faulty absorption or failure of function of the other vitamins. In that case, the morphologic changes observed in vitamin B_1 deficiency are not the primary effects but the secondary, the primary effects being on other vitamins. In any event, in species other than the pig the morphologic changes are the results of B_1 deficiency whether primary or secondary. The reaction of the central nervous system may be similar to different kinds of insults; for example, fasted rats (229) and pigeons (618) suffer essentially the same structural changes in the nervous system as animals deprived of vitamin B_1. Yet, as mentioned above, biochemically the tissues of starved animals do not respond to the presence of thiamin by an increased oxygen intake.

Whereas in a prolonged deprivation of vitamin B_1 in man the neurologic changes are among the prominent clinical features, an acute deficiency would be more accurately described as producing personality changes (1006, 1007, 354). Such symptoms are unmistakable and easily reproduced experimentally by restricting the thiamin content of the diet. When this was done on human beings, the subjects became irritable, depressed, and fearful that some misfortune awaited them. They complained of a number of subjective symptoms: headache, inability to tolerate painful stimuli, and sensitivity to noises. Further confirmation that the symptoms were caused by lack of vitamin B_1 is the fact that all the patients revealed abnormal pyruvic acid metabolism.

Reviewing the data, we may summarize with the following points: (1) vitamin B_1 is necessary for the oxidation of pyruvic acid, an obligate of carbohydrate metabolism; (2) pyruvic acid accumulates and oxidations diminish in avitaminotic cerebral tissues; (3) human beings suffering from vitamin B_1 deficiency exhibit a hyperpyruvemia. These three points seem to be in favor of the conception that a low AVO_2 difference is likewise an expression of an impaired cerebral metabolic rate in avitaminotic B_1 human beings. If this is the case, then we have found a basis for both the symptoms and the structural disturbances in the central nervous system manifest in a vitamin B_1 deficient diet.

We are left with the unexplained fact that the intravenous administration of cocarboxylase produced no significant change in the cerebral AVO_2 difference of the pellagrins with vitamin B_1 deficiency within a period of three hours (see page 84) (522). The lack of response to cocarboxylase is surprising when we recall how quickly the normal metabolism was restored on the addition of cocarboxylase to tissues excised from acutely avitaminotic animals. Probably a longer time is required in patients with chronic deficiency for the re-establishment of normal carbohydrate metabolism. In one patient, at least, AVO_2 difference was raised to normal one week after the administration of coarboxylase. This delayed recovery is in accordance with the observation of Wortis, Bueding, Stein and Jolliffe (1022) who showed that pyruvic acid metabolism may not be restored to normal even after several days of specific therapy. The clinical symptoms of peripheral neuropathy require even a longer time, for they may not be completely corrected even after four months of continuous and intensive treatment (1005).

C. Acute destruction by exogenous agents

We have shown that various forces active in organic psychoses, growth, and avitaminosis, affect the oxygen utilization of the brain. We will now

discuss still another condition in the brain which may have a bearing on the
C.M.R., one in which cerebral tissues have been destroyed by exogenous
agents. This injury to the brain interferes with normal activities as indicated by clinical symptoms described below. Is brain metabolism also
affected by the action of these agents?

Hypoglycemic destruction. As discussed in Chapter 3, the brain possesses
two sources of foodstuff: blood sugar and cerebral glycogen. During profound hypoglycemia true blood sugar approaches zero and the brain must
draw on its intrinsic glycogen stores. When both sources are exhausted and
there is not enough carbohydrate to maintain metabolism at $\frac{1}{4}$ of the normal rate (sect. II, C, this chapter) the minimum necessary for maintaining
the structure of the brain as a whole and the operation of the vital centers
of the medulla oblongata, brain damage ensues. Irreversible changes occur in
the brain only because energy is no longer obtainable from carbohydrate.
If non-carbohydrates afford any energy, the supply is too small to save the
brain from injury.

The effect of such a protracted deprivation of carbohydrate (478) was
seen in a patient who was receiving insulin for diabetes complicated by a
localized infection in his left great toe. Gradually his dose of protamine
zinc insulin was increased in order to overcome the insulin resistance resulting from his infection. When this infection was eliminated by surgical
intervention, the patient's insulin resistance disappeared. But unfortunately the physician failed to decrease the dose of protamine zinc insulin.
The patient was, therefore, thrown into a profound hypoglycemic coma and
finally developed a series of recurrent epileptoid convulsions. These con-
sisted of severe extensor spasms followed by violent clonic movements.
During each convulsion, this muscular activity prevented normal respiration and caused livid cyanosis. Despite subsequent intravenous injections
of dextrose, which raised the level of blood sugar to 250 mg. per cent, the
convulsions persisted until the patient succumbed from exhaustion. Two
sets of blood samples taken between convulsive episodes revealed an
average AVO_2 difference of 2.8 vol. per cent, a value much reduced when
compared with the average normal. Carbohydrate had been administered
too late to prevent cerebral damage, which inevitably happens when a
person has been allowed to remain in the fifth stage of a hypoglycemic
coma beyond a limited time. (See Chapter 10 on Symptoms of Insulin
Hypoglycemia). The low AVO_2 difference in this patient was therefore the
result of a smaller number of viable cerebral cells. Cerebral metabolic rate,
then, was depressed because a portion of the brain was destroyed.

Carbon monoxide destruction. Two patients who had been exposed to
carbon monoxide gas were admitted to the hospital in deep coma (478).
The first patient was flaccid, with depressed reflexes. She was examined on

three successive days before her death, and an average AVO_2 difference of 3.1 vol. per cent was observed. The second patient had extensor spasticity, a picture resembling decerebrate rigidity. His oxygen utilization was 1.8 vol. per 100 cc. of blood passing through the brain.

In these patients we see the end results of the deprivation of oxygen from the brain. Carboxyhemoglobin had been formed during the inhalation of carbon monoxide; oxygen was temporarily prevented from combining with hemoglobin, and the brain was bereft of its oxygen supply. Gradually the carbon monoxide was released from the hemoglobin, but by that time the brain of these patients had been permanently damaged, and the condition could not be ameliorated even though the oxygen content of the arterial blood was sufficient to assure a plentiful supply of oxygen to the brain. When these biochemical observations were made, both patients were virtually free of carbon monoxide. These patients may well be compared with the one in irreversible hypoglycemic coma. In both cases the cause for cerebral destruction had been alleviated too late to restore the brain to normal.

Syphilitic destruction. A patient revealed symptoms referable to destructive processes in the brain especially the cerebral hemispheres, a result of inflammation of the brain due to syphillis (499). His symptoms included loss of cerebral functions, and release of subcortical mechanisms; he was not in contact with his environment and exhibited forced grasping, forced sucking and cogwheel rigidities. It was suspected that the condition was due to niacin deficiency but this diagnosis was rejected when the patient did not improve after receiving niacin intravenously. The cerebrospinal fluid Wassermann test was strongly positive and his AVO_2 difference, 3.3 vol. per cent, was approximately half the normal value. This reduced cerebral oxygen intake in conjunction with a high content of the venous blood, 15.6 vol. per cent, suggests that the brain failed to utilize the available oxygen because it had suffered degenerative impairment. The high oxygen content of the venous blood in this patient is therefore the result of cerebral damage and not the cause of the brain pathology.

In the four patients just described it is probable that the degree of depression of cerebral AVO_2 difference indicated a decrease of C.M.R. It is not likely that the small cerebral AVO_2 differences could be attributed to a faster blood flow because cerebral circulation would have to increase from 2 to 4 times the normal rate to cause such falls in the AVO_2 difference if C.M.R. remained normal. At least in two of the patients, the one flaccid with carbon monoxide poisoning and the other with syphilis, both of whom were lying quietly in bed, there is no indication that cerebral blood flow could have been accelerated at all. Characteristically cerebral blood flow is slowed in neurosyphilis (783a).

D. *Some types of mental deficiency*

In the previous discussion of undifferentiated mental defectives it was found that their particular type of deficiency was not distinguished by any variation from normal in their cerebral arterio-venous differences. Results obtained on other mental defectives, however, are not necessarily the same. These persons are described as having additional stigmata to that of low intelligence, and they reveal distinct modifications in brain metabolism. In this section we shall discuss 6 types of mental deficiency: mongolism, cretinism, phenylpyruvic oligophrenia, amaurotic familial idiocy, hydrocephalus, and microcephalus. A descriptive word on each will be supplemented as respective results are discussed.

Mongolism, cretinism, and phenylpyruvic oligophrenia. Mongolism is the name given to that kind of mental deficiency characterized by elevated outer canthus of the eyes, from which the mongoloid derives his peculiar facies and his name (563). The body, like the mind, is dwarfed; the joints are hyperflexible, and complete sexual maturity is never attained. Cretins are born without functioning thyroid tissue. In the absence of the stimulating hormone, thyroxin, growth is not completed, leaving both body and mind infantile. A rarer form of mental deficiency has been termed phenylpyruvic oligophrenia (562). The members of this group are incapable of oxidizing phenylalanine, an inborn error of metabolism, and consequently excrete most of it in the urine, after deamination by the kidney, as phenylpyruvic acid. Some of it however is recovered in the form of phenyllactate and a portion escapes deaminization and appears unchanged as phenylalanine.

These 3 classes of mental defectives were studied at all stages of their life span, but the largest number of observations was made in patients 20 years old and over. This age-group was sufficiently large to furnish enough data for satisfactory statistical comparison with the AVO_2 differences of normal individuals. The average values for mongoloids, cretins and phenylpyruvic oligophrenics (498) are practically identical, and considerably lower than those of normals, 6.7 vol. per cent and of undifferentiated mental defectives, 6.6 vol. per cent (498). Or, to be exact, the average AVO_2 difference of 30 mongoloids (494, 498) between the ages of 20 and 45 was 5.6 vol. per cent. As for the phenylpyruvic oligophrenics (494, 498), it was possible to study only 9 patients between 20 and 37 years with this rare disease, though this number included all that were available st such a large institution as Letchworth Village. Their average cerebral AVO_2 difference was 5.5 per cent. The study of cretins (486, 498) was made on only 6 persons between the ages of 22 and 31; nevertheless, each individual was examined more than once and on separate days, making a total of 17 observations which averaged 5.5 vol. per cent oxygen utilization. This low

GIGI → L.H.H. Lon

metabolism of the cretin seems to be in keeping with a generally low metabolism as exemplified in their B.M.R. The undifferentiated mental defectives differ significantly from the mongoloids and from the cretins and probably differ significantly from the phenylpyruvic oligophrenics, according to Fisher's t test (327).

There is no reason to suspect a cerebral blood flow faster than normal in any of these 3 types of mental deficiency; in fact, in the mongoloid and cretin the flow may even be slower. In patients with myxedema a slowed C.B.F. and a diminished C.M.R. have been demonstrated (848b). With this in mind, as well as their low values for oxygen exchange, it appears that these 3 groups of mental defectives have a subnormal cerebral metabolic rate. In other words, their mental diseases are associated in some way with an inadequate elaboration of cerebral energy.

Amaurotic familial idiocy. This infantile idiocy (456) is marked by an abnormal accumulation in the brain of a lipid substance, which Klenk names "substance X",[11] and as a result of this accumulation, there is widespread cerebral atrophy. Eleven observations of the AVO_2 differences were made on 3 such patients between 1 and $1\frac{1}{2}$ years of age (498). The average of 6 observations in which the blood was collected from the internal jugular vein was 5.7 vol. per cent, while 5 observations with venous blood drawn from the fontanel averaged 7.5 vol. per cent. The values for the AVO_2 differences in the patients with amaurotic familial idiocy are higher than could be expected from other infants at that age, and are more nearly like those of newborn babies. The average of 12 observations of mongoloids three months to five years of age is 3.4 vol. per cent and of five moderately severe hydrocephalics from $\frac{1}{2}$ year to five years of age, 4.7 vol. per cent (498), both values of which are considerably lower than those for amaurotic idiots. Because the actively respiring grey matter is supplanted by the lipid material which is probably relatively inert from a respiratory standpoint, it is probable that despite a high AVO_2 difference, brain metabolism is depressed in this disease. If the cerebral blood flow were slower than normal, it would solve the unexplained high AVO_2 difference in the brain.

Hydrocephalus and microcephalus. When the cerebrospinal fluid which is secreted by the choroid plexus finds its escape from the cerebral ventricles blocked, it is retained at increased pressure. The resulting abnormality is termed hydrocephalus and its essential feature is destruction of brain tissues under the influence of this excessive cerebrospinal fluid pressure. If we consider the age of the patients, only 1 of 6 with hydrocephalus had an AVO_2 difference significantly reduced (first patient in Table 19). In

[11] "Substance X" is composed of a cerebroside (containing sphingosin, fatty acid and galactose) and neuramic acid, a nitrogen containing organic acid (613, 614).

that one patient the cerebral AVO_2 difference was 2.2 vol. per cent in an observation made one day before the brain ruptured (498). Autopsy revealed that the thickness of the remaining cerebral cortex was reduced to 2 mm., which is proof that the brain tissue was badly destroyed, and accounts for the small oxygen consumption. Unless such destruction is extensive, however, no decrease of the cerebral AVO_2 difference is observed; in fact, in the other five patients with hydrocephalus the differences are what might have been expected at their respective ages. If these five patients also suffered a depression of brain metabolism, which is probable, then cerebral blood flow must have been retarded in order to maintain the normal AVO_2 difference.

Though mcrocephalus may arise from many causes, the observations to be described are concerned with mental defectives suffering from essential

TABLE 19

Cerebral arterio-venous oxygen differences in mentally defective patients with hydrocephalus or microcephalus

HYDROCEPHALUS		MICROCEPHALUS	
Age	AVO_2 Diff. vol.	Age	AVO_2 Diff. vol.
	per cent		per cent
Less than 1 year	2.2	5 years	4.1
Less than 1 year	4.6	8 years	3.1
Less than 1 year	4.8	15 years	6.2
3 years	4.4	22 years	6.5
5 years	3.8		
5 years	5.7		

microcephalus, the type for which there is no apparent cause for the small cranial capacity other than failure of cerebral growth (74). We have four observations of patients with this form of microcephalus, and their AVO_2 differences all fall within normal limits according to their ages. Irrespective of a normal AVO_2 difference, the total cerebral metabolism must be less than normal because of the reduction in the size of the brain.

Cerebral respiratory enzymes and mental deficiency. We have said that cerebral metabolic rate is an expression of the activity of cerebral respiratory enzymes. Since these two phenomena increase simultaneously with growth, would it not seem that the basic reason for a decreased C.M.R. in some kinds of mental deficiency could be traced to an impaired development of the enzymatic system in the brain? An analysis of the various types of mental deficiency indicates that in general there are at least two causes for such an impairment in the enzyme concentration: a relentless action destroying the cerebral tissues containing these enzymes, as seen in hydrocephalus and amaurotic familial idiocy, or, failure of the enzymes to develop normally, as in mongolism and cretinism. In the patient in the terminal stages of hydrocephalus, pressure atrophy of cerebral tissues was widespread, and no doubt a destruction of respiratory enzymes also occurs in amaurotic familial idiocy where grey is replaced by lipid matter. It is well known that the metabolic rate of grey matter is much higher than that of the white (535), presumably because of a higher concentration of respiratory enzymes in the grey. The distribution of the lipid matter may explain why the blood drawn from the internal jugular vein had a smaller oxygen content than that collected from the fontanel. According to Hassin (456) though the lipid matter accumulates throughout the central nervous system in a diffuse manner in this disease, it is especially obvious in the optic thalamus. Such a differential distribution of pathologic infiltration may account for an oxygen utilization lower in the blood collected from the internal jugular vein, representing the return flow from the

TABLE 20

Average cerebral arterio-venous oxygen differences (vol. %) in mongoloids and undifferentiated mentally defective persons

AGE	UNDIFFERENTIATED	MONGOLOIDS
Less than 10	4.7 (30)*	4.4 (21)
10 to 19	5.4 (55)	5.9 (17)
20 and over	6.6 (45)	5.6 (30)

* Numbers in parentheses indicate the number of observations from which the average values were obtained.

entire organ including the optic thalamus, than from the fontanel which contains the venous blood coming chiefly from the cerebral hemispheres.

Whereas in hydrocephalus and amaurotic familial idiocy, the grey matter and its constituent enzymes were destroyed, in mongolism the trouble lies in the fact that the grey matter may never attain normal concentration. Morphologic studies reveal that mongoloids exhibit degeneration of brain tissue, loss of nerve cells and atrophy of the cortex (224, 733, 73). These differences between mongoloids and normal subjects are most marked after 19 years of age, as indicated by failure of the cerebral AVO₂ difference to rise after that time (Table 20). When the oxygen differences are compared in the first two decades of life, no significant divergence is apparent between the mongoloids and the undifferentiated mental defectives. It would seem that the enzyme concentration which should increase along with the growth of the body is arrested 10 years earlier in the mongoloid than in the normal person. Presumably, the cerebral metabolic rate of the mongoloid is also stunted at this early age. This conclusion is supported by the observation of Benda who found that the growth and development of the mongoloid brain does not continue to maturity but is arrested at an early age (73).

In the cretins, like the mongoloids, a low C.M.R. may be attributed to an incomplete development of cerebral enzymes. If this conception is correct, then the subnormal brain metabolism in athyrotic cretins may be charged to a sparse concentration of respiratory enzymes. Such an interpretation is supported by experiments on newborn rats indicating that thiouracil, an agent which prevents the formation of thyroxin, impairs growth and the concentration of the cerebral enzyme, carbonic anhydrase (849) as well. We are not aware of any reason for the depression of cerebral metabolism in patients with phenylpyruvic oligophrenia, but we do know that they lack the enzyme necessary for the oxidation of phenylalanine.

We may conclude that in relation to cerebral metabolism there are two types of mental deficiency, one with a normal cerebral metabolism and the other with a reduced metabolism. It is suggested that C.M.R. is normal in the undifferentiated mental defectives, but is below normal in patients with mongolism, cretinism, phenylpyruvic oliogophrenia, advanced hydrocephalus, microcephalus, and perhaps amaurotic familial idiocy. We might also mention one observation made on a patient with gargoylism,[12] mental deficiency accompanied by certain physical stigmata, a rather large rounded head with bulging forehead and wide mouth making a striking resemblance to a gargoyle (437, 564). Corneal opacities, bony deformities and an enlarged liver and spleen are frequently associated with gargoylism. The mental deficiency is a result of destruction of the cytoplasm within the nerve cells as they are crowded by the deposition of granular material. But whether this abnormal storage is lipid or polysaccharide in character is not decided. The patient studied had an AVO_2 difference as low as 4.8 vol. per cent. If his cerebral blood flow was not accelerated that value suggests a slow metabolic rate. It should be interesting to determine whether mental defectives possessing a normal brain metabolism have no apparent defect other than low intelligence while patients with a reduced metabolism suffer from either anatomic, physiologic or biochemical stigmata. Whether or not such a startling relationship holds true for all mental deficiencies cannot be said until many observations are carried on along this line.

At any rate, it is apparent that mental deficiency may or may not be associated with deficiency of cerebral energy exchange. Even though the brain of undifferentiated mental defectives appeared to be supported by a normal metabolism, the energy is made available to cerebral tissues incapable of adequate function. When mental deficiency is accompanied by depressed brain metabolism, there are three possible relationships between

[12] Unpublished observation of the author.

the two phenomena: the mental deficiency may be a result of diminished brain metabolism; or, it is possible that deficiency and the impairment of cerebral oxidations are independent effects of the same underlying cause, i.e., enzyme deficiency. And third, the depression of cerebral metabolism and mental deficiency may be two entirely unrelated phenomena. At present a decision among these possibilities would be merely conjectural.

E. *Interference of cerebral oxygen supply*

Until now we have stressed the fact that various intracerebral changes, physiologic and pathologic, affect the oxygen intake of the brain. Our present interest is in the reverse process: how would the extracerebral interference of the oxygen supply affect the metabolic processes of the brain? Just as C.M.R. is depressed by lack of sugar in the blood, so it may be depressed by lack of oxygen in the circulating fluid, for both factors are necessary for cerebral oxidations. Oxidative processes are the first support of cerebral activity, for the ability of the adult brain to obtain energy anaerobically is too limited to maintain nervous function adequately for any but the shortest period (see Chapters 7 and 10 for discussion of anaerobic cerebral metabolism).

Before we recount the data on the effects of anoxia on C.M.R., it will not be out of place to describe the various types of anoxia responsible for depression of brain metabolism. These may be classified as follows: (1) anoxic anoxia (47), characterized by incomplete saturation of arterial blood leaving the lungs. This may be caused by diminished pressure of oxygen in the inspired air, obstruction of the respiratory passages, pulmonary disturbances and depression of respiratory centers. (2) Anemic anoxia (47), due to a shortage in the amount of hemoglobin available for the carriage of oxygen, as manifested in anemia, carbon monoxide poisoning, and methemoglobinemia. (3) Stagnant anoxia (47), the result of a slackening of the blood flow as in cardiac failure and shock. (4) Histotoxic anoxia (786), failure of cellular respiratory functions caused by some poisonous agent such as cyanide. This last form will be treated in the next chapter.

Anoxic anoxia. A frequent cause for anoxic anoxia is ascent to high altitudes (17), and there are numerous observations showing that the higher one goes the more pronounced is the fall in oxygen content and pressure. Under these conditions of reduced oxygen pressure in the arterial blood, if the same amount of oxygen is to be delivered to the brain as at sea level, it can be done only at the cost of a lower oxygen pressure within the brain, since an equilibrium has been found to exist between the oxygen pressure in the blood and in the brain. This fall of cerebral pressure is important because it is likely to enhance defective functioning of the brain.

In order to determine the effects of high altitude on the cerebral AVO_2 difference, two sets of blood samples were drawn from each of two men in a decompression chamber. The first pair of samples was collected while the subjects breathed the sea level pressure of air with the doors of the chamber open. The second samples were drawn when they were respiring oxygen via a mask at simulated altitudes of 35,000 or 37,000 feet. They were allowed 30 minutes under these conditions before the second pair of blood samples was drawn. The first subject exhibited an arterio-venous difference of 6.0 vol. per cent (art. 19.7 vol. per cent and ven. 13.7 vol. per cent) at sea level, and when he was exposed to a reduced pressure in the chamber equivalent to that of 35,000 feet, this value remained the same within the error of the method, 5.8 vol. per cent (art. 17.3 vol. per cent and ven. 11.5 vol. per cent), both arterial and venous oxygen content falling approximately by the same amount. The oxygen exchange of the second subject was 8.0 vol. per cent at sea level, (art. 20.7 vol. per cent and ven. 12.7 vol. per cent). When an altitude of 37,000 feet was simulated, his difference fell to 6.7 vol. per cent (art. 18.6 vol. per cent and ven. 11.9 vol. per cent), in this case arterial blood decreasing more than the venous.

These are two different responses[13] to high altitude, but in both instances the content and pressure of oxygen in the blood are reduced, reductions reflected throughout the body with immediate consequences in the brain. Because this organ is forced to labor under a low pressure of oxygen, it does not receive enough energy and this provokes alterations in the behavior of the subject. These modifications in personality are well known, and are not unlike those resulting from the ingestion of alcohol. Usually temporary, they are alleviated by restoring a cerebral oxygen pressure which exists at sea level. Occasionally, however, these disturbances may be

[13] The first type of response is regularly observed at altitudes less than 10,000 feet above sea level when the subject is breathing air. In the second, a compensatory accleration of the blood flow diminishes the cerebral AVO_2 difference, a reaction similar to that which usually occurs only with a degree of anoxia more severe than that suffered by the second subject, apparently hypersensitive to oxygen lack. He was in an atmosphere equivalent to that of a man breathing air at 8,000 feet, but he responded with circulatory adjustments like those occurring at greater heights, adjustments which served to lift somewhat the low cerebral oxygen tension. When an aviator, for example, in an unsealed cabin, climbs rapidly to altitudes of over 10,000 feet while breathing air, or more than 40,000 feet inhaling oxygen (17), compensatory reactions take place: (1) the velocity of cerebral blood flow is quickened; (2) the brain therefore absorbs less oxygen from each unit of blood; (3) the oxygen content and pressure in the venous cerebral blood is raised and (4) the arterio-venous difference becomes smaller (485). Since the cerebral venous oxygen pressure is in equilibrium with that of the brain, this rise (in the venous blood) acts as a partial corrective, heaightening the oxygen pressure in the brain (197).

of more serious nature. For instance, Cournand, Richards and Maier (194) describe a patient with tuberculosis who was given artificial pneumothorax as a therapeutic measure but then developed a psychosis with personality changes and delusions. Striking improvement of the psychosis followed re-expansion of the lungs and in four days the patient was free from mental symptoms. The saturation of hemoglobin in his arterial blood going to the brain was reduced drastically to 58 per cent, equivalent to that observed at an altitude of 22,000 to 25,000 feet, while the patient exhibited delusions, and rose to 90 per cent when he returned to a stable mental condition.

Anoxic anoxia is frequently produced in the operating room as part of the process of anesthesia. It has also been used as a therapeutic measure in schizophrenia. In both instances the oxygen content of the arterial blood may become so low and the brain so depleted of oxygen that the patient is rendered unconscious. For example, in nitrous oxide anesthesia the oxygen content of the arterial blood was reported as low as 4.4 vol. %, and in the nitrogen inhalation treatment as low as 2.1 vol. %. In such instances the cerebral AVO_2 differences must necessarily be greatly reduced. (See Chapter 10, p. 273, 11, p. 308, and 12, p. 349).

Anemic anoxia. The supply of oxygen to the brain is decreased not only when there is a lack of oxygen in the inspired air but it is also lessened when the amount of hemoglobin, the oxygen carrier of the blood, becomes insufficient. Mental changes in patients with pernicious anemia were noted by Addison in his classic description of the disease in 1885. Various observers (see ref. 315 for literature) have reported that from 25 to 64 per cent of their patients show cerebral symptoms. It is true that mental symptoms of sufficient severity to be classified as a psychosis are relatively rare, but less conspicious disturbances such as accentuated irritability and stubbornness are often apparent. The literature contains a striking example (499) of cerebral AVO_2 differences on a patient with pernicious anemia before and after successful liver therapy had increased his red blood cells and hemoglobin. The first two observations on the patient were made before liver therapy was instituted. At that time the patient was disorientated, confused and incoherent, and his mental condition reflected his average AVO_2 difference which was reduced to 2.5 vol. per cent. Other laboratory findings made before therapy was begun include a red blood cell count of 995,000 and a hemoglobin of 3.2 gm. It is probable that the mental symptoms were caused by inadequate oxygen supplies to the brain. Evidence in favor of this conclusion is afforded by the third observation which was made after the patient had reacted successfully to therapy and had lost all of his mental symptoms. The oxygen content of the arterial blood going to

the brain rose from 4.6 vol. per cent to 13.9 vol. per cent; his cerebral AVO_2 difference was restored to 7.4 vol. per cent, red blood cell count to 4,700,000, and his hemoglobin to 13.2 gm.

Another patient studied by the author and not hitherto reported, resembles the one just described both as to mental condition and hematology. When the patient was first seen, he was confused. Because of his concentration of hemoglobin, 4.5 gm., in conjunction with his low arterial carrying power, 6.6 vol. per cent, he was able to remove only 2.4 vol. per cent of oxygen from the blood. When his mental status first began to clear, his brain was removing a much larger amount of oxygen from the blood, 6.5 vol. per cent, made possible by the hemoglobin concentration which had risen to 8.5 gm. and an arterial capacity of 11.1 vol. per cent. These are not isolated instances of alleviation of a disturbed mental status when the anemic condition is ameliorated by liver therapy. Bowman (104), as well as Herman, Most and Jolliffe (464) also reported improvement of psychosis in patients with pernicious anemia after treatment. Measurements of cerebral metabolic rate are at hand on 7 patients with anemia secondary to chronic loss of blood. Scheinberg (848c) observed a reduction of AVO_2 difference but cerebral blood flow was proportionally increased and cerebral metabolic rate was therefore maintained. In pernicious anemia however the acceleration of cerebral blood flow could not compensate for the great reduction in the oxygen carrying power of the blood so that 5 of 6 patients suffered striking decreases in cerebral metabolic rate. No wonder then that a psychosis may develop in a susceptible individual. The curtailment of the oxygen supply is therefore one factor involved in the complex development of the mental condition.

Stagnant anoxia. In stagnant anoxia the oxygen in the inspired air is of normal pressure, the amount of hemoglobin in the blood is ample, but the rate of blood flow is so reduced that the brain does not receive sufficient oxygen in a given interval of time. The decreased cerebral blood flow is an expression of a general retardation of blood flow throughout the body, and symptoms referable to the brain are frequently but not invariably seen accompanying cardiac decompensation. They may assume the character of a neurosis or more rarely of a psychosis. But they are always associated with an episode of cardiac failure. Among the symptoms of cardiac neurosis are weakness, insomnia, sighing respirations, faintness, dizziness, nervousness, irritability and flushes. The psychosis which develops is characterized by an anxiety state, confusion and delusions of persecution.

The cerebral AVO_2 difference of a cardiac patient whose decompensation precipitated psychotic symptoms was studied in order to estimate his brain metabolism. His average AVO_2 difference soared above the normal to a value of 11.0 vol. per cent (499). That these changes were caused by slow cerebral blood flow is indicated by a circulation time, determined by the potassium cyanide method, of 30 seconds, almost twice as long as the normal. This patient did not respond to cardiac therapy and his psychosis showed no improvement during his stay at the hospital. Wortis, however, has observed patients with psychosis developing during cardiac decompensation in whom relief of the cardiac condition was followed by restoration to a normal mental status (1024). A reduction in cerebral metabolic rate is reported by Scheinberg (848d) who observed a 40% decrease in cerebral blood flow producing a 13% diminution in cerebral metabolic rate in patients with heart failure. These observations afford a quantitative basis for one factor responsible for the mental changes which develop in some patients with cardiac decompensation.

The problem of the intensity in the cerebral energy turnover has also been attacked by Romano (829) and Engel (279), who used the EEG as their method of approach. In a group, including patients suffering from anoxia due to pulmonary disease, pernicious anemia, and cardiac decompensation, these workers were able to compare the severity of the disturbances in consciousness, though not in the character and the expression of anxiety, with the degree of dissolution in the electrical patterns. Their observations support the conclusion that the depression of C.M.R. occurs in these conditions and that a restoration to a more rapid metabolic rate may follow, in many instances, either the inhalation of oxygen or the amelioration of the disease.

In the three types of anoxia just discussed, the brain receives less oxygen than the normal amount and cerebral oxygen pressure is thereby reduced. There is evidence that the brain functions best at a definite pressure of oxygen, the pressure which is found in the brain at sea level (see Chapter 6, p. 110). In all these types, the oxygen content of the cerebral venous return is below the normal, which indicates a low oxygen pressure in the venous blood and in the brain.

What, then, is the underlying cause for the irregular cerebral function in the types of anoxia which we have just been discussing? It is not so much that the oxygen supply to the brain is not adequate since that may be compensated for to a certain extent by a more rapid blood flow. The chief reason for the decline of cerebral function is dependent upon the fact that during anoxia of whatever type the brain is forced to labor under a reduced oxygen pressure. That the cerebral oxygen tension is reduced at high altitudes is a well known fact, but it must be recognized that similar reductions also occur in anemic and stagnant anoxia.

A comparison of the results from anoxia and brain destruction reveals that in these patients the oxygen content of the cerebral venous blood may be used as an indicator to determine whether the cerebral changes underlying acute mental episodes are either of intracerebral or extracerebral origin (499). A low oxygen content of the venous blood for the patients described with pernicious anemia and cardiac decompensation would indicate that the depression of brain metabolism is secondary to some extracerebral cause which interferes with the oxygen supply to the brain. A high oxygen content suggests that the pathologic change in the brain is the cause of the metabolic disturbance. This increase of the venous oxygen content applies especially to patients with acute cerebral destruction. When the destructive process in the brain is relatively slow in developing, an adaptive reaction in the form of a retarded cerebral circulation takes place (834). As a result of this prolonged circulation time, the brain removes more oxygen from each unit of blood and the cerebral venous oxygen content may drop towards the normal value.[14]

Cerebral metabolic rate and mental disturbances. A review of the diseases discussed in this chapter reveals that a normal C.M.R., as in schizophrenia, does not rule out mental disorder, but a retarded brain metabolism frequently indicates a cerebral disturbance. It is not surprising, however, that the observation of a slow energy turnover is not adequate to single out the particular aberration in any given patient, for the relation between impaired cerebral oxygen intake and mental malady is a varied one. In some illnesses cerebral metabolic depression is secondary to destructive changes in brain and, more rarely, to failure in the proper development of that organ. Examples of the former are general paresis, severe hydrocephalus and irreversible hypoglycemic coma, and of the latter, cretinism and mongolism. In other instances, the anoxia may be either the primary or the precipitating cause of the mental derangement as observed in healthy persons at high altitudes or in patients with pernicious anemia and cardiac decompensation. But here also the disease picture is not invariable. The energy deprivation acts upon an individual and upon a central nervous system possessing characteristic patterns of activity, and the type of reaction to anoxia will vary accordingly. For example, some patients with congestive heart failure are relatively resistant while others respond more readily with disturbances which may be either neurotic or psychotic in character. The greater the susceptibility of the organism to disease, the less the intensity of anoxia required to produce disorder. But when the cerebral metabolic depression becomes profound, as in a man at an altitude of 12,000 feet, breathing air unreinforced by oxygen, impairment of reason, memory and judgment as

[14] See Chapter 6, p. 119 for discussion of the relation between cerebral AVO$_2$ difference and cerebral blood flow.

well as a loss of emotional control are the rule. Hence, it is important to recognize the fact that though in many instances cerebral oxygen consumption is decreased, the clinical picture varies with the personality structure of the affected individual. The oxygen studies reveal only one facet, though an important one, of a complex problem.

Therapeutic suggestions. The therapeusis of anoxia is by far too broad a topic for this chapter, but a few angles not frequently discussed may be interjected, and for a more complete treatise of the subject, the reader is referred to Armstrong's book on aviation medicine (17) and the work of Barach on inhalational therapy (44).

The therapeusis of anemic anoxia will be merely indicated by the suggestions that transfusions of whole blood in emergency situations as well as measures to increase regeneration of blood and to diminish the loss of blood should be undertaken.

We are more interested in the remedial measures for patients in a state of anoxic anoxia and stagnant anoxia. Barach (43) and others have demonstrated that patients with anoxic anoxia may be benefited by inhaling oxygen. One aspect of this principle may be seen in the aviator whose anoxia is managed by the inhalation of oxygen. This same treatment may be given to patients whose anoxic anoxia is a result of pathologic conditions; for example, acute lobar pneumonia and broncho-pneumonia (43). Because inhalational therapy improves the oxygenation of hemoglobin in the lungs, the patient's tissues receive more oxygen, his labored breathing is relieved, and he is made more comfortable. Stagnant anoxia whether generalized as observed in congestive heart failure and shock (40, 41), or localized, as in acute coronary thrombosis and cerebral thrombosis, can be greatly improved by employing oxygen (44). In stagnant anoxia, arterial oxyhemoglobin is normal and the effective therapeutic factor is the increment of oxygen dissolved in the blood.

Aviators breathe undiluted oxygen at the reduced pressures of high altitudes with consistently good results (181). Pressurized cabins and breathing oxygen at positive pressures (361) are two other notable advances for improving arterial oxygen in flyers. In a similar fashion at sea level, almost every patient who is undergoing a spell of anoxia can achieve relief from his symptoms by inhaling a 50 per cent oxygen mixture. But this favorable response to oxygen therapy does not necessarily hold for patients who have suffered from chronic anoxia (42), for they may react adversely at first (42). Patients with pulmonary emphysema or pulmonary fibrosis, or cerebral arteriosclerosis occasionally exhibit transient mental disturbances upon inhaling oxygen. Lassitude, depression and headache are among the milder symptoms. Rarely, periods of irritability or coma are observed. More to be feared are tensions of oxygen above normal, up to 4 atmospheres (71). The mechanism underlying the neurological altera- tions of oxygen poisoning is not entirely understood. One factor involves the retention of carbon dioxide due to the retarded pulmonary elimination of that gas (386). The difficulty with carbon dioxide originates in the failure of oxyhemoglobin to yield its quota of oxygen on passage through the capillaries because the large volume of oxygen retained in physical solution is adequate to supply the needs of the tissues. For example, at a pressure of 3 atmospheres the oxygen held in solution would be more than sufficient to satisfy metabolic requirements. For that reason the decrease in the oxygenation of hemoglobin usually observed in the venous blood cannot take place. Thus there could be little increase of oxyhemoglobin in the lungs and since that increase aids the unloading of carbon dioxide, the volume of pulmonary carbon dioxide eliminated is dangerously reduced. The resulting accumulation of carbon dioxide as such, as well as the acidosis created by that acid metabolite, must be taken into consideration in evaluating the toxic effects of oxygen at high pressure (see ft. p. 274 for a description of the narcotic and convulsant effects of excessive carbon dioxide) (172).

Another etiological factor is interference with the respiratory enzymes (67), a paradoxical histotoxic anoxia not observed when oxygen pressure is maintained within normal limits. Such an enzymatic inactivation could be effective in depressing cerebral metabolic rate. If the central nervous system is thus deprived of energy, we may recognize a nervous site for the toxic action of oxygen at high pressures. Stadie, Riggs, and Haugaard (907) ob- served that an entire hour elapsed before oxygen intake of cerebral tissues excised from a rat was halved. This delay is indicative of inactivation of the sulfhydryl (—SH) groups in enzymes. Several workers (236, 707) concur in laying the basis of the nervous symptoms on the ability of oxygen at high pressures to oxidize and thus inactivate essential —SH groups and especially so of the protein moiety of the pyruvate oxidase system. This interpretation accounts in a fundamental way for the neurological changes because the oxidation of carbohydrate goes through a pyruvate stage.

Yet a valid objection to this metabolic explanation arises out of the ob- servation that at high pressures of oxygen the nervous signs occur more rapidly than do the *in vitro* changes. Moreover neurological alterations come on at pressures of oxygen which exert little depression on the oxygen intake of excised cerebral tissues. One factor which deserves consideration in accounting for the rapid onset of the pathological behavior at high pressures of oxygen is cerebrovascular constriction (622a) which if sufficiently intense reduces cerebral blood flow and perhaps cerebral metabolic rate. However, the brain *in situ* may be more sensitive to enzymatic intereference than after excision. A similar phenomenon has been observed with the barbiturates which are also more effective in the intact organism. With the barbiturates too, functional impediment is excessive in comparison with the depression in cerebral metabolic rate (see Chapter 12, pages 345–349). Animal experimentation shows that after repeated exposures to high pressure, the nervous disturbances lose their reversibility and permanent crippling motor dysfunction is produced because of damage to the central nervous system (66).

The central nervous system, thus, is at a disadvantage not only with low oxygen but also with an excess. May a similar comparison be drawn with blood glucose? Is hyperglycemia as disastrous as hypoglycemia? Theoretically this is so—a high level of blood sugar will eventually interfere with cerebral function—but in a practical sense, it is of little importance since blood sugar, *per se*, assumes pathologic influence only at extremely high levels, even much higher than those attained in the most severe diabetes. The coma sometimes seen in diabetes, therefore, has no direct connection with the fact that blood sugar has accumulated in quantities above the normal. Experimentally, with the aid of a pump for the infusion of large amounts of glucose, Wierzuchowski (999) was able to produce enormous concentrations of blood sugar in dogs; but, except for some slight narcotic action, not until a concentration of 2,000 mg. per cent (about 20 times the normal value) did he observe any abnormal neurologic signs; and 3,000 mg. per cent brought on tonic and clonic convulsions. The central nervous system is dehydrated due to the hypertonicity of the blood and the motor neurones, both in the cord and brain, are rendered hyperirritable. Death comes at levels of 37,000 to 38,000 mg. per cent, too high for any bodily functions to continue.

Of greater practical significance are the reciprocal effects of oxygen and glucose for to some extent a deficiency of one can be made up for by a moderate excess of the other. In fasting men the ingestion of glucose results in a considerable amelioration of the visual impairment (722) caused by oxygen deficiency. Because an elevation of blood sugar confers such improvements upon performance as well as gains in altitude tolerance it is possible to understand why preflight and inflight meals of relatively high carbohydrate content have been suggested for aviators (603). In a similar fashion the inhalation of 100 per cent oxygen during hypoglycemia has proved to be advantageous. For example, the decrease in visual sensitivity observed during moderate hypoglycemia is reversed by respiring undiluted oxygen (723). In the last analysis it is the maintenance of the cerebral metabolism whether by the use of oxygen or sugar which is the predominant therapeutic directive for these treatments.

TABLE 21

General table of data on human brain metabolism

CONDITION	CEREBRAL METABOLIC RATE

A. C.M.R. values in various conditions

CONDITION	CEREBRAL METABOLIC RATE
Normal adult	3.3 cc oxygen/100 g./min. (2.5–3.7) 46 cc oxygen/min. (35–52)
Schizophrenia	Normal
Essential hypertension	Normal
Moderate changes in inspired O_2 and CO_2	Normal
Pregnancy	Normal
Eclampsia	Reduced
Lobotomy, postoperative	Reduced
Depression	Normal
Arteriosclerosis	Reduced
General paresis	Reduced
Injection of aminophylline	Reduced or Raised
Coma	
Hypoglycemia	Reduced
Diabetes	Reduced
Brain Tumor	Reduced

B. Preliminary results

CONDITION	CEREBRAL METABOLIC RATE
Coarctation of aorta	Above Normal
Idiopathic epilepsy	Normal
Parkinsonism	Reduced

C. C.M.R. values not proved because of inadequate data on C.B.F.

CONDITION	CEREBRAL METABOLIC RATE
Psychoses associated with	
Pernicious anemia	Reduced
Cardiac decompensation	Reduced
Pneumothorax	Reduced
Pellagra with B_1 deficiency	Reduced
Changes with age	Lowest in newborn, increases to maturity, decreases in senium.
Mental deficiency	
Undifferentiated	Normal for respective ages
Microcephalus	Reduced
Hydrocephalus	Reduced
Mongolism	Reduced
Cretinism	Reduced
Phenylpyruvic oligophrenia	Reduced
Amaurotic familial iodiocy	Reduced
Gargoylism	Reduced

IV. SUMMARY

The data presented in this chapter are presented in Table 21. The average AVO₂ difference for normal adults is 6.7 vol. per cent and for normal newborn is 8.6 vol. per cent.

Adult brain metabolism is referred to a standard of 46–53 cc. of oxygen per minute and is thus defined as C.M.R. Like B.M.R. this measurement is the energy required in the state of physical rest and mental relaxation compatible with wakefulness. In general it may be said that brain metabolism is raised above this level by greater activity and depressed below it by deprivation of foodstuff or oxygen, and by destructive processes. While C.M.R. in normal newborns is not established, it seems to be lower than in the adult.

Complete data for the calculation of C.M.R. are available in patients with schizophrenia and they are found to possess an AVO₂ difference and a total brain metabolism which are within normal limits. In profound hypoglycemia, however, their brain metabolism falls significantly. Another group of patients studied from one to three weeks after lobotomy also exhibited a reduction of C.M.R.

In depression C.M.R. may prove to be unchanged while it is retarded in the organic psychoses, cerebral arteriosclerosis and general paresis.

Three anoxic conditions were viewed with regard to their relation to brain metabolism. Several illustrative cases were added substantiating the point that all kinds of anoxia may reduce C.M.R. Mental symptoms in these cases were associated with the representation of low cerebral metabolism.

Coma, whether due to diabetes, hypoglycemia or brain tumor, is always associated with a reduction in C.M.R.

In other abnormal conditions we possess data only on cerebral AVO₂ differences and the C.M.R. is merely suggested. The AVO₂ differences and probably C.M.R. are reduced in patients suffering from acute destructive changes in the brain, whether caused by hypoglycemia, carbon monoxide or syphilis. Pellagrins with an uncomplicated niacin deficiency or a niacin and riboflavin deficiency exhibited AVO₂ differences within normal levels, but pellagrins who also had a vitamin B₁ deficiency suffered a reduction in their cerebral AVO₂ difference, and perhaps in their cerebral metabolic rate.

The observations on undifferentiated mental defectives reveal an increasing cerebral AVO₂ difference in the 4 age-groups from 6 to 29, and no change thereafter. Brain metabolism may rise along with the AVO₂ difference and be normal for their respective ages.

The mental defectives with microcephalus and hydrocephalus exhibit normal cerebral AVO₂ differences but one patient in the terminal stage of hydrocephalus showed a greatly reduced AVO_2 difference. Mongoloids, cretins, and phenylpyruvic oligophrenics 20 years of age and older, disclosed a low cerebral AVO_2 difference in comparison with the normal. Mongoloids were studied at various ages and they exhibited an AVO_2 difference which rose from the first to the second decade, but not in the third as was seen in the undifferentiated. The AVO_2 differences in amaurotic familial idiots were unexpectedly high, but in this group as in all the defectives except the undifferentiated, the brain metabolism is probably reduced.

Therapeusis for anoxic states was touched upon and oxygen poisoning discussed.

A summary of the influence of various conditions on CMR is presented in Table 21. Because of recent quantitative determinations the positions of pernicious anemia and cardiac decompensation should be removed from category C and placed under category A of that table (see pages 218 and 219 respectively). Cretinism is also found under C but a reduction of CMR has been measured quantitatively in patients with myxedema (see page 146).

CHAPTER 9

THERAPEUTICS AND THEIR APPLICATION TO BRAIN METABOLISM

I. INTRODUCTION

The main theme of this chapter is the presentation of data on the influence of therapeutic procedures on the cerebral metabolic rate of human patients. The procedures and drugs enumerated in the outline have been previously studied both in the clinic and in the laboratory, studied for their effect on the nervous system, on the cardio-vascular apparatus, and for their influence on the equilibria of the body, i.e., the levels of oxygen, carbon dioxide, and glucose in the blood stream, the acid-base balance, and temperature control. This work will not be reviewed in detail, but because the brain is sensitive to these factors, they must be considered in order to substantiate the principal theme, that is, the response of the brain to elective medical interference.

Some drugs and therapeutic procedures are used by physicians chiefly for their effect on the brain, as for example, the depressant drugs to produce sleep or anesthesia. Other procedures call forth generalized responses from the whole body, but an important therapeutic effect is on the brain. Illustrations are fever therapy for general paresis, thyroxin in hypothyroidism, and shock therapies for some of the psychoses. Needless to say, it is important for the physician to know the effects of these procedures on cerebral metabolic rate in order to understand and administer rational therapy, to achieve the most effective results, and to avoid any injury to the patient.

The reaction of the brain to such therapeutic measures permits us to divide them into three classes: those which *increase* the rate of metabolism in the brain, those which *decrease* the rate, and a third group whose action as yet has not been completely analyzed.

II. THERAPEUTIC PROCEDURES WHICH INCREASE BRAIN METABOLISM

A. *Fever therapy and general paresis*

We are indebted to Wagner-Jauregg (964) for the brilliant discovery of a therapeutic method which leads to the amelioration of general paresis in a large proportion of the cases. General paresis may be defined as an infection by the spirochaeta pallida which lodges in the brain causing chronic and progressive degeneration within that organ and its enveloping meninges. The symptoms are characteristic: frequently the disease begins with a change of personality; the usual adjustment to the environment may give way to one of indifference or apathy; or just the reverse, to a display of unbounded egoism. Among the early motor features which precede the onset of mental symptoms are muscular tremors which interfere with fine co-ordination making writing difficult and speaking slow and blurred; the pupils are unequal and no longer respond to light. The deep reflexes such as the knee jerk may be either hyperactive or diminished. Finally, as the motor symptoms progress, exultation and excitement become extreme and acute maniacal states develop. It is at this stage that delusions of grandeur are marked. This expansive delirium does not always occur, but instead there may be a deep melancholia and a peculiar stolidity in which the patient is passive and inattentive to his surroundings. For a further and more complete description of this disease, the reader is referred to any standard textbook on neuropsychiatry.

The discussion of patients in the advanced stages of general paresis, in the preceding chapter, indicates that they exhibit a subnormal cerebral energy exchange. It might seem superficially that any elevation of this low metabolic rate would have its effect on alleviating the symptoms detailed above, but since we still can give no acceptable explanation as to how fever therapy cures the victims of general paresis, it is not safe to say that any change in cerebral metabolic rate is the primary factor in the cure. Any additional information, then, which might solve this therapeutic riddle is eagerly welcomed.

Inasmuch as fever is a method used in the treatment of general paresis, it seems logical to begin with a description of the mechanisms causing deviations from the normal temperature control. *Fever is essentially a condition of imbalance between heat production and heat loss.* Under the influence of the heat regulating centers in the hypothalamus these two processes are balanced so that we maintain a temperature subject only to minor diurnal variations. Ranson and his co-workers (68, 817) have disclosed bilateral centers in the anterior portion of the hypothalamus which control heat loss (sweating and panting) (462). In the posterior portion they have shown the presence of centers controlling heat production (muscular and glandular work) and heat conservation. The amount of blood in the skin is important in heat conservation. It is obvious that when the skin is pink because its capillaries are distended with blood, there is an excessive amount of heat being given off; on the other hand, if the capillaries have squeezed out the blood from the surface, the skin is left cold and white and therefore loses less heat to the environment. Thus, the amount of blood in the skin is instrumental in determining the extent of the heat loss from the body by conduction, convection and vaporization.

Speaking broadly, from a point of view of causation, there are three kinds of fever. In the first (469) the thermoregulating mechanisms are intact and working properly, but the atmospheric temperature becomes hotter than the body temperature, and elimination of heat both by conduction and radiation is prevented. If vaporization cannot cope with this situation, the temperature in the body must mount. Such a condition, of course, is prevalent in the torrid zone, but the heat regulating mechanisms of our body can be disturbed in any section of the globe if the regulating scales are tipped against the dissipation of excess bodily heat. A subdivision of this type of fever is manifest when the rate of heat formation exceeds the capacity of the body to dispose of it, and this is exemplified when the body is deliberately heated by electrical currents as in the inductotherm therapy for general paresis, or by the administration of the drug, dinitrophenol.

In the second type of fever, according to Liebermeister (666), the thermoregulating mechanisms of the central nervous system are forced, under the influence of a toxic agent, to operate at a higher temperature than normal. Not only is more heat manufactured in the body, but less is given off. This condition prevails in infections of any kind, or when the physician creates such a fever at will by the injection of foreign proteins into the blood stream.

The third kind of fever need not long detain us at the present moment because it is not employed in fever therapy. Acute and profound dehydration drains the body of water and cuts down considerably the total volume of blood. Consequently, less blood can be spared from the vital organs for perfusing the periphery of the body, leaving a relatively bloodless and cold body surface which cannot readily get rid of heat (505).

In the treatment of general paresis either the first or second type of fever is used. By one method, that of the inductotherm, the body is overheated by electrical currents passing through it. During this operation the patient is wrapped in warm blankets preventing the escape of heat, and any desired increase in body temperature can be effectively brought about and maintained. Fever is produced according to the second method by the injection of protein or dead typhoid bacilli, or living malarial parasites. The action of these injections causing the thermoregulating apparatus to fix the body temperature at a higher level is facilitated because here too, the patient is warmly clad to prevent heat leakage.

Brain metabolism in humans. In experiments conducted to determine the effects of fever therapy on brain metabolism, the inductotherm or the injection of typhoid-paratyphoid vaccine or malarial parasites were used to induce fever (479). Irrespective of the method of raising the temperature, the conduct of the experiments was the same. Rectal temperature, circulation time,[1] blood pressure and pulse rate were recorded. Blood samples were drawn simultaneously from the internal jugular vein and an artery to determine the oxygen, sugar, and lactic acid contents of the cerebral blood before, during and after fever therapy. A typical example is the response of patient 11 in Table 22 to the injection of typhoid vaccine. As his rectal temperature climbed from 98° to 106°F., his cerebral arterio-venous oxygen difference likewise rose from 5.2 vol. per cent to 9.1 vol. per cent. His circulation time was accelerated from 17.6 to 7.4 seconds.

TABLE 22

Observations made during three types of fever therapy

PATIENT NO.	TEMP. °F.	OXYGEN A:V DIFF. VOL.	CIRCULATION TIME SECONDS	BLOOD PRESSURE MM/HG	PULSE RATE /MIN.	ARTERIAL	
						Lactic acid	Sugar
Inductotherm							
		per cent				*mg. per cent*	
2	100.8	6.9	15.4	156/110	100	16	97
	103.8	11.0	11.8	147/75	160	25	101
Typhoid vaccine							
8	98.6	7.8	20.0	126/94	80	15	95
	105.0	15.8	17.0	138/86	120	36	119
11	98.0	5.2	17.6	158/106	78	20	97
	100.4	6.6	11.0	156/96	108	20	92
	102.0	6.6	10.0	155/70	96	27	84
	104.4	7.6	13.0	140/62	130	17	102
	106.0	9.1	7.4	125/70	140	27	129
Malarial parasite							
15	99.0	3.6	17.0	116/70	84	..	122
	102.0	6.2	14.2	104/70	100	..	159
	104.2	9.3	12.6	110/50	100	..	141

Pulse rate, lactic acid and glucose all rose. In this particular experiment blood pressure fell though this was not typical of all the patients. The significant point is that in 11 of the 15 patients treated by the inducto-therm, the oxygen difference increased at least by 2 vol. per cent during fever.[2] This elevation in the cerebral AVO_2 difference, significant though

[1] Circulation time may be defined as: the number of intervening seconds from the time 0.35 cc. of 2 per cent sodium cyanide solution is injected into the antebrachial vein until it impinges on the chemosensitive receptors in the carotid body, capable of initiating impulses which stimulate the medullary respiratory centers, thus evoking a reflex gasp from the patient (824).

[2] Dr. William R. Thompson has kindly made a statistical analysis to test the significance of the apparent increases in AVO_2 differences of this research. A pair of

it may be, does not by itself indicate an increase in brain metabolism unless we can show that the circulation rate through the brain is maintained or at least does not drop. In the table we see that circulation time is not only maintained but in all cases is accelerated; and furthermore, there is no consistent drop of blood pressure to indicate a decrease in cerebral blood flow. Grollman finds that cardiac output is also increased during fever (426). It would therefore seem that the brain takes part in the over-all increase of metabolism.

Unlike the results of the author and his associates, subsequent work by Looney and Borkovic (687) revealed no increase in the AVO₂ differences, and these observers concluded that brain metabolism was unchanged by hyperpyrexia. They examined 12 patients who were given the diathermic fever treatment for general paresis. Blood was sampled before and during fever and the average values for cerebral AVO₂ differences were substantially the same throughout. These workers write that the rate of blood flow was "markedly accelerated" during the period of fever. If the brain took part in this faster blood flow through the body, then we may conclude that brain metabolism also rose, since as we have already explained, C.M.R. is the product of blood flow multiplied by arterio-venous oxygen difference. We therefore find that a higher brain metabolism is produced by fever therapy. Other investigators in this field also concur that brain metabolism rises in fevered patients (455, 212). This conclusion is in keeping with DuBois' work (256) on basal metabolic rate in fever of any kind. He observes that for each degree Fahrenheit the basal metabolic rate of the entire body rises 7 per cent. Since this is true of the body as a whole, it is not unreasonable that it should also apply to the brain.

The effect of temperature on brain metabolism has been demonstrated

---

observations were taken from each of 15 patients in the study. The first was the control before fever therapy, and the second was the first value obtained after the rectal temperature had reached 103°F. This gave a set of 15 differences which may be arranged in the following ascending order: (X_k) −2.69, −0.94, 0.95, 1.08, 2.01, 2.08, 2.26, 2.46, 2.67, 4.08, 4.26, 4.31, 5.02, 5.78, and 8.07. If these may be considered as a random sample of results obtainable in this manner, it is simple to give confidence ranges for their median value, M (i.e., the value such that half the observations would be greater). As shown elsewhere (942) the probability that the median is less that X_k, the k-th observation in the ascending order is given by:

$$P(M < X_k) = (\tfrac{1}{2})^{15} \sum_{\gamma=0}^{k-1} \binom{15}{\gamma}$$

Thus, $P(M < 0.95) = 0.0037$ approximately, and thus the apparently positive median difference may be regarded as significant. Furthermore, ordinary Fisher's t test applied to the set of differences gives t = 4.005 and accordingly P is about 0.001. The increases of cerebral AVO₂ differences during fever therapy in these patients (Table 22) are therefore significant.

not only with increases above normal but also with decreases below. Blood was sampled from dogs anesthetized with pentobarbital and packed in ice until rectal temperature fell from approximately 38° to 26°C. Their AVO_2 difference decreased and did so despite a circulation time which progressively lengthened (308). It is therefore probable that cerebral metabolism was greatly depressed (355).

Examination into the processes underlying metabolic changes in the brain: Excised cerebral tissues. Another method of studying metabolism and fever

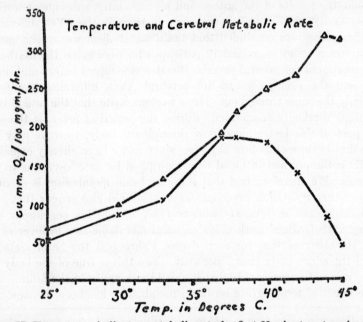

FIG. 37. Upper curve indicates metabolic rate for first 20 minutes at various temperatures. Lower curve indicates metabolic rate from 50th to 60th minutes.

is to expose excised cerebral tissues to various temperatures. This procedure has the advantage of measuring oxygen intake quantitatively in the Warburg apparatus, and eliminates one of the two factors for estimating the metabolic rate of the brain *in situ*, that of blood flow. This method, of course, is subject to the general criticism leveled at *in vitro* experiments in that the tissues are removed from all the normal bodily influences. Dixon (242) studied the effect of temperature on excised rabbit brain and observed an increment with higher temperatures. The author and his co-workers (479) tried minced rat brain, the results of which are arranged in Fig. 37. The metabolic rate of the brain increases consistently as the temperature climbs from 25° to 44°C. during the first 20 minutes of a 60-minutes observation. Above 44°C. or 111°F. this increase is not maintained. The lower curve of the chart pictures the observations made between the 50th and 60th minutes and reveals a rapid fall of oxygen intake as temperature raises above 40°C. It is obvious that two processes are operating: most prominent in the first 20 minutes of the experiment is an increase in brain metabolism, but as the high temperatures are endured, some harmful process interferes with cellular function, ultimately leading to a depression in cerebral metabolism (320, 321). This reduction of energy formation in the brain, if of sufficient severity, may eventually work destruction on the brain tissues.

Morphology. Among those who have examined the gross and minute structure of brain tissues which have been subjected to fever therapy was Hartman (455), who used both canine and human subjects. His morphologic work disclosed degenerative changes similar to those observed after a period of intense anoxia. Hartman's explanation involves two factors: increased demand for oxygen in the cerebral tissues in response to the stimulation of fever, and an impaired oxygen content of the arterial blood. The latter may be ascribed to a faulty pulmonary exchange; for example, a dog with an arterial oxygen saturation of 59 per cent during hyperpyrexia revealed, upon autopsy, hemorrhagic consolidations in both lungs. An ineffectual gaseous exchange, however, is not the rule and with high body temperatures, respiration is usually stepped up, oxygen supply is ample, and carbon dioxide is pumped out of the body, leaving the patient in a state of alkalosis. As observed by Cullen, Weir, and Cook (212), in patients rendered febrile as a result of treatment in a heated cabinet, the alkalosis diminishes oxygen pressure. Such a diminution causes a smaller flow of oxygen into the tissues, even if the oxygen content of the arterial blood is maintained. The clinical observation that patients with fever do better by breathing oxygen instead of air may be therefore ascribed to a twofold compensation: raising the oxygen pressure when reduced by the alkalosis resulting from overactivity of normal lungs and an increase in the oxygen content in those patients who acquire pulmonary lesions in the course of hyperpyrexia.

So far, the foregoing data point to two distinct directions in which cerebral metabolism reacts to fever therapy: (1) a primary increase in brain metabolism, and (2) a succeeding fall which, in the intact animal is imputed partly to unavailability of oxygen, and in excised tissues entirely to the irreversible damage incurred by hyperpyrexia. Guided by these two generalizations, we are in a better position to unravel the physiologic processes underlying brain metabolism during fever. (Other effects of high temperatures on cerebral metabolic rate may be found in Chapter **7**, section on temperature).

Enzymology. In an attempt to understand what has occurred in fevered cerebral tissues, whether excised or *in situ*, we must recall the processes of cellular metabolism which were presented in Chapter 5. If we consider the three variables of metabolism—blood sugar, oxygen, and respiratory enzymes—the first two may be eliminated because neither the small rise of glucose and most certainly not the fall of oxygen pressure, could exert such pyretic effects. One variable, therefore, remains to account for the observed rise in metabolism: the respiratory enzymes. An acceleration of their activity might explain the mysterious surplus of energy in fever. How can we connect an accelerated enzymatic activity with the excess metabolism present in fever? We know that various hydrogen acceptors are pyrogenic. These acceptors step up the activity of the dehydrogenating enzymes, energy turnover is accelerated, and this process provokes fever. Among these acceptors are methylene blue, dinitrophenol and pyocyanin. Thionine, cresyl blue and dinitrocresol act in a similar fashion.

In fever therapy where hydrogen acceptors are not employed it is probable that the activity of all members of the respiratory enzyme systems are accelerated and it would be difficult to know whether any one enzyme system is speeded up more than the others.

This is in accordance with van't Hoff's classic law that a rise in temperature of 10°C. increases the rate of chemical reactions between 100 and 200 per cent (534). If the oxygen supply is not sufficient to provide for this unusual spurt of enzymatic action, as suggested by Hartman (455) and Cullen, Weir, and Cook (212), then the brain *will suffer* from anoxia and will respond, as it always does to anoxic conditions, first with a temporary and reversible disability and later with permanent damage (852). This, however, is only a part of the story. For what happens in the Warburg apparatus where oxygen is abundant even at high temperatures and cerebral damage is still apparent (479)? In this case the damage cannot be attributed to a scarcity of oxygen, but to destruction of the enzymes by heat. It is probable that the protein portion of enzymes are thermolabile and under a high temperature the proteins are coagulated. Until this critical degree is attained, the delivery of energy for cerebral metabolism is accelerated, but after the proteins are coagulated by the heat, the enzyme can no longer take part in the delivery of cerebral energy. Hence, stripped of their catalytic agents, the cells must finally die. (For further discussion on the effects of high and low temperatures on metabolism, see ref. (321)).

Discussion. As we stated at the beginning of this subject, there is no generally acceptable explanation for the beneficial effect of pyrotherapy. The suggestion that the spirochaeta are destroyed by the excessive heat has been rendered unlikely by experimental trial, which has proved that the spirochaeta may survive the high therapeutic temperatures (775). Since this suggestion for the action of pyrotherapy is not satisfactory, it is necessary to seek some other explanation more in line with the physiologic events taking place during fever therapy. For this explanation, we must recall the histologic picture of general paresis, which shows that though the disease process is diffuse throughout the brain, its intensity varies greatly even in adjoining areas. If the abnormal behavior of the patient is caused by the malfunction of the cells which have been more intensely attacked by the spirochaeta, and if these cells are especially vulnerable to excess heat, then it seems likely that they would be the first to be destroyed when subjected to fever therapy, leaving the normal cells and those less intensely affected to carry on.

Some[3] say that the tissues develop a non-specific defense against the spirochaeta pallida, a generalized tissue response to fever as evidenced by the increased protein content and by a multiplication of cells in the cerebrospinal fluid, signs of a stronger resistance of the host to the invader. Patients who exhibit such a reaction have a more encouraging prognosis and will derive more benefit from fever therapy. If we know that an increase in temperature accelerates all biologic processes, it seems likely that the reactions of the body against the invading spirochaeta would also be intensified by fever, and if so, it is this catalyzing effect of fever to which the therapeutic success may be attributed (476). At this stage in the development of syphilology it is impossible to decide the exact mechanism for the cure, whether it can be traced to a single process, or a combination of those suggested, or yet to other factors still undetermined.

Though the foregoing observations were made largely on patients with general paresis and animal experimentation, it is logical to expect that the same cerebral progress—at first stimulating, later harmful—would be evident in patients irrespective of the disease for which they are receiving therapeutic hyperpyrexia. Furthermore, any fever, whether therapeutically induced or the result of pathologic processes, would probably affect the metabolism of the brain in much the same way as observed in the paretics. Though the usual response to moderate fever is to accelerate cerebral metabolism without significant deleterious action, still excessive fever may injure the brain beyond repair, thus explaining the lethal terminus which sometimes follows in patients succumbing to heat stroke, acute infection and severe dehydration, all different forms of fever. In any form of hyperpyrexia all parts of the body suffer, but the loss of the organizing and regulating influence of the central nervous system is important in the fatal conclusion.

[3] Personal communication from Dr. Carl W. F. Lange.

B. *Thyroid therapy in cretinism*

Hormones are important not because they initiate any action of their own, but because they influence the rate of various physiologic processes in the body. They are therefore like catalysts—by themselves they have no effect, but they do change the rate of reactions already in progress. Thyroxin, like any other hormone, catalyzes certain specific physiologic processes. Its characteristic activity is to facilitate cellular oxidations, and thus maintain the normal metabolic rate of the body. Secondary to this capacity is its more apparent influence to hasten the functions of all the organs, and this capacity can be most clearly discerned when it is exaggerated by more than a sufficient amount of thyroxin in the body or by its failure in the absence of the hormone. In immature children, absence of thyroxin hinders the growth and differentiation of both body and brain. At all ages a deficiency of this hormone diminishes metabolic rate. Cardio-respiratory, gastro-intestinal, and nervous activity are all abated. The reverse of the above condition is that of hyperthyroidism.

Though we have many data on the influence of thyroxin on *basal* metabolic rate, the studies of this hormone on *cerebral* metabolic rate are scarce. We will delay our discussion of patients to mention the work on excised tissues of hyperthyroid and hypothyroid animals. It seems agreeable to all workers in this field that the metabolic rates of excised tissues other than brain are similar to those of the intact organism (that is, below normal in a thyroidectomized animal and above normal in thyroid-fed animals), but unfortunately, the conclusions on excised *cerebral* tissues are discordant. Cohen and Gerard (175) and Macleod and Reiss (700) argue in favor of a rise in metabolism in the brain of animals rendered hyperthyroid. But against their conclusions are those of Spirtes (903), Gordon and Heming (412) and Fazekas (305) who found no significant change in the metabolism of such tissues. This discrepancy has not been resolved for excised tissues but *in vivo* studies failed to disclose a significant increase of C.M.R. in patients with hyperthyroidism (848b). In contrast patients with myxedema revealed a reduced C.M.R. and one moreover which was restored to normal with therapy. These observations made with the nitrous oxide technic are essentially in agreement with previous ones obtained with the thermo-electric flow recorder (486).

In the preceeding chapter data were presented disclosing that the average cerebral AVO_2 difference of cretins above the age of 20 is 5.5 vol. per cent. This value is significantly lower than that of normal controls in the same age group, and data in Chapter 8 indicate that cretins have a subnormal C.M.R. In this chapter we shall relate the events which occurred following the administration of desiccated thyroxin to cretins in experiments to determine whether the C.M.R. of these persons can be raised by replacement therapy. It should be pointed out that if thyroxin *can* produce an increase in C.M.R., the best experimental condition is the low metabolism of the cretin's brain which makes the therapeutic results more readily discernible, since the effect of thyroxin is magnified when administered to an athyrotic individual. This work was done on 11 cretins ranging from 9 to 31 years of age (486) and the results of 8 studied most

TABLE 23

Changes of total metabolism, cerebral blood flow, cerebral arterio-venous oxygen differences, and cerebral metabolism during thyroid therapy

1	2	3	4	CEREBRAL ARTERIO-VENOUS O$_2$ DIFFERENCE			8
				5	6	7	
PATIENT	AGE	INCREASED BODILY O$_2$ INTAKE,	BLOOD FLOW RATIO	Before	After	After corrected	INCREASED CEREBRAL METABOLISM
		per cent		Vol. per cent	Vol. per cent	Vol. per cent	per cent
C. B............	22	22	1.48	5.2	4.2	6.2	18
M. K............	19	19	1.65	7.1	5.6	9.3	31
G. S............	31	8	1.40	5.9	4.8	6.8	15
A. C............	22	44	1.81	4.6	4.2	7.7	68
G. A............	29	13	1.51	4.8	4.4	6.7	39
B. S............	9	19	1.45	5.0	5.4	7.8	56
R. C............	15	23	1.71	5.7	4.0	6.8	19
R. G............	22	29	1.52	7.3	5.4	8.3	13
Average......	21	22	1.57	5.7	4.8	7.4	32

Each value is the average of several observations. They include the percentage changes of oxygen intake for the entire body, (column 3) taking the premedication value as a base line, the ratios of the cerebral blood flow after therapy to the flow before treatment (column 4), the averages of the cerebral arterio-venous oxygen difference before thyroid therapy (column 5), and after (column 6), the latter values corrected for blood flow (column 7). Column 7 is obtained by multiplying the values of column 4 by those of column 6. Column 8 contains the per cent increase in cerebral metabolism as a result of thyroid therapy. This increase is obtained by dividing the values of column 5 into those of column 7.

intensively are presented in Table 23. In order to secure adequate control measurements, the administration of all thyroid therapy was omitted for two months, at the end of which time repeated determinations of AVO$_2$ references, cerebral blood flow (Chapter 2, footnote p. 14) and basal metabolic rate were made. Using these values as controls, thyroid medication was initiated and a constant watch was kept of the basal metabolism. As soon as a definite increment in the basal was observed, a second series of observations was made on the cerebral oxygen utilization and the rate of blood flow, thus permitting a comparison of the values before and after therapy.

It may be seen from the table that the increase of 22 per cent in oxygen intake for the entire body was the average of values whose two extremes were 8 per cent and 44 per cent. In all instances there is a large and constant acceleration of cerebral blood flow averaging 57 per cent over the control. The average cerebral AVO_2 difference decreased from 5.7 vol. per cent[4] to 4.8 vol. per cent, but when the latter value was corrected for cerebral blood flow, it was greater than the original. The percentage increase of C.M.R. was found to be between the limits of 13 per cent and 68 per cent, yielding an average of 32 per cent over the control. It would be interesting to determine whether such a rise in C.M.R. produces any changes in the function of the brain.

The latter was accomplished by electroencephalographic and psychologic examinations made on these same patients, and performed along with the biochemical determinations. A comparison of the electroencephalographic records before and after the initiation of thyroid therapy shows that the patients exhibited an increase in the energy level of the brain waves in certain frequencies ranging from 7 to 11 cycles per second. The spontaneous electrical activity of the brain cells therefore reveals a greater release of energy. In the psychologic tests efforts were made to determine steadiness, speed of tapping and memory. An appreciable decrease in steadiness was noted. Though speeds of tapping and of verbal production were slightly increased, any improvements in perception and learning were of questionable significance in the higher mental processes. It may therefore be concluded that the greatest changes both electrically and psychologically were noted in processes closely related to energy expenditures. As for the quality of psychologic activity, it became more rapid but not improved, so that the patient remained at his previous low level of mentality despite therapy. Most of these patients had been cretins for many years, and their brains had probably undergone irreversible damage which could not be improved by specific therapy. Of course, in the athyrotic infant, replacement medication is more effective and may be relatively successful. The stimulating influence of thyroxin finds its expression in terms of behavior and the person with hypothyroidism who has received successful therapy no longer exhibits the delay and listless action characteristic of a sluggish cerebral metabolic rate. It is surprising to the author that C.M.R. has not been found to be higher than normal (848b) in patients with hyperthyroidism. The error of the nitrous oxide technic however increases as C.B.F. is accelerated. Furthermore the effect of equal doses of thyroid becomes progressively smaller as C.M.R. is raised from

---

[4] It is true that some normal subjects may have values below 5.7 vol. per cent'
but it must be remembered that 5.7 vol. per cent is the *average* value for cretins while
the *average* for normals is 6.7 vol. per cent, one whole volume per cent higher.

subnormal values. In such a case it would be difficult to establish significant differences on comparing the patient with hyperthyroidism and the control.

We shall now turn our attention to the more fundamental aspect of this problem, specifically, how does thyroxin raise metabolism? A conception which may explain the acceleration of metabolic rate in most organs of the body is a denser concentration of enzymes and as we shall see, this is the one determinant in the action of thyroxin. Though the evidence quoted earlier (175, 700, 903, 412, 305) reveals that the effect of thyroxin on cerebral enzymes is controversial, this lack of agreement does not hold for other organs. Klein (605) who worked on rat liver states that the administration of thyroid hormone increases the concentration of the colloidal protein carrier of some oxidative enzymes. He observed an enhanced activity of the d-amino acid oxidase as a result of thyroid feeding. Remembering that this enzyme is composed of riboflavin and a protein colloidal carrier, and that the total riboflavin is unchanged as a result of thyroid therapy, Klein concludes that some riboflavin which hitherto had been free is now able to combine with the protein component of the oxidase. Other evidence indicates that the thyroid hormone may stimulate the synthesis of the prosthetic group as well as of the protein moiety of enzymes (945).

In the reverse condition, myxedema, brought about by thyroidectomy, Dye and Waggoner (265, 267) have reported a marked diminution of the enzyme, indophenol oxidase, in several non-nervous tissues. But more important from the viewpoint of the brain are experiments in which thiouracil prevented the normal increase of cerebral enzyme, carbonic anhydrase, in young growing rats (849). Though thiouracil inhibits the production of thyroid yet a direct relationship between thyroid function and the concentration of cerebral enzymes is not proved. The influence of the thyroid gland may be indirect and the smaller concentrations of enzymes an expression of the general retarded growth. (See Chapter 7 for changes in enzyme activity during early development).

Indirect effects on brain metabolism must also be considered because reflex stimuli can spur cerebral enzymes to greater speed, irrespective of their concentration. Since the time of Magnus-Levy (256) the effect of the thyroid gland has been imputed in part to the acceleration of intrinsic cerebral oxidations and partly to mechanisms involving the organization of the entire animal. Factors that may be concerned in raising cerebral metabolism include a change in blood constituents and an intense bombardment by nervous stimuli. An example of the latter is the excited function of the sympathetic nervous system during hyperthyroidism, and this is the one cause for the rapid heart rate of the patient. Stimuli from overactive organs pass more frequently to the nervous centers and in return motor impulses issue therefrom more rapidly. It is apparent that all portions of the central nervous system including the autonomic and somatic divisions take part in the general speeding up of the bodily functions and nervous enzymatic action is hurried in this reflex manner. These indirect influences are necessarily absent in studies of excised cerebral tissues.

In the last analysis we may say that the administration of thyroid accelerates cerebral metabolic rate. This hypothesis has proved to be effective only for cretins and patients with myxedema. Though it seems reasonable to expect a similar, though quantitatively much milder influence on the brain of normal individuals yet measurements made on patients with hyperthyroidism revealed C.M.R. within normal limits.

III. DRUGS AND PROCEDURES DECREASING BRAIN METABOLISM

Brain metabolism may be depressed by depriving the brain of either oxygen or glucose. In this section we shall deal with procedures and drugs, exclusive of the narcotic reagents, which depress brain metabolism by creating an anoxia. The consideration of narcotic medicinals and of glucose deprivation will be reserved for Chapters 12 and 10 respectively. Some of these drugs exert an anoxic effect on the brain by displacing the oxygen of the inspired air, while others induce anoxia as a secondary result of their violent stimulating action on the central nervous system (663). Such methods of attack on mental disease are not new and the use of nitrous oxide and electrical currents was reported in 1871 (750a) and 1872 (9a) respectively.

It has been pointed out that at present all the so-called "shock" therapies (insulin hypoglycemia and convulsant therapies) involve an element of metabolic depression in the brain (496). According to some psychiatrists (845) insulin is especially effective in the treatment of schizophrenia, particularly of the paranoid type and in early cases. The convulsants are of greater value in the affective psychoses and especially so in the agitated depressions peculiar to older patients (730, 79, 151, 659, 575, 72, 472). At this time we do not intend to enter into a discussion on the controversial question of whether these shock therapies are curative, and if so, whether depression of cerebral metabolism is an essential step in the cure. Rather, we shall employ these therapies purely as experiments to study brain metabolism. Even though the observations are made on abnormal subjects, the results not only throw light on the pathologic brain but also reveal certain fundamental characteristics of the healthy brain.

A. *Anoxiants*

Asphyxia is produced whenever the normal exchange of the respiratory gases is abolished, demonstrable in strangulation, or when any part of

Pituitary

TEMP. REG. CTR.

the respiratory tract is blocked. Anoxia is not the same as asphyxia, and Gellhorn (374) differentiates between these two frequently interchanged terms. Lack of oxygen is a prominent feature in both anoxia and asphyxia, but in the latter there is a retention of carbon dioxide coupled with a lack of oxygen. Hence, we have substituted the new name "anoxiant", descriptive of those anoxic drugs which do not hold back carbon dioxide, in place of the older, less explicit term, "asphyxiant".

In the course of an operation anoxia is all too frequently the result of carelessness on the part of the anesthetist. Using the closed system of administering anesthesia, where no contact is made with room air and where carbon dioxide is reabsorbed and not allowed to accumulate, the anesthetist assumes the responsibility for regulating the supply of oxygen to satisfy the patient's requirements (See picture on "nitrogen procedure" Fig. 38 in next section).

Cyanide. Anoxia may also be produced by cyanide which interferes with the process of cellular respiration, and particularly with the activity of the enzyme, cytochrome oxidase (582, 921). This form of anoxia is designated histotoxic (786) and was mentioned in passing in the previous chapter.

Cyanide was perhaps the first anoxiant to be used in the treatment of schizophrenia, reported by Loevenhart and his co-workers as early as 1918 (675). But there are other reasons for studying the effect of cyanide on brain metabolism: it is a frequent cause of death whether by accident or with suicidal intent. In small non-toxic doses, however, it is used to determine circulation time (see footnote 1 p. 230). Because of this diagnostic use, and in view of its lethal possibilities, it is important to broaden our knowledge on the effect of cyanide in various quantities and its action on brain metabolism, and thereby direct the treatment of its toxic effects into the proper channels.

Cyanide in the concentrations used for diagnostic purposes has little significance for brain metabolism. It would be difficult to determine the effects of a lethal dose on a human being because in such a contingency the only concern of the physician is to save his patient's life. Inasmuch as research on man must necessarily be limited, some experiments were carried out on dogs, injecting potassium cyanide either into the carotid artery or the femoral vein (304). Though non-lethal doses were administered, it may be seen from a typical experiment (Table 24) that the brain practically ceased to remove oxygen from the blood, at least for a short time; in other words, the venous oxygen content so closely approached that of the arterial as to make the difference between them insignificant. It would seem impossible to have an increase of blood flow through the brain of sufficient magnitude to account for this wiping out of the AVO$_2$

difference, so it must be attributed in large part if not entirely to a profound depression of brain metabolism, which is caused by the temporary inactivation of the cyanide-sensitive oxidase system, (temporary because the non-lethal dose permitted the detoxication of cyanide and the reestablishment of the AVO_2 difference).

When excised cerebral tissues are examined for their reaction to cyanide (503), it is found that the activity of cytochrome oxidase is obstructed, and that cyanide inhibits cerebral metabolism *in vitro*, a fact which supports the conclusion derived from *in vivo* observations. Evans' calculations (296) show that the respiration of excised tissues is inhibited by approximately the same concentration of cyanide as is lethal to the intact organism (296), and to an extent that is almost complete. This work reveals that most, but not all, oxidations are catalyzed by a cyanide-

TABLE 24

Effect of potassium cyanide on cerebral respiration

OXYGEN, VOLUMES PER CENT			RELATION OF TIME BLOOD WAS DRAWN TO INJECTION OF KCN IN CAROTID ARTERY
Arterial	Venous*	Difference	
15.9	7.0	8.9	3 min. before
16.9	16.3	0.6	2 min. after 20 mg. of KCN injected
16.4	15.7	0.7	18 min. after injection
15.7	20.0	4.3	1 hr. 32 min. after injection

* The venous blood was collected from the superior longitudinal sinus of a dog under pentobarbital anesthesia.

sensitive enzyme though not necessarily to the same degree. Resting muscle[5] for example was shown to be less affected by cyanide injections than the brain (304). Since the brain is deprived of oxidative support it must draw upon anaerobic resources for maintenance and function. The anaerobic mobilization is speeded up when cyanide induces convulsive

[5] Stannard (909) used sodium azide to which cytochrome oxidase is even more sensitive than it is to cyanide and found that the respiration of resting muscle was not inhibited by azide, but that any increment in respiration above the resting level caused by electrical or chemical stimulation was specifically checked. Thus both cyanide and azide inhibit the respiration of "active" muscle while only cyanide works on "resting" muscle. Apparently, the increase of cellular respiration which is brought about by the stimulated activity is catalyzed by an azide-sensitive enzyme. These results indicate that at least two different enzyme systems of muscle are cyanide-sensitive. In addition to cytochrome oxidase, cytochrome C may combine with cyanide (540). Another explanation for these diverse effects also takes into consideration the conception that both inhibitors act on the oxidized form of cytochrome oxidase and in addition two other characteristics are suggested for cyanide: to increase the apparent association constant between oxygen and cytochrome oxidase and to combine with another unidentified enzyme (1014).

activity (611) as brain glycogen, glucose, adenosine triphosphate rapidly diminish and yield energy while lactate, adenosine diphosphate and inorganic phosphate accumulate (777).

It is not surprising that Geppert (382) who first showed that cyanide prevents the cells from removing oxygen from the blood came to the conclusion that the symptoms of cyanide poisioning are essentially similar to those seen in acute oxygen lack. More recently, Ward and Wheatley (977) have found that the order of the electrical changes of cyanide poisoning duplicate the neurophyletic regression observed in anoxia, starting in the cerebral hemisphere and gradually descending the neuraxis. In both instances oxygen is no longer available for cerebral cellular metabolism. Their distinction lies in the basic analysis of their action; in the case of anoxic anoxia, oxygen does not reach the brain, and in cyanide poisoning, though the oxygen is safely transported to the brain, the cells are not able to utilize it.

Nitrogen. Of the many effects of nitrogen inhalation on the body we will mention only the two most important. In the first place, it may displace oxygen in the inspired air, serving as an anoxiant. Secondly, it may be the cause of the caisson disease, or as it is commonly referred to, "the bends". The origin of this disease is rooted in the solubility of nitrogen, which is greater in lipid than in aqueous solution (436). When the pressure surrounding the diver is increased as he descends below sea level, nitrogen accumulates in great concentration in the lipid portions of the central nervous system. Then, when the pressure is abruptly reduced, as when the diver ascends quickly to sea level, or when an aviator suddenly rises from sea level to high altitudes (17), more nitrogen leaves the lipid tissues than those predominantly aqueous. The blood and other aqueous tissues are not able to retain the relatively large amount of nitrogen in solution and therefore bubbles of this gas form within them. Oxygen and carbon dioxide have less tendency to form bubbles because carbon dioxide is readily soluble and eliminated through the lungs, and oxygen is utilized by the tissues. In cases of caisson disease with motor paralysis or severe pain in one or another region of the body, the bubbles are obstructing the circulation, damaging the involved tissues. A not uncommon symptom is itching of the skin as nitrogen bubbles accumulate in the skin capillaries. It has also been suggested that nitrogen at high pressure exerts a narcotic action (70) but this idea has been seriously questioned (66). Our main interest, however, lies in the capacity of nitrogen to displace oxygen and the opportunity to study this problem presented itself in the nitrogen inhalation therapy for schizophrenics.

Undiluted nitrogen is employed either alone (668, 72), or administered as an adjuvant to insulin hypoglycemia (439). In this technic the

244   ENERGETICS

nitrogen (9) is administered much the same way as any gaseous or volatile
narcotic, that is, by the closed system method in which a mask is fitted
tightly to the face of the patient, a canister of soda lime is inserted to
remove carbon dioxide and to this is attached a 5-liter rebreathing bag,
all connected in a chain-like series (Fig. 38). To this closed system the
gases, either oxygen or nitrogen, are admitted by way of the face mask;
an exhalation valve at the end of the rebreathing bag permits the excess

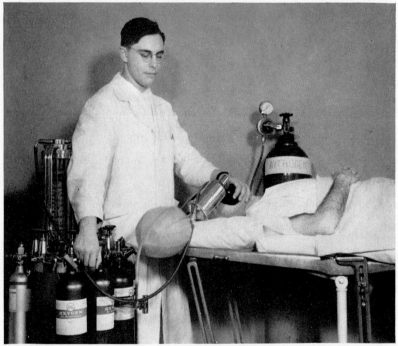

Fig. 38. Apparatus for the nitrogen treatment assembled and in use.

gases to spill over into the air. After the mask has been closely adjusted
to the face of the patient and the apparatus has been flushed with oxygen,
the oxygen supply is shut off and undiluted nitrogen is released into the
mask. When the anoxia is sufficiently profound, usually by the fourth
minute, (see Chapter 10 for signs of acute anoxia), the nitrogen control
valve is closed and oxygen is readmitted. While the patient is exposed to
the nitrogen, the oxygen content of his arterial blood rapidly decreases
(496); normally this value may be 19 vol. per cent, but as a result of
nitrogen inhalation it may be forced down to as low as 3 vol. per cent.
As can be seen from Table 25 the oxygen content of the arterial blood
which is low, 5 vol. per cent, at the time the patient loses contact with

his environment, falls to still lower levels, 2.5 vol. per cent, before the inhalation of nitrogen is terminated. The involuntary motor activity of the patient during this procedure complicates any attempt to draw samples of internal jugular venous blood, but the AVO_2 difference has been determined on amytalized dogs respiring nitrogen and it usually falls to a value less than 1 vol. per cent (518). So little oxygen is absorbed by the brain that it cannot continue its elaboration of energy.

Concomitant with the biochemical transitions taking place during the nitrogen procedure are vascular and neurologic adaptations. In the chapter on cerebral circulation (Chapter 6) the point was made that as anoxia deepens, systemic blood pressure rises, the cerebral vessels dilate and brain blood flow is faster. Therefore, during the inhalation of nitrogen, which is essentially an anoxic episode, the cerebral blood flow must have been increased. This increase is only incidental, the main

TABLE 25

Effect of progressive anoxia on hemoglobin saturation of patient with schizophrenia receiving nitrogen inhalation treatment

CONDITION	OXYGEN CONTENT	OXYGEN CAPACITY	HEMOGLOBIN SATURATION
	vol. per cent	*vol. per cent*	*per cent*
Loss of contact......................	5.0	18.2	22
Before termination with oxygen........	2.5	18.2	13

point being that the blood going to the brain is low in oxygen. During the time that the patient is out of contact with his environment, he passes through a number of neurologic phases which arise in a definite sequence, and will be described in Chapter 10. When the patient is again permitted to breath either oxygen or air, the biochemical and neurologic events are recapitulated, and all within a moment or two. The whole performance can be explained by the successive deprivation and restoration of oxygen to the brain.

A clear distinction between the action of the two anoxiants—nitrogen inhalation and cyanide poisoning—is revealed by an analysis of cerebral blood samples. In anoxic anoxia, or in nitrogen inhalation, the oxygen content of the arterial blood is greatly reduced; in histotoxic anoxia, or cyanide poisoning, venous blood is highly oxygenated. In both conditions the cerebral AVO_2 difference is reduced.

B. *Convulsants*

The convulsants used therapeutically are included among the drugs and procedures which diminish brain metabolism, and in this section we propose to explain why they have been so classified. Our data have been gathered from patients subjected to convulsive therapies for mental diseases.

Metrazol. The modern advent of convulsive therapy began with von Meduna's (730) use of camphor and metrazol, but since that time camphor has been discarded because of the uncertainty of its action. Metrazol, more widely used, is injected into the antebrachial vein and the patient undergoes a series of clinical manifestations: a short period of mild clonic movements followed by a violent tonic spasm, beginning with a gaping mouth and immediately succeeded by a rigid extension of the extremities. During this time respiration ceases, and respiratory movements remain in abeyance throughout the next clonic phase. The latter is the longest phase of the convulsive episode and is marked by violent rhythmic jerkings of the body musculature. The skin which exhibited a pallor at the beginning of the convulsion assumes a livid cyanosis, gathering intensity as the clonic phase progresses. When the convulsive movements cease, respiration is re-initiated and the skin assumes its natural coloring. During most of the convulsion the patient is unconscious, regaining contact with his environment a few minutes after the convulsion has subsided.

In a group of patients receiving this metrazol convulsive therapy, samples of arterial blood were drawn and in all instances the oxygen content was reduced (496). A decreased saturation of hemoglobin to 50 per cent or less was observed during some of these convulsions. With such a drop in oxygen, the pressure in the arterial blood may fall from an original value of 95–100 mm/Hg to 25–30 mm/Hg. The volume of oxygen entering the brain will therefore be diminished. This fall in oxygen content of the arterial blood is caused by the violent seizures which interrupt respiratory movements. Proof of this effect of the spasms on respiration is afforded when the seizures are eliminated by employing a paralyzing drug like curare, in which case, the oxygen content of the arterial blood can be maintained at the normal level if artificial respiration is given (663).

Several modifications of the metrazol therapy have been introduced. Fabing (301) anesthetizes his patients with nitrous oxide before he injects metrazol, in this way eliminating the apprehension of the patient, and at the same time, intensifying the factor of anoxia. A further discussion of nitrous oxide and its effect on brain metabolism will be discussed in Chapter 12.

Two other modifications of metrazol have been introduced in an effort to avoid, or at least mitigate the untoward complications of dislocated joints and bone fractures. This has been accomplished by diminishing the severity of the muscular spasms. Curare has been used by Bennett (79) and erythroidin by Rosen, Cameron and Ziegler (833) both with success. Despite this constraint of the muscular spasms, an examination of the arterial blood of patients subjected to these modified treatments, discloses an equal, if not a greater depression of oxygen going to their brain (496). The combination of metrazol and erythroidin in adequate doses (Table 26) depresses the oxygen content of the arterial blood more than metrazol alone, whenever the combined treatment is followed by a postconvulsive apnea. Even though this apnea may be treated by an injection of prostigmine, until respiration is re-established the O_2 content of arterial blood may decrease to values below 1 vol. per cent, which of course cannot be withstood for a long time. Under these conditions the oxygen deprivation of the brain is much greater than in the unmodified metrazol convulsion.

TABLE 26

Effect of metrazol convulsions modified by erythroidin

NO. OF PATIENT	OXYGEN CONTENT	OXYGEN CAPACITY	HEMOGLOBIN SATURATION	TIME BLOOD WAS DRAWN IN RELATION TO CONVULSIONS
	vol. per cent	*vol. per cent*	*per cent*	
1	18.5	19.2	97	Before
	16.6	....	86	After
2	13.9	16.1	86	After
3	11.4	16.6	69	During
	6.2	....	38	Later
	8.9	....	53	After
4	8.0	17.5	46	During Clonic
	5.7	....	32	During Clonic
5	11.3	15.3	74	During Tonic
	4.6	....	30	During Clonic
	2.0	....	13	Postconvulsive apnea
6	1.7	16.4	10	Postconvulsive apnea
	0.7	....	4	Postconvulsive apnea
7	0.4	17.0	2	Postconvulsive apnea
	3.6	....	22	Immediately after prostigmine

The use of curare, a drug having a similar pharmacologic action to erythroidin, relieves the severity of convulsive spasms but also tends to produce apnea after the fit. Consequently, the arterial blood is desaturated (Table 27) (496). Patient 2 illustrates best a progressive decrease in the oxygen content of arterial blood as the convulsion comes to a climax.

Electroshock. There is another form of convulsive therapy in which cerebral AVO_2 difference was also determined. Cerletti and Bini (151) first introduced this therapy because of its advantages of easier administration and a finer regulation of dosage. The treatment consists of applying an electrical current to the head, thus inducing epileptoid convulsions which resemble those elicited by metrazol, except perhaps for a greater frequency of postconvulsive apnea as also occurs in the metrazol treatments modified by the use of either curare or erythroidin. Table 28 contains results on the oxygen content of the arterial blood of 10 patients receiving the treatment (496). It is seen that both in the incomplete or

TABLE 27

Effect of metrazol convulsions modified by curare

PATIENT NO.	OXYGEN CONTENT	OXYGEN CAPACITY	HEMOGLOBIN SATURATION	TIME BLOOD WAS DRAWN IN RELATION TO CONVULSIONS
	vol. per cent	vol. per cent	per cent	
1	17.7	18.6	95	Before
	12.9	....	69	During
2	17.5	18.4	95	Before
	16.1	....	87	Early
	15.1	....	82	Middle
	7.8	....	42	Late

TABLE 28

Effect of electroshock convulsions

PATIENT NO.	OXYGEN CONTENT	OXYGEN CAPACITY	HEMOGLOBIN SATURATION	REACTION	TIME BLOOD WAS DRAWN IN RELATION TO CONVULSIONS
	vol. per cent	vol. per cent	per cent		
1	13.8	14.9	91	Incomplete	Early
	11.6	....	78	Incomplete	Late
2	3.2	17.6	43	Incomplete	Late
3	6.9	17.1	40	Incomplete	Late
4	2.7	18.6	14	Major seizure	Late
5	9.6	....	..	Major seizure	Late
	4.4	....	..	Major seizure	Late
6	10.1	19.9	50	Major seizure	Middle
7	9.1	21.7	42	Major seizure	Late
	1.7	....	8	Major seizure	Postconvulsive apnea
8	16.8	17.5	91	Major seizure	Early
	11.5	....	60	Major seizure	Late
9	7.0	19.3	36	Major seizure	Middle
	4.5	....	23	Major seizure	Late
10	8.5	18.0	41	Major seizure	Late
2	13.1	16.3	80	Major seizure	Early
	10.8	....	67	Major seizure	Late
7	6.7	21.3	32	Major seizure	Late
	17.4	....	80	Major seizure	After

subconvulsive reaction and in the major seizure or convulsive episode, the oxygen content is depressed and reaches its lowest point in the period of postconvulsive apnea.

The oxygen pressure within the brain during convulsions was first studied by Davis, McCulloch, and Roseman (227). By completely paralyzing their animals with erythroidin while employing artificial respiration, they were able to circumvent any decline in arterial oxygen which might be caused by convulsive muscular activity. In this way the arterial oxygen supply was kept constant and any change in cerebral oxygen pressure was a key to how much oxygen the brain used. Seizures were induced electrically and also by intravenous injections of caffeine, aminophylline, coramine, metrazol, picrotoxin or strychnine. In all cases there was a marked fall in the oxygen pressure within the brain which tells us of anoxia in that organ, a condition brought about by the exalted (226) utilization of oxygen as measured by Schmidt, Kety and Pennes (856) as well as Davies and and Rémond (226). Even though the action of erythroidin prevented any decrease in arterial oxygen supply, still there was not enough oxygen to satisfy entirely the great demands of the brain under such extreme stimulation. After the fit, the oxygen pressure within the brain began to rise towards the preseizure level and temporarily surpassed it, a sign of impaired oxygen consumption. This secondary depression of cerebral oxidations is in accordance with the high degree of oxygen saturation in the cerebral venous return from a locus of epileptic convulsion as was observed by Penfield (785) and previously mentioned in Chapter 6, page 104. One of the first effects of the administration of a convulsant apparently is to stimulate cerebral functions to such an extent that the oxygen supply, though maintained constant by the use of erythroidin, becomes inadequate to satisfy the heightened demands of the overactive cerebral tissues. These observations of Davis, McCulloch and Roseman (227) and Schmidt, Kety and Pennes (856) bring further support to the conclusion of Himwich and Fazekas that all the shock therapies contain an element of cerebral metabolic depression (496).

With the failure of the oxygen supplies to support adequately the induced convulsive activity of the brain its anaerobic sources of energy are tapped. Evidence for recourse to anaerobic stores was obtained on dogs immobilized with erythroidin and maintained by artificial respiration. Despite the excellent oxygenation of their arterial blood lactate accumulated and phosphocreatin broke down within the brain (917). In cats, similarly treated, the invasion of the anaerobic deposits went even further for not only did lactate accrue and phosphocreatin, an energy-rich phosphate substance, undergo depletion but another energy-rich phosphate compound, adenosine triphosphate, was diminished and after brain glycogen was impaired (611). It is not known whether the human beings paralyzed by erythroidin and artificially ventilated would exhibit the more moderate reaction of the dog or the more severe one of the cat. But the convulsing psychotic patient is subjected to a grave decrease in arterial oxygen (496) just at the time when his energy turnover is maximal. Even in a nonconvulsing individual a brief period of anoxemia evokes an increase of lactate while inorganic phosphate rises at the expense of phosphocreatin (916). The coupling of the curtailment in the oxygen available to the brain with the excessive cerebral requirements would therefore make for more serious inroads into the anaerobic resources of that organ. On this basis inhalation of nitrogen or injection of cyanide should be less taxing to the anaerobic cerebral mechanisms of the patient than convulsions induced by such stimulants as metrazol or an electric current.

The injection of thiopental before the application of the convulsant is ameliorative because the barbiturate limits the depletion of energy-rich phosphate bonds within the brain (656a) and perhaps this is the reason for the diminution in the severity of the muscular hyperactivity (see Chapter 13, page 365). Even though the brain with the rest of the body is further handicapped by an anoxemic factor, aggravated by the thiopental (292), yet it might be expected that this oxygen lack may be more than compensated for by a reduction in the tremendous expenditure of energy which usually accompanies convulsions for C.M.R. is inhibited (528) and the utilization of energy-rich phosphate bonds is opposed by that drug (656a). Clinically the pre-convulsant administration of thiopental serves to allay the apprehension of the patient but it intensifies somewhat the post-convulsant depression. This depressant or soporific action is prolonged when a longer acting barbiturate, like pentobarbital is injected after the fit is completed.

It is not to be supposed that the tremendous intrinsic utilization of oxygen, as well as the cutting off of the oxygen supplies, is limited to *induced* convulsions. The same effects on brain metabolism probably occur irrespective of the cause of the convulsions—in epilepsy, meningitis, uremia and gastro-intestinal disturbances in children. It is well to remember that convulsions induced for therapeutic reasons are relatively controllable and of short duration and evidence of brain destruction is controversial.

Thirteen patients with depression who received the electroshock therapy were examined for cerebral AVO_2 difference before treatment was instituted and after it was completed. Their average AVO_2 difference before treatment was 6.6 vol. per cent and afterwards 6.1 vol. per cent (141). Since the average cerebral AVO_2 difference was not significantly changed as a result of the therapy, if there are any alterations in the brain produced by electroshock, they are not of sufficient magnitude to be detected by this method of study. It is interesting that electroencephalographic changes wrought by this treatment are largely transitory (781) and in a control series of experiments on monkeys histologic studies of the brain did not reveal any changes that were different from those obtained in other monkeys not subjected to electroshock (56). However, in status epilepticus or prolonged convulsions due to any cause, a protracted deprivation of oxygen will produce cerebral damage (see Chapter 10).

As a concluding point, it might be added that though all the therapeutic procedures discussed in this section involve a factor of anoxia, the convulsants and anoxiants each have their characteristic pathogenesis. In general, all anoxic conditions are due to an imbalance between supply and utilization of oxygen. Whether the supply of oxygen becomes insufficient or whether the utilization of oxygen is excessive depends upon the drug or procedure responsible for the anoxia. If a physician wishes to use an *anoxiant* form of therapy, he will know that the anoxia of his patient is created by a niggardly supply of oxygen. Or, if the patient has been injected with a *convulsant* drug, the physician may look to an excessive cerebral consumption of oxygen as the primary cause of the anoxic condition. In passing, it should be said that the stimulating effect of the convulsants on the central nervous system produces greater muscular activity than do the anoxiants. It is the convulsants, rather than the anoxiants, which sometimes cause dislocations and fractures.

New convulsant drugs. One group of convulsant drugs depends for its activity on the inhibition of cholinesterase and consequent accumulation of acetylcholine. Though the anticholinesterases are employed therapeutically in a variety of conditions: glaucoma, paralytic ileus, atony of the urinary bladder and myasthenia gravis, yet in large doses they may produce convulsions. Eserine (physostigmine) and prostigmine, which in small amounts accentuate muscarinic parasympathetic activities, such as pupillary constriction, cardiac slowing, urinary bladder contraction and gastro-intestinal stimulation, in toxic doses yield nicotinic responses, fibrillary twitchings and other uncoordinated muscular movements as the neuromyal junction becomes hyperexcitable. In addition to these peripheral actions the central nervous system is stimulated to such a point that convulsions occur. Di-isopropyl fluorophosphate (DFP) is another member of this group of convulsant drugs (342) but instead of inhibiting cholinesterase in a reversible manner, as for example eserine does, the inactivation appears to be irreversible, recovery from DFP depending in large part on the production of new cholinesterase in the body. If eserine is administered just prior to DFP, the latter deprived of its point of attack on cholinesterase by the eserine, fails to combine with that enzyme and is eliminated from the body before it can exert its irreversible effects (616, 622). The treatment for an overdose of this drug requires the control of all its manifestations. The visceral responses to DFP may be managed by atropine sulfate, the peripheral muscular by magnesium sulfate and those on the central nervous system by barbiturate, atropine (727, 751), trimethadione (487) and some antihistamines including Dramamine, Benadryl, Phenergan and Lergigan (286, 564a).

Among the new convulsant drugs which do not exert their primary effect on cholinesterase are the rodenticides, hexachlorocyclohexane (gammexane) and methyl fluoracetate (MFA) and the insecticide, 2,2 BIS (p-Chlorophenyl)-1,1,1 Trichloroethane (DDT). Because of the efficacy of these noxious substances they will be widely used in campaigns against pests. Though it is known that barbiturates symptomatically control the convulsions produced by these toxic agents a knowledge of their mode of action is necessary in order to discover specific antidotes to be used in the case of poisoning in man.

The nervous changes of dogs and cats induced by the intravenous injection of MFA include repeated tonic convulsions. In agreement with the tonic character of these fits rhythmic electric discharges are observed in subcortical areas: thalamus, hypothalamus and reticular formation of the pons. According to Ward (975) the cortical petit mal pattern occasionally seen (162) with fluoroacetate is only indirectly related to the phenomena observed in the subcortical structures, emphasizing the subcortical origin of the tonic contractions.

Following the intravenous administration of DDT emulsions into cats and monkeys characteristic periodic electrical manifestations are observed in the cerebral cortex and cerebellum. Fast waves appear in increasing frequency until electrical seizures, grand mal in character, supervene (208). A detailed description of the type of convulsions induced by gammexane still awaits accomplishment (726).

In regard to the action of MFA we have the clue of interference with brain metabolism due to inhibition of pyruvate (548) or acetate (62) oxidation. The oxidation of both these substances may be inhibited via a common pathway, the tricarboxylic acid cycle, since fluoroacetate may give rise to fluorocitrate and thus interfere with the further progress of the tricarboxylic acid cycle (see Chapter 5 Fig. 12) (273). Even less information is available for DDT and gammexane, but a correlation between metabolic electrical and clinical changes wrought by these poisons is a necessary step in establishing a basis for their effects in the body.

IV. SUMMARY

In this chapter the influence of therapeutic procedures on brain metabolism has been described in the hope that an understanding of the cerebral effects will aid in the proper use of these therapies. First were considered 2 procedures which raise the C.M.R.: fever therapy for general paresis and thyroid medication for cretinism. It has been shown in the case of fever therapy that the brain takes part in the general increase of metabolism which is impelled by high body temperatures, but that when a high temperature is prolonged, there is danger of destroying the cerebral tissues. During thyroid therapy C.M.R. rises, as does B.M.R. But unfortunately, in patients who had been cretins for some years, this increment of cerebral energy turnover only speeded up their psychologic activities, and did not improve them. Comparing the methods by which fever and thyroid therapies increase C.M.R., we saw that both have in common the ability to accelerate enzymatic activity, the former as a result of heightened temperature, the latter in response to a flood of nervous stimuli. In addition, the thyroid augments the concentration of enzymes in most organs. Whether or not such a direct effect applies to the brain is controversial.

The drugs which depress C.M.R. were divided into 2 groups: anoxiants and convulsants. Nitrogen and cyanide were classified as anoxiants. The inhalation of nitrogen displaces oxygen from the inspired air and prevents its entrance into the body. Brain metabolism therefore suffers from failure of the arterial oxygen supply. Cyanide impedes cerebral oxidations *not* by interfering with the transport of oxygen by the blood to the brain, but by interrupting its path of cellular oxidation at the cytochrome oxidase stage.

The convulsive therapies—injection of metrazol and the use of electroshock—produce cerebral anoxia in 2 ways: as a result of the stimulating effect of the metrazol (or electroshock) the demand for oxygen exceeds the supply, thus reducing the oxygen tension in the brain. The second factor promoting the anoxia is initiated as the respiratory movements are disrupted by the convulsion, preventing the oxygenation of the blood in the lungs and thus diminishing the oxygen supply. The additive effect of these two factors makes it probable that the cerebral anoxia would be more intense under a convulsive drug than with an anoxiant, since the former involves the combined action of both factors, while an anoxiant being relatively unhampered by convulsions is concerned for the most part with the oxygen supply to the brain.

PART II

Patterns of Nervous Activity

CHAPTER 10

THE SOMATIC[1] DIVISION OF THE CENTRAL NERVOUS SYSTEM:

Studied through the symptoms of hypoglycemia and acute anoxia

I. INTRODUCTION

A young school teacher had been a diabetic of some duration, thriving on regular doses of insulin. One day, she returned to her home at 6:30 p.m., behaving queerly probably because of the long interim since her lunch. Her family called a physician, who arrived 30 minutes later. By this time, the young woman was unconscious and in a state of violent convulsions. The physician, unable to obtain a urinary specimen, assumed the coma to be of a diabetic nature, and therefore injected 200 units of insulin during the night. The following morning her blood showed an alarmingly low concentration of sugar, and in a desperate attempt to raise it, the physician administered quantities of glucose. Although he succeeded in elevating the patient's blood sugar well above normal, it was of no avail. The woman died shortly (568).

A man 76 years old had been a diabetic for 5 years. Arriving at a friend's home after a long railroad journey in the late morning, he drove about the country, sight-seeing, and probably was without food several hours longer than usual. Just before lunch, he began acting queerly, and before long became violent, finally lapsing into unconsciousness. When he did not recover from small doses of glucose, the physician, mistaking him to be in a diabetic coma, administered a "good shot" of insulin. Death occurred five days later (568).

* * *

What are the symptoms of insulin coma? How is a physician to differentiate between a diabetic and an insulin hypoglycemic coma? The above deaths are only 2 of a vast number of similar cases, published and unpublished, which might easily have been prevented had the physician understood the symptoms of hypoglycemia. It is true that the mistreated diabetic, and the patient with an overdose of insulin are both in coma. But

---

[1] In employing the word "somatic" to describe the division of the central nervous system which controls the movements of the limbs, trunk and head, we are following the terminology of Tilney and Riley (944). Because this definition has been widely accepted by neurologists, neuroanatomists and neurophysiologists, we have retained it despite the fact that another interpretation of the word is associated with the body as a whole (skeletal muscle and viscera) in contrast with the mind.

at this point, the similarity between the two ceases. The history of a patient in diabetic coma (in contrast to hypoglycemic), shows that too much food has been ingested and too little insulin injected. Physical examination reveals that the skin is dry rather than moist, tremors are absent, the eyeballs are softer than normal, and blood sugar is too high, rather than too low. Sugar is profuse in the urine, while it is absent in hypoglycemia. A thorough knowledge of the symptoms in insulin hypoglycemic coma seems to be the best weapon for avoiding a mistaken diagnosis.

Until recently, our understanding of the symptoms attending hypoglycemic coma was confused and nebulous. Today, we have been able, guided by Hughlings Jackson's theory (558) on the phyletic organization of the central nervous system (see Chapter 1), to divide and segregate these symptoms into five separate and easily distinguishable phases. These may be said to apply to acute anoxia, as well, but for the sake of certain peculiarities, we have treated each separately.

Important as it is to recognize the symptoms of hypoglycemia, it is also advisable at the same time to apply this knowledge to many unanswered questions on the construction and operation of the central nervous system. We have, therefore, placed a special emphasis on the role which Hughlings Jackson's theory of phyletic regression may play in this analysis and arrangement of symptoms.

II. The five stages of symptoms in insulin hypoglycemia

The first favorable opportunity to study the symptoms of hypoglycemia was created by the discovery of insulin (39). The protean character of the clinical picture was then perceived. Many heterogeneous symptoms were recognized, and these were found to be referable directly to the central nervous system and to its effector organs—muscles and viscera. In the central nervous system the abnormalities were manifested by visual disorders, coma followed by amnesia, and behavioristic disturbances (1002): neurologic and psychotic in character and occasionally leading to delinquency and crime (1001, 7). Muscular responses took the form of weakness, tremors, tonic and clonic convulsions and paralysis. Visceral disturbances included salivation and hunger, nausea and vomiting, sweating and chilliness, and deviations from the normal heart rate.

The second step, the segregation of these symptoms into groups, was made possible by Sakel's insulin treatment of schizophrenics (845). To study the symptoms of hypoglycemia when a diabetic patient is precipitated into such a condition would be a precarious undertaking. A physician is not in a position to make studies at this crucial time, his one desire being to free the patient from danger. On the other hand, an excellent opportunity is afforded to study the symptoms when this condition is regularly produced as a therapeutic measure in the insulin hypoglycemia treatment of schizophrenia. There is no indication that these symptomatic changes take on a different form in the non-schizophrenic. It must be remembered that many of the symptoms are transient and some last but a short time. Moreover not all that are described below appear in any one hypoglycemic episode. Nevertheless by observing the time relationships between the symptoms, von Angyal (15), and especially Frostig (350), were able to show that they do not arise in a haphazard fashion but arrange themselves in symptom-complexes which follow a definite sequence. If the patient is given an adequate dose to bring on coma, the average length of time for the insulin treatment is from 4 to 5 hours, depending upon the magnitude of the dose, a small one delaying the coma and a large one hastening it, but nevertheless, the span of each phase is sufficiently long to lend itself to careful observation and study of the patient's behavior. In general, the symptoms seem to appear in constellations which, as a working hypothesis, may be said to be linked with the functional patterns of different levels of the neuraxis. As these symptom-groups are described, we notice a striking similarity to those which would arise if a series of successive sections were made through the various phyletic layers of the brain. The behavior resembles to some degree the focal symptoms of neurologic impairment of the layer in question. Of course, such a conception cannot receive a final stamp of approval until we are able to allocate each symptom to some special portion or portions of the brain.

A. *Cortical phase*

After the injection of insulin there is a latent period of about one-half hour before the first group of symptoms becomes evident. As the cortex is depressed by the hypoglycemia, the dominant pattern of human nervous activity loses its hold, and the fine balance between sensory stimulation and motor response in muscle and organs begins to break down. The first sign of this dissociation is an overactivity in the parasympathetic branch manifested by watery sweat, salivation and a slow heart rate, observed if the patient happens to go off quietly to sleep. More frequently, however, and especially if the patient is restless, or is stimulated by some act or movement of the attendants, the sympathetic signs of thick viscid perspiration and salivation assume prominence.[2] Muscular changes take the form of muscular relaxation, hypotonia and tremors, all symptoms of joint cortical and cerebellar origin (250). Visual disturbances develop, speech is slow, and the execution of voluntary muscular activity becomes more and more imperfect. All this is accompanied by a gradual clouding of consciousness. The patient's orientation as to time and place in which he lives

[2] For further analysis of autonomic changes, see Chapter 11.

becomes poor. He is inattentive, his speech is incoherent and his understanding of what is going on around him defective. Both perception and
thinking grow difficult as exemplified in the vague and incoherent response
to simple questions. These signs gradually become more marked as somnolence deepens, and are finally succeeded by complete loss of contact
with the surroundings. Sometimes a state of wild excitement marks the
end of the first stage.

B. *Subcortico-diencephalic phase*

Loss of contact may be regarded as the onset of coma and the beginning
of the second group of symptoms, which may be localized in the subcortico-
diencephalic portion of the brain. On watching the patient in the second
phase, we notice that the integration of the cortical level has broken down
completely, and in its place we find an entirely different interaction of the
sensory, motor and visceral phenomena. Sensations become less discrimi-
native, but more intense, and the motor reactions they evoke are correspondingly changed: reflex activity is more generalized and less adapted to
the specific stimulus, while the visceral component of this uncontrolled
motor behavior reaches its height in maximal sympathetic function.

Briefly reviewing this layer anatomically, we find that it is comprised
of the sensory thalamus, the visceral hypothalamus, and the motor striatum. This is not to imply that each of these functions is allocated to a
single cerebral area, and none other. Though the thalamus is closely associated with sensation, the hypothalamus also receives afferent impulses,
though these probably do not attain awareness. In a like manner, visceral
reflexes are resident not only in the hypothalamus, but also in the thalamus
and striatum (995). And motor patterns are mediated by other subcortical nuclear masses as well as the striate body. But, for simplicity in
the following presentation, these various components of neural activity in
the second layer will be referred to their most important center.

When the subcortical motor nuclei are freed from cortical influence,
stereotyped movements become apparent. These are primitive movements
such as involuntary grasping[3] and sucking, both of which may be spontaneous or may be elicited by placing an object either in the hand or between the lips of the patient. Other primitive movements which may appear
at this time are protrusion of the tongue, kissing, snarling and grimacing.
During this time the patient exhibits aimless motions known as "motor
restlessness". Fine myoclonic twitches of the small muscles are observed

[3] Kennedy (587) in discussing the changes of behavior observed in monkeys subjected to insulin hypoglycemia suggests that in this primate too the grasp reflex is
a sign of cortical release. Surgical extirpation of area 6 in monkey and lesions of that
area in man may lead to forced grasping (528a).

and if they become generalized and more vigorous, lightning-like in character, and seize the large muscles of the neck, shoulder and hip girdles, they assume a clonic form and may be the precursors of a fit. Rarely are these convulsions seen in hypoglycemia, but if they do appear, it is almost always in the second phase.

Any response to stimulation of the body throughout this period is like that to a painful protopathic stimulus since the fine discriminatory capacity of the cortex is lost in the second phase. Any irritation whatsoever evokes an abnormally large reaction whether in terms of brain waves (63) or muscular contractions. The release of the sensory thalamus from higher control is responsible for this hypersensitivity. For example, the normal response on stimulating the sole of the foot from the heel to the toe is flexion of all five toes and moderate retraction of the fore-leg. A patient in the second stage of hypoglycemia has lost his ability to localize a stimulation, and so he responds by withdrawing his whole leg and moving his body agitatedly as if in extreme pain.[4]

The release of the hypothalamus brings about signs of preponderance in the sympathetic nervous system expressed periodically in waves of activity as the heart rate accelerates, the pupils dilate and exophthalmos is observed, the eyeballs bulging from their sockets. The face is flushed and the body is drenched in viscid perspiration.[5] The pupils still react to light. When these motor, sensory and autonomic symptoms begin to disappear, it is a fairly accurate sign that the patient is entering the third phase of his episode.

Though convulsions are comparatively rare in the course of hypoglycemia and seldom are fatal, still they are sufficiently dramatic to warrant further description. They may be evoked by stimulating the patient who is hyperirritable at this time, but usually they are spontaneous. As we have said, they almost always occur in the second phase, and in that portion of the phase when the release of the medial thalamic nucleus, an end-station for protophathic sensitivity, and of the hypothalamus responsible for sympathetic hyperactivity, attains a climax. The actual convulsions may be preceded by conjugate deviation of the eyes and myoclonic twitchings as the

[4] The normal response, flexion of the 5 toes (29, 359), depends upon the integrity of the cortico-spinal tracts, starting from the cerebral cortex down to its endings in the motor nuclei of the spinal cord. A break in these paths results in extension of the great toe and fanning of the other 4 toes—the sign of Babinski.

[5] The old clinical observation that there are two kinds of sweat, viscid and watery, has received experimental support from Haimovici (434b). Though the sweat glands are innervated by fibers which are sympathetic from a morphological viewpoint, functionally they are not necessarily so. In addition to the well known cholinergic fibers, stimulated by pilocarpine and inhibited by atropine, there are also adrenergic ones excited by adrenaline and depressed by dibenamine.

subcortical nuclei are liberated. The twitchings then are intensified and become more generalized, finally spreading throughout the body musculature in clonic spasms to complete the convulsive episode. The latter lasts but a minute or two. Completely exhausted by the fit, the patient lies prostrate, with an ashen pallor, a thready pulse, and shallow breathing. The patient's coma is, as a rule, lightened after one of these convulsive fits (see Chapter 3, p. 29, for explanation), and before he can again relapse into deeper coma, the physician terminates the treatment by glucose, obviating any chance of a second convulsion. The great majority of patients is never seized by one of these fits, but instead passes directly to the third phase.

C. *Mesencephalic phase*

After the activities of the second "layer" have been completely suppressed, the third, or mesencephalic, layer is left in uninhibited control over the remaining active portions of the central nervous system. The primitive movements distinctive of the second phase cease, the patient is less responsive to external stimuli, but more so to those arising within the body itself. Signs of parasympathetic activity reappear as pupils contract and pulse slows down. This parasympathetic reign is repeatedly overcome, usually in response to stimulation of any kind when for short periods he, exhibits the strenuous spasms which are pathognomonic of the mesencephalic phase. During each spasm the integration of the somatic (skeletal muscle) and visceral activities of the third layer is seen by an accelerated heart rate, raised blood pressure and dilatation of the pupils accompanied by failure to react to light at each dilatation. The spasms are built upon a growing hypertonia and are of 2 types: tonic and torsion. In the tonic spasms agonistic and antagonistic muscles contract simultaneously, so that the limbs and trunk are held taut. This increased tonus is displayed in a postural distribution throughout the body, that is, in the upper extremities the flexors are dominant over the extensors so that the arms are partially crooked at the elbow, and in the remainder of the body the extensors are prepotent causing the trunk to be arched and the legs rigidly extended. The other motor symptom is the torsion spasm, where the body rotates along its own long axis as the shoulders and trunk twist on the pelvis and legs.

Sometimes towards the end of this phase the eyes no longer act in an associated manner but reveal movements independent of each other, a symptom explained by the fact that the midbrain houses the nuclei of the third and fourth nerves, which together with the sixth nerve control ocular movements. As the functions of the medial longitudinal bundle connecting these nuclei and the layers above the midbrain are struck out of operation, the unregulated activities of the extra-ocular movements are observed. An important sign of the inhibition which is lost as the upper portions of the brain are depressed is the Babinski, most easily but not exclusively elicited in the mesencephalic phase.

D. *Premyelencephalic phase*

We are aware that the premyelencephalic phase is approaching when the tonic spasms of the third phase give way to extensor spasms. In this type of spasm, the back and lower extremities are arched as in the tonic, but the difference is in the position of the arms. Instead of being flexed, as they were in the mesencephalic period, they gradually work themselves upward and backward until all four extremities are extended at full length. Like many spasms, these are recurrent and each one lasts but a short interval, at which time the visceral accompaniments of motor activitiy are seen. The pupils dilate and do not react to light and the pulse rate increases, as the sympathetic temporarily overcomes the parasympathetic. During the transition in postural tone from the tonic pattern to the extensor, the reflexes of Magnus and DeKleyn (702) may be elicited in this way: rotation of the head, whether spontaneous or passive, is accompanied by extensor spasms of the extremities on the side toward which the chin points, and flexor spasms of both extremities on the side towards which the back of the head turns, a fundamental figure and one often seen in interpretive dancing. In many ways, this whole fourth phase resembles the picture of decerebrate rigidity which Sherrington (874) studied on a brain sectioned through the mesencepahlon below the red nuclei but above the vestibular nuclei. All of these symptoms may therefore be allocated to the rostral portion of the medulla oblongata, hence, the term premyelencephalic. This stage, while not dangerous in itself, gives warning of the succeeding and perilous myelencephalic phase, and if the physician is inexperienced it is advisable to terminate the coma at this point.

E. *Myelencephalic phase*

The fifth stage, or myelencephalic, is risky and constitutes the most dangerous point in the coma. It should not be allowed to continue more than 15 minutes or so, in fact, the instant it is recognized, glucose could be administered. This phase is marked by a predominance of parasympathetic signs; the patient's respiration is shallow, his heart rate slow, his skin pale and bloodless and the pupils are pin-point, no longer reacting to light. His perspiration takes on a water consistency and the body temperature, which has been falling constantly after the end of the first phase, now reaches its lowest point (715). The patient's muscles are relaxed in extreme hypotonia, tendon jerks are depressed, and the corneal reflex is lost entirely.

TABLE 29

Table of hypoglycemic symptoms

GROUP	SYMPTOMS	LOCALIZATION
First	Perspiration Salivation Muscular relaxation (hypotonia) Fine tremor Somnolence Clouded consciousness Excitement	Depression of activities of cerebral hemispheres and cerebellum

Second	Loss of environmental contact
	
	Motor phenomena
	  Primitive movements
	  Forced grasping
	  Myoclonic twitchings
	  Clonic Spasms
	  Motor restlessness
	Sensory changes
	  Increased sensitivity to stimulation
	Changes in the autonomic nervous system
	  Increased sympathetic activity
	  Periodic exophthalmos
	  Dilatation of pupils; still react to light
	  Fast heart rate
	  Perspiration
	  Salivation
	  Flushing of the face
		Release of subcortico-diencephalon
		1. Subcortical motor nuclei
		
		2. Thalamus
		
		3. Hypothalamus

Third	Diminished sensitivity Tonic spasms Torsion spasms Independent movements of the eyes Babinski reflex	Release of midbrain
Fourth	Extensor spasms	Release of medulla 1. Upper 2. Lower

Fifth	Increased parasympathetic activity
	  Pin-point pupils
	  No light reaction
	  Slow heart rate
	  Pallor
	  Depressed respiration
	Muscular flaccidity
	  Depressed reflexes
	Loss of corneal reflex	

One gets the impression that all the life processes are slowed down to a minimum, but in truth it is actually the brain which is suffering most. Indeed, any further cerebral depression would not be compatible with a complete recovery (see Table 29 and Fig. 39).[6]

III. RECOVERY

Recovery from insulin coma follows as definite a plan as its development, but the symptoms occur in the reverse order. If glucose is administered at any time up to and including the first 15 minutes of the fifth phase, the

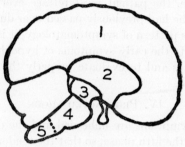

FIG. 39. Transverse section of brain revealing the five layers to which the symptoms of hypoglycemia have been allocated. (1) Cortex, the depression of which brings on the cortical phase in hypoglycemia; (2) the subcortico-diencephalon, responsible for the symptoms of release in the second phase; (3) the mesencephalon involving the symptoms of the third phase; (4) the pons and the rostral portion of the medulla (upper) and (3) the caudad portion of the medulla (lower), releasing the premyelencephalic and myelencephalic symptoms, respectively. The cerebellum is left unnumbered, for it has anatomic connections with all parts of the brain, and in its function has associations especially with the spinal cord, medulla and cerebral hemispheres. It seems logical that the many and varied symptoms of the cerebellum should be active in accordance with the metabolic state of their respective phyletic layers.

patient retraverses the hypoglycemic path, a process requiring only a few minutes for complete restoration. Once glucose is again available to support cerebral metabolism, the various phyletic layers are brought back into function, one by one, this time in a rostral direction. The vagotonic symptoms of the fifth phase immediately disappear. The extensor spasms of the fourth phase may last for a brief moment before the tonic spasms of the third phase are substituted in their place. The "motor restlessness" of the second stage follows directly and the clouded consciousness of the patient gradually clears as he regains contact with his environment.

The rate of awakening depends upon the method of administering the carbohydrate. When glucose is given by stomach tube, the awakening is

[6] Tyler (951) observes that it is necessary to maintain cats in the medullary phase of insulin shock to produce clinical symptoms of brain damage.

slow since a ten- to thirty-minute period is required for absorption. But if glucose is given intravenously, the patient rouses quickly, often while receiving the injection. A second factor influencing the rate of recovery is the depth and duration of the depression at the time the hypoglycemia is terminated. The later the termination, the greater the number of stages to be retraversed. For example, when sugar is given, deep in the second stage, primitive movements persist for a little while, and the patient may be drowsy and disoriented (symptoms of the first stage) before he returns to his habitual state. If termination takes place during the deep coma at the end of the fifth stage, the patient must retrace every step of the hypoglycemic road which he had previously passed over during the shock.[7]

With the aid of this pattern of symptomatology, it is not difficult for the physician to appreciate the early symptoms of hypoglycemia, to recognize and fear the later ones and to evaluate properly the prognosis of insulin coma.

IV. PROTRACTED SHOCK

If the medullary symptoms are unheeded and the depression is allowed to endure too long in the fifth phase, so that the tendon jerks are depressed and corneal reflexes disappear, recovery is delayed and perhaps may be incomplete, or even entirely impossible—depending upon the duration of this dangerous period. The delayed administration of carbohydrate may result in a recovery, which instead of taking place in a few minutes, may require hours or even days, and this is commonly called a protracted shock (353). Irrespective of the duration of this sequela, the path of symptoms to recovery is always the same, and just as constant as when the patient is falling into the coma, but in the opposite direction.

The symptoms of the patient in protracted shock denote depression of the formerly hyperactive medullary centers, and this despite the administration of carbohydrate. He continues to lie motionless but his slow pulse becomes fast and irregular, his pin-point pupils dilated, not reacting to light and his shallow respiration further depressed and Cheyne-Stokes in type. Then the extensor spasms return and are even more violent than in their original appearance during the fourth phase, but the previously observed integration between the somatic and autonomic divisions of the central nervous system fails. This failure is demonstrated by comparing the autonomic accompaniments of the motor symptoms of protracted

[7] The word "shock" is not used here in the sense of medical or surgical shock connoting collapse with fall of blood pressure and rapid heart rate, but rather with the meaning applied by Sakel who employs this term to describe profound hypoglycemia, and this use has been subsequently extended to the convulsive therapies, metrazol and electroshock, for mental disorders.

shock with those of the fourth phase. Instead of a pulse rate and blood pressure which grow faster and stronger with each extensor spasm only to return to lower levels between times, the pulse rate and blood pressure gradually fail as the violent muscular effort continues but both regain some strength after the spasm is over. If the lack of co-ordination between the somatic and autonomic divisions results from depression of the medullary visceral centers, then we may ascribe the fast heart rate and dilated pupils of protracted shock to impulses emanating from the inframedullary sympathetic centers in the cord and passing to the pupils and the heart through the sympathetic cervical ganglia. The color of the patient which becomes intensely cyanotic as his respiration is impeded by each paroxysm turns ashen-grey between spasms when he lies completely exhausted with shallow respiration and thready pulse. These symptoms of protracted shock were seen in a patient described in Chapter 8, p. 208, who succumbed in the fourth phase from exhaustion. This is not the rule, however, and usually the patients recover activity of the medullary autonomic centers and are able to withstand the extensor spasms to enter the third phase of tonic and torsion spasms.

After the patient passes through this phase successfully, the tonic and torsion spasms disappear and they are eventually replaced by the characteristic motor activity of the second phase. Localized mycolonic contractions appear, and various forms of primitive movements, forced grasping and sucking, may persevere for many hours or even days. The patient tosses and thrashes around the bed heedlessly throwing his arms and legs in a violent fashion. Arriving at the first stage, he sometimes has outbursts of wild excitement as though he were enraged, a sign which occurs at the borderline between absolute loss of contact and the clouded consciousness which finally leads to recovery. He may exist for some time in this disoriented haze, not quite able to execute a purposeful movement. The attending physician offers an object, but the patient cannot marshal his co-ordination to grasp it. Or, his perception may be dulled; he has not the faculty to interpret correctly what he hears and sees. When he has fully recovered, questioning reveals that he has complete amnesia for the entire episode.

Rarely is recovery so incomplete that neurologic symptoms take root and persist for a number of days. These may range from a facial palsy to a paralysis of large muscle groups, or impairment of any sensation governed by centers in the cerebral hemispheres (500). If the destruction of the brain is widespread, death will ensue despite any treatment. Such an outcome, fortunately, can be avoided through care and attention to the course of the coma.

V. OTHER CONDITIONS WHERE THE SAME HYPOGLYCEMIC
SYMPTOMS PREVAIL

The classification of hypoglycemic behavior into five progressive phases is a useful working hypothesis not only because it simplifies the clinical picture of the treatment, affords criteria for the depth of cerebral depression, and provides a rational basis for the prognosis of the coma, but also because this same pattern of symptoms applies to hypoglycemia irrespective of its cause. In Chapter 3 we presented the mechanisms involved in maintaining the level of blood sugar in our bodies, reviewed the function of the liver in supplying glucose to the blood stream, the role of insulin prompted by the vagus to accelerate the use of carbohydrate, and the complicated neuroendocrine organization which prevents an excessive fall in blood sugar. Keeping these points in mind, we may condense the causes for hypoglycemia into a tri-partite classification: (1) hepatic failure, (2) excessive insulin of endogenous origin, and (3) a defect in the general endocrine defense against hypoglycemia.

A. *Failure of the liver*

Since it is a function of the liver to release glucose continuously into the blood steam, it follows that failure of this organ should lead to hypoglycemia. Conn (182) reports a case of hepatogenic hypoglycemia in a laborer, aged 47, with periodic attacks of unconsciousness, occurring usually from 9 to 12 hours after his evening meal. The attacks were characterized by perspiration, drowsiness, and disorientation followed by unconsciousness with vomiting and incontinence of urine and feces. There were no convulsions. Feeding would end his attack almost at once, and after arousal, he was always unaware of his episode. The level of his blood sugar before breakfast was low and the glucose tolerance test curve prolonged. After various tests it was thought that this condition was due to malfunctioning of the liver. An X-ray film of the gall bladder revealed gall stones. The patient, therefore, underwent an operation to remove his gall bladder. During the operation the pancreas was examined carefully and found to be normal, but the liver was pale and granular, with surface nodules. The gall bladder was distended and contained several large stones and some thick yellow pus. Histologic examination of the minute structure of the liver revealed inflammation of the bile ducts, which in turn had poured their pus into the gall bladder. It is to this inflammatory process that the impaired liver function must be attributed. Proof for this interpretation came when the gall bladder was removed, and normal function of the liver returned in the postoperative period. It was apparent that the pre-operative prolongation of the glucose tolerance test was the fault of the liver in not being able to store glycogen, and this paucity of glycogen was also responsible for the hypoglycemia observed between meals.

Sometimes the liver is damaged so severely that the condition cannot be remedied and it seems reasonable to assume that if the patient succumbs, he has been permitted to pass through the fifth phase. This has been reported in patients with chloroform poisoning (908), or atrophy of the liver (811). In the laboratory hypoglycemia has also been observed when hepatic damage has been effected by phosphorus (1009), carbon tetrachloride (747), guanidine poisoning and yellow fever (965).

B. *Excessive insulin of endogenous origin*

The syndrome of hyperinsulinism as it appears spontaneously in the body was first described in 1924 by Harris (449). He pointed out that the symptoms are identical with those reported from the injection of overdoses of insulin in treating diabetes. The sweating and weakness which occur before mealtime or during the night belong to the first stage of hypoglycemia. In more severe cases the second stage is achieved with attacks of unconsciousness and convulsions. Occasionally, the entire gamut of symptoms may unfold, even protracted shock terminated by death. Hyperinsulinism may be caused by organic or functional ailments in the islands of Langerhans. The severity of the organic abnormalities may range from adenoma to carcinoma. Surprising enough, these diseased cells continue to secrete insulin but do so without the usual bodily regulation. Hence, insulin is liberated in excessive amounts and hypoglycemia must be contended with. Hanno and Banks (444) report a case of cancer of the pancreas in which the symptoms first noted were cold sweats accompanied by marked weakness in the early morning before the patient had a chance to breakfast. Though never unconscious, on one occasion the patient could not speak. His wife would give him milk and bread and he would feel much better. An operation revealed the cancerous condition of his pancreas. Glucose intravenously either every 4 hours as a 50 per cent solution, or continually as a 10 per cent infusion was necessary to prevent severe hypoglycemia. Nevertheless, the patient finally succumbed in shock. In 50 per cent of organic hyperinsulin cases resection of parts of the pathologic pancreas has relieved the condition (449).

Functional hyperinsulinism is an overactivity of the normal island cells. The Finneys (326) report a woman who had attacks in which she seemed dazed, could not concentrate or think clearly and occasionally would see double. The attacks at first would last but a few minutes with no aftereffects. They grew in intensity and frequency, becoming almost a daily occurrence, and usually before breakfast. At times she would scream and throw herself about violently as if in uncontrollable rage, (*apparently the excitement which we have catalogued at the deepest portion of the first phase*[8]). Other times the attack would unfold beyond the first phase, her eyes becoming fixed in a stare, (*may be interpreted as the conjugate deviation of the eyes which foretells a second-phase convulsion*[8]), and then her head and body beginning to jerk and roll from side to side. There was never any biting of the tongue nor any physical injury during an attack, nor any loss of sphincteric control. Memory of the attack was hazy, and she was left exhausted. It was discovered that such episodes might be aborted at any time if, at the first warning of their approach, food was taken. Blood sugars varied from 20 to 30 mg. per cent, sufficiently low to account for the attack. Even though the pancreas was proved normal on operation, about ⅔ was removed in an attempt to diminish the amount of insulin secreted. On the ninth post-operative day her blood sugar started to fall again and signs of another hypoglycemic attack were averted by the administration of glucose. According to the Finneys, the evidence pointed to a functional disorder of the pancreas since they could discover no apparent disturbance of the pituitary gland, adrenal glands or thyroid. In view of the apparent influence that the operation had upon the blood sugar level—for although it did not return to normal, it was considerably higher post-operatively than pre-operatively—the authors concluded that it would not be unreasonable to suppose they were dealing with a patient who had functional hyperinsulinism.

C. *Defect in the endocrine defense against hypoglycemia*

The organization of the neuroendocrine defense against hypoglycemia encompasses the sympatho-adrenaline apparatus, thyroid and posterior pituitary glands, all three accelerating the release of hepatic glucose to the blood stream. The anterior pituitary and adrenal cortex are also constituents of this mechanism. Their contribution to raise blood sugar is twofold: to accelerate the new formation of carbohydrate from protein, and at the same time to prevent the use of glucose by inhibiting the glucokinase reaction (see page 80, Chapter 5). Because several endocrine glands are involved in preventing hypoglycemia, it cannot be expected that the failure of only one of these glands should precipitate a fatal attack. The sympatho-adrenaline system, the chief defense against the emergency of a fall in blood sugar, is rarely rendered completely inactive by disease. In the laboratory, however, it is easy to demonstrate the fatal hypoglycemia which is incurred after injections of insulin in animals with one adrenal gland extirpated and the other denervated by cutting its splanchnic nerve (491). The same principle of this reduplication of defense is effective in preventing grave

---

[8] Italics are the author's.

hypoglycemia in myxedema. In patients with hypothyroidism post-absorptive blood sugars tend to be low, but the degree of hypoglycemia is mild and of little clinical importance (363). By the same token, lesions destructive of the posterior pituitary would probably not lead to a significant decline of blood sugar. But, when the cortex of *both* adrenal glands is completely destroyed, as occurs sometimes in Addison's disease, the hypoglycemia is more severe, and may even lead to decided personality changes, with unexplained bursts of anger and periods of amnesia and unreality (278). In this disease not only is the cortical effect to intensify the anterior pituitary inhibition of the glucokinase reaction lost, but also the ability to accelerate the formation of new carbohydrate from protein. Welty and Robertson (991) among other authors, cite two proved cases of Addison's disease which showed evidence of marked hypoglycemia with coma relieved by dextrose administration. One of these patients was a colored woman who had been complaining of weakness, loss of weight, and malaise for about a year. She consulted a physician because of what appeared to be a perverted appetite for sweets. He told her that her diet contained too much carbohydrate and advised her to take one consisting chiefly of vegetables, which she followed faithfully. The patient appeared to be well until one day when her family found her unconscious. Her blood sugar at this point was only 50 mg. per cent. Following an intravenous injection of glucose, the patient improved but only temporarily. She again became stuporous and died six days after admission to the hospital.

Another exception to this rule (that the multiplicity of defense prevents a grave hypoglycemia) may be found when the anterior pituitary gland is destroyed, as seen in Simmonds' disease. Mogensen (752) reports a female patient who presented this syndrome in typical form with premature senility, loss of weight, gonadal atrophy, and who had been nervous and irritable for some time. One morning about 5:30 a.m. she suddenly became restless and in time, delirious. Her condition was interpreted as an acute psychosis, though we would regard it as the "first-stage" excitement. She was given a sedative and grew quieter, but at 8:30 a.m. she was again restless and confused, and this time hypoglycemia was suspected. Her blood sugar was found to be only 38 mg. per cent and glucose by mouth relieved the attack. The next morning at the same hour she had a similar but more violent attack. Her blood sugar was 43 mg. per cent and she was relieved this time by glucose given intravenously. From then on she received food every 3 or 4 hours in the day and night, and in this manner succeeded in avoiding other attacks except for the milder forms of hypoglycemia, giddiness, headache with strange transient psychotic episodes sometimes with delusions. Apparently she never reached the second stage of hypoglycemic reaction.

In Simmonds' disease hypoglycemia is likely to be profound because more than one endocrine element is impaired. As we know, not only can the

TABLE 30

Comparison of the symptoms of hypoglycemia and acute anoxia

INSULIN SHOCK THERAPY SYMPTOMS	CEREBRAL LOCALIZATIONS	NITROGEN THERAPY SYMPTOMS
	First phase	
Perspiration Salivation Motor Excitement Clouded consciousness	Depression of cortical and and cerebellar activity	Salivation Motor Excitement Clouded consciousness Slight cyanosis
	Second phase	
Loss of consciousness Myoclonic twitchings Clonic spasms Motor restlessness Dilated pupils Tachycardia	Release of subcortico-diencephalic region	Loss of consciousness Myoclonic twitchings Clonic spasms Motor restlessness Dilated pupils Tachycardia
	Third phase	
Bradycardia giving way to tachycardia during spasms Tonic spasms Torsion spasms	Release of midbrain	Uninterrupted tachycardia Tonic spasms Torsion spasms
	Fourth phase	
Extensor spasms Dilated pupils Bradycardia except during spasms	Release of upper medulla oblongata	Extensor spasms Dilated pupils Tachycardia (uninterrupted)
	Fifth phase	
Bradycardia Respiratory depression	Release of lower medulla oblongata	Bradycardia Respiratory depression Marked cyanosis

Note that the symptoms of anoxia closely adhere to the hypoglycemic pattern except for the marked cyanosis and the fact that the heart rate is continually fast gathering momentum until the vagotonic symptom of the fifth phase manifests itself.

anterior pituitary depress the glucokinase reaction but it occupies a central position of influence over the other glands. It follows therefore that any destruction to this gland would naturally concern the welfare of other organs of the body, such as the thyroid and the adrenal cortex which will suffer a secondary degeneration. When the trophic hormones cease emanating from the anterior pituitary gland, and the thyrotrophic and corticotrophic hormones no longer maintain the function of their appropriate glands, the latter undergo regressive changes, and in general, the degree of hypoglycemia depends upon the extent of their regression. The basis upon which the entire endocrine defense rests is the anterior pituitary; therefore, any injury to this all-important organ would effect a more serious hypoglycemic condition than would result from malfunctioning of any other one gland, with the possible exception of the adrenal cortex.

VI. A COMPARISON OF ACUTE ANOXIA AND HYPOGLYCEMIA

Anoxia and hypoglycemia have in common the characteristic of decreasing the brain metabolism. During anoxia, the oxygen content of the arterial blood falls, severely reducing the volume of oxygen available to the brain (see Table 7, Chapter 7).

The neurologic changes of acute anoxia present a striking similarity to those of hypoglycemia both in the nature of the symptoms and in the order of their appearance (9). Many of the phenomena of hypoglycemia may be seen in anoxia, though they are more difficult to study in the latter because any form of acute anoxia progresses on a much faster time-scale. Despite the fleeting character of the neurological picture, it nevertheless points clearly to a descending depression of the neuraxis during anoxia and a retracing of this pathway on the subsequent respiration of air. The comparison of some of the outstanding symptoms of anoxia and hypoglycemia is presented in Table 30.

Just as the insulin treatment of schizophrenia presents the opportunity to study hypoglycemia, so the nitrogen therapy for the same disease similarly creates a favorable occasion to study the symptoms of acute anoxia (470).[9] The method of procedure in producing anoxia has been

[9] Several investigators have used the inhalation of anoxiant mixtures to make exploratory observations in the management of the psychoses and the psychoneuroses. Like the author and his co-workers (9, 72), Fogel and Gray (332) brought patients with schizophrenia to a state of deep anoxia but used nitrous oxide instead of nitrogen. Lehmann and Bos (642) diminished the severity of the treatment by limiting the depth of the anoxia to a level just beyond the loss of environmental contact. These workers were concerned with the symptomatic control of the manic patient and used 9% oxygen in nitrous oxide (see Chapter 12 for description of the pharmacologic action of nitrous oxide in the brain). The patients with depression treated by Gurevitch, Sumskaya and Khachaturean (431) presumably did not lose consciousness

described in Chapter 9, page 244. Among the first symptoms of anoxia is a motor excitement where the patient moves his hands, legs and head voluntarily; when the second stage commences and the patient has lost contact with his environment, fine myoclonic movements begin as twitchings appear about the face, usually in the corners of the mouth. These are followed quickly by clonic contractions of all four extremities for a period of 20 to 30 seconds. During this time the pupils are dilated and the gradually increasing tachycardia becomes evident. Violent convulsions are never seen during an anoxic episode brought about by the respiration of nitrogen, but brief, mild tonic and clonic seizures have been reported (836) when a temporary cerebral asphyxia is effected by arresting circulation to the brain, and these resemble the fit sometimes seen in the second stage of hypoglycemia.

In the third, or mesencephalic symptom-complex, these movements give way to tonic spasms and sometimes to torsion spasms. When the latter occur, they are usually preceded by conjugate deviation of the eyes. Finally the fourth, the premyelencephalic stage, is attained, and at this time the postural reflexes of Magnus and DeKleyn (702) may be elicited as in insulin coma. Characteristic of the fourth phase, spasms develop either emprosthotonic or opisthotonic in type. With the former, the legs are flexed at the hip joint and thrust upward from the table upon which the patient lies, and the arms extended forward with the hands in a tetani posture, all typical of a high decerebration in the human. This position may give way to opisthotonos, or extensor spasms, as the legs are extended at all joints and the arms are gradually brought back above the head, true to the picture of low decerebration. These spasms are an important clue of the fourth phase. Oxygen is withheld until this time. If the patient passes

---

for they were subjected to only a moderate deprivation of oxygen produced by the inhalation of oxygen-nitrogen mixtures.

Meduna (729) recently revived the use of high concentrations of carbon dioxide and employed them in the convulsant treatment of the psychoneuroses. The effect of carbon dioxide are complicated: physiologically, that substance accelerates cerebral blood flow while stimulating the respiratory centers. In higher concentrations however, pulmonary respiration and cellular metabolism are inhibited (66). Both actions are associated with the excess of carbon dioxide as well as the accompanying acidosis which together probably account for the rise of threshold for nervous activity as well as for the narcosis induced by the inhalation of that gas. In view of the metabolic inhibition exerted by carbon dixode the epileptiform convulsion may be regarded as a subcortical release phenomenon resulting from cortical depression. The pathologic neuromuscular activity moreover is facilitated by carbon dioxide which has the power to accelerate recovery after nervous activity. This restorative action makes for the continuation and repetition of the fit. Both the rise in threshold and the rapid recovery are based on the ability of carbon dioxide to increase the membrane potential of nerve (691).

beyond to the fifth phase with depression of the medullary centers, automatic respiration may cease, but it is easily restored by the physician conducting the treatment and no fatalities have been reported. When oxygen is again inspired, the patient recapitulates the same series of symptoms in an amazingly rapid succession, but not too fast to see that they are directly reversed, almost identical to a hypoglycemic awakening. Extensor spasms are replaced by tonic and torsion spasms and these are followed first by clonic and then by myoclonic twitchings just before contact with the environment is regained.[10]

An excellent study of a series of men revived from threatened asphyxial death reveals the same recapitulation of symptoms (923). One of these was a patient in a psychopathic hospital who succeeded in hanging himself, but remained suspended only from 5 to 10 minutes before he was freed from his position. He was found to be in complete respiratory arrest. Artificial respiration and stimulants were therefore administered until spontaneous respiration was reestablished. When examined a few hours later, the patient was unconscious, in profuse perspiration, and exhibited violent extensor spasms. The postural reflexes of Magnus and DeKleyn (702) were elicited. Then clonic convulsions developed and the grasp reflex was found to be active. The next day these symptoms had disappeared as improvement continued, but clouded consciousness and myoclonic twitchings were still present. He showed difficulty in articulation, and the words which he did manage to form were repeated over and over again. A period of excitement preceded the regaining of consciousness and there was amnesia of the entire episode. Ten days later the neurologic picture returned to normal.

This striking similarity between anoxic and hypoglycemic symptoms has as its common denominator a brain, which in both conditions is stripped of energy (480, 496). Hypoglycemia singles out the brain because of the place

---

[10] Another line of approach to mental disease, employing the principle of anoxia, consists in the intravenous injection of sodium cyanide (720a). The initial dose of .6 mg/kg is gradually increased until convulsions occur. The injection brings on hyperpnea, probably due to carotid body stimulation. Unconsciousness, a sign of the subcortico-diencephalic phase, is initiated during the latter part of the hyperpneic period. The mesencephalic flexion of the arms and their premyelencephalic extension are well developed as the clinical picture of decerebrate rigidity is produced: for opisthotonos is followed by flexion of the arms and extension of the legs, and finally both arms and legs exhibit strong tonic extension (672).

Whether the anoxia is produced by the inhalation of nitrogen gas or the injection of cyanide the cellular deprivation of oxygen must be sudden and profound in order to produce fits. When cyanide poisoning is brought about by the slow absorption of that substance, coma and death may supervene without manifestations of increased muscular activity (438). Similarly, the effects of chronic anoxia as seen for example in the decompensated cardiac patient do not include the convulsions resulting from acute anoxia.

occupied by carbohydrate in maintaining cerebral function. Anoxia makes no such qualitative distinction; anoxia affects every organ of the body to some extent, though its greatest quantitative insult is on the brain. This predilection of the brain for oxygen is made evident when circulation is interrupted even for a few seconds by a sudden fall in blood pressure, for unconsciousness rapidly supervenes. The reason for the sensitivity of the brain to anoxia is twofold, as far as we know: (1) the energy demands of the brain are large, larger even than those of the beating heart when the body is in repose. The heart consumes 10 per cent of the total basal oxygen requirement of the body while the brain may use as much as 18 per cent (Chapter 8) or more. The kindey, per gram of tissue, has an oxygen consumption higher than the brain, but the manifestations of anoxia most evident on inspection are those affecting the central nervous system. (2) Of less importance, but still a mentionable factor, is the small supply of cerebral glycogen, limiting the anaerobic production of energy (310). The glycogen content of the brain is somewhat less than 0.1 per cent (589, 164) while the heart is not so handicapped by anoxia because it can resort to anaerobic energy from a larger store of glycogen, 0.6 per cent (211). For these two reasons the brain is one of the organs most sensitive to anoxia.

The symptoms of hypoglycemia and anoxia bring to bear additional strength for the phyletic conception of the central nervous system proposed by Hughlings Jackson, and reviewed in Chapter 1. Using Jackson's terminology, we have witnessed the "dissolution" of the brain under the dissection scalpels of hypoglycemia and anoxia; at the termination of these treatments we have seen a resynthesis of this neural breakdown, in truth, a recapitulation of the "evolution" of the nervous system. It would seem that the anatomic construction and functional organization of the brain arise in an embryologic process consisting of five stages of accretions, each built upon its predecessor, and each exercising characteristic functions. The integrative action of the brain depends upon an ordered co-operation of these five layers. When this harmonious interplay is dissolved for want of cerebral energy, the release of the activities inherent in any given layer reveal the loss of the inhibitory influence emanating from the layer immediately above it. It is this inhibitory capacity which permits the exercise of finer discrimination in the higher layers. And when energy is restored we again see this phyletic organization in operation, this time in the opposite direction, as the brain regains its co-ordination and each lower section is again subjected to the inhibitory and reinforcing powers of its superior. It is this reinforcing quality which facilitates expression of a more or less primitive structure, when such an expression is useful to the organism. Top-most in this nervous scale, and over all other members, are the cerebrhemispheres, exercising the highest discrimination and regulating the motor activity of all sections beneath.

VII. THE RELATION OF OTHER FACTORS TO THE CLINICAL SYMPTOMS

A. *Blood sugar, oxygen consumption and the EEG during hypoglycemia*

We have shown that the symptoms of hypoglycemia and acute anoxia occur in a definite order. In an effort to determine why they are grouped so, further observations were made on these same schizophrenic patients subjected to hypoglycemia to determine blood sugar levels, cerebral oxygen utilization and the electrical activity of their brain. Each of these measurements was not done independently, but instead simultaneously and repeated at various intervals during the insulin therapy.

Blood sugar. During the first two hours after insulin was given, blood sugar falls (512) and during this time the patient's mind becomes increasingly clouded. Any temporary interruption of the downward course in blood sugar is accompanied by signs that the symptomatic progression has been halted and for the time being, is partially reversed. In the same manner, when the blood sugar continues to fall, the progress towards coma is again resumed. But once the low level is established (20 to 30 mg. per cent) towards the end of the first two hours, the minor variations in the glucose curve thereafter probably do not affect the conduct of the patient nor break up the succession of his symptoms. The consensus of opinion of most observers is that, except for the initial drop in blood sugar until the patient loses contact with his environment, there is little correlation between the symptoms of hypoglycemia and the amount of glucose in the blood. Since these studies did not offer an adequate explanation of the symptomatic enigma, additional work was done to ascertain the oxygen intake and the electrical potentials of the brain.

Oxygen consumption. The observations on the oxygen removed from the cerebral blood proved to have much more bearing in regard to explaining the march of the symptoms than did the glucose level. Blood was sampled from several patients (512) and the following averages calculated: before the patients received insulin, their oxygen intake was 6.8 vol. per cent. Two hours later when they had lost contact with their environment, the bloods revealed a tremendous drop in the oxygen utilization to 2.6 vol. per cent. It appears as though a great fall in cerebral metabolism is necessary before the second phyletic phase envelops the patient. Continuing our observations, we found that this figure was to fall even lower when the later phases ensued until an extreme value of 1.8 vol. per cent was observed just before glucose was injected. The relationship between the amount of oxygen the patient's brain can consume and the neurologic symptoms at each point along the coma is further demonstrated by the fact that the AVO₂ difference returned to 5.1 vol. per cent at the moment of awakening. Because fluctuations in cerebral blood flow during hypoglycemia are, for the main part, within the experimental error of the method,[11] the cerebral AVO₂ difference may be considered as an indicator of oxygen consumption, demonstrating that the brain uses less and less oxygen as the phyletic phases unfold.

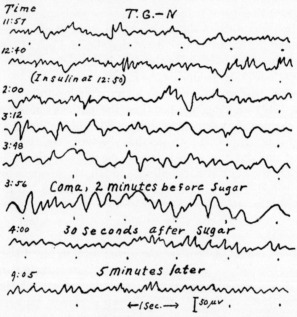

FIG. 40. Brain waves during insulin treatment. Note that the alpha waves become somewhat less rapid after the injection of insulin and are finally displaced by slow waves as the patient becomes comatose. Note also disappearance of slow waves immediately after sugar, and reappearance of alpha frequency.

The EEG. The brain waves, like the cerebral AVO₂ difference, are another reliable indicator of the hypoglycemic state of the patient. As can be seen from Figure 41 (530) long before the patient becomes comatose significant changes take place in the EEG as the waves become somewhat less rapid (512, 282). Our own observations disclosed that the rapid waves vanish approximately at the time when the functions of the cortex are completely suppressed and contact with the environment can no longer be maintained (508). The cessation of the alpha electrical rhythm has a fairly distinct endpoint. The clinical method for determining loss of contact has no such distinct break. By this method, it is customary for the physician to try to

[11] See Chapter 8 for observations on C.B.F. during hypoglycemia.

obtain an appropriate response to a stimulus—such as shaking the patient and calling him by name to see if it excites recognition. It is obvious that this or other clinical methods of ascertaining consciousness might be inaccurate by a margin of 15 to 30 minutes. If, however, we keep this margin

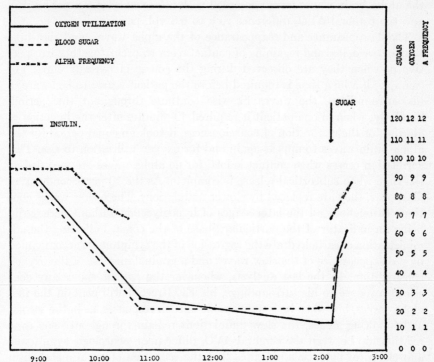

FIG. 41. The cerebral arterio-venous oxygen difference, blood sugar, and brain waves during insulin hypoglycemic treatment for schizophrenia. After insulin effect takes hold, the alpha frequency decreases, the same as cerebral arterio-venous oxygen difference and blood sugar. At the time when the alpha frequency has disappeared, the cerebral arterio-venous difference and blood sugar have fallen to a low level, and the patient is no longer in contact with the environment. During the subsequent period of hypoglycemic coma, the arterio-venous oxygen difference falls somewhat, and blood sugar remains low. When the treatment was terminated by the oral administration of sugar, the alpha waves reappeared, cerebral arterio-venous oxygen difference and blood sugar rose, and the patient aroused.

in mind, we can say that the disappearance of the 10 per second waves on the EEG is simultaneous with the lapse into unconsciousness.

Taking Figure 41 as a specific example (512), let us follow its pattern through and attempt to explain its significance in connection with the hypoglycemic symptoms. The patient starts with the pre-insulin frequency of 9.5 per second and an oxygen utilization of 9 vol. per cent, and when contact was lost the alpha brain potentials had disappeared and the oxygen intake had diminished to 2.8 vol. per cent. This value dropped even lower 3 hours later to 1.6 vol. per cent. Thirteen minutes after the coma was terminated by the administration of glucose, the patient roused and simultaneously the alpha brain waves were reinstated with a frequency of 8.8 per second, and the cerebral AVO_2 difference rose to 6.8 vol. per cent.

The disappearance and reappearance of the alpha waves, and the shuttling between loss and regaining of contact seem to occur together irrespective of when they are observed during the course of hypoglycemia. For example, if a long time is required before the patient ceases to be aware of his surroundings, the waves likewise continue throughout this period. Similarly, when in one patient it required 40 minutes after the injection of glucose for the restoration of consciousness, it took an equal period for the alpha brain waves to appear again and for oxygen utilization to rise. This correlation ceases when contact is lost, for no alpha waves are recorded at the time when subcortical release is complete. As the 10 per second waves disappear, they are replaced by slower undulations. These slow waves continue throughout all the later stages of hypoglycemia without necessarily being an indicator of the particular phase of the coma. Following the administration of carbohydrate the regression of the symptoms is accompanied by a disappearance of the slow waves and a gradual increase of the oxygen consumption. In the last analysis, whenever the patient shows any conscious response to his surroundings, his EEG record will contain the fast alpha waves, but when he is not capable of such responses, as in the second and following stages, the slow undulations remain throughout. The time relationship between the cerebral AVO_2 differences, neurologic symptoms, and electrical potentials indicates that the reduction of brain metabolism during hypoglycemia is a prime cause for the electrical pattern as well as for neurologic symptoms. It is true that for short periods there may be discrepancies between the metabolic rate of the central nervous system and its functional activities. Over long periods, however, as in the insulin treatment for schizophrenia, the correlation is close.

Patient M. W., 9/13/38 in Table 31 (508) tells the whole story of the interrelationship of the metabolic, electrical and neurological changes during hypoglycemia: as the cerebral AVO_2 difference declines from 7.4 vol. per cent to 3.3 vol. per cent, the fast electrical potentials starting at 9.7 per second and 9.9 per second ultimately disappear completely, to be replaced by the slow waves. At the same time the clinical features of the patient give evidence that his cerebral depression is progressing downward through the neuraxis. This particular patient had a spontaneous but temporary lightening of his neurological symptoms, and his record shows that the electrical activity of the slow waves fades as they are finally replaced by

TABLE 31

Temporal correlation of the hypoglycemic phases with the biochemical and electrical changes

TIME IN HRS.	PHASES	BLOOD SUGAR	AVO₂ DIFF.	ALPHA WAVES P.S.
		mg. per cent	vol. per cent	
	Cortical	75	7.4	9.7
1				9.9
				8.9
2				7.6
				6.7
				3.9
3	Subcortico-diencephalic			
				5.3
4		34	3.3	0
5	Mesencephalic			
6	Cortical (Spontaneous Awakening)	29	7.1	8.3
	Subcortical & Mesencephalic	26	1.7	5.5
7	Termination with glucose			

The cortical phase with clouding of consciousness takes place over a period of $2\frac{3}{4}$ hours. Simultaneous with loss of contact and initiation of the subcortico-diencephalic phase, motor symptoms develop: primitive movements, forced grasping, myoclonic twitchings and sympathetic overactivity. The mesencephalic phase is marked by tonic spasms at $4\frac{1}{2}$ hours. At 5 hours they are the most prominent feature and at this time the sign of Babinski is elicited. After $5\frac{1}{4}$ hours the patient commences to show signs of a spontaneous regression of symptoms. The Babinski disappears, tonic phenomena give way to hypotonia (subcortico-diencephalic) and then partial consciousness is regained (cortical). The patient responds to questions, though his answers are not appropriate. The spontaneous awakening lasts for $\frac{3}{4}$ hour, then contact is again lost and soon thereafter the subcortical motor symptoms again reappear, followed by the tonic spasms and the Babinski. After $7\frac{1}{2}$ hours the treatment is terminated by tube feeding.

the alpha waves with a rate of 8.3 per second. At the same time, the AVO_2 difference returned practically to the pre-insulin value, 7.1 vol. per cent. The point is, therefore, that whether or not glucose is administered, the alpha waves only return when contact with the environment is regained. This patient, being without the benefit of injected gluocose, again fell into a subsequent deepening of the coma, and this was paralleled by a second disappearance of the alpha waves and a drop in his cerebral metabolic activity.

The exact temporal coincidence in the behavior of the patient and the alterations of his electrical activity during insulin coma permit us to conclude that at each point of the hypoglycemic journey, the oxygen utilized by the brain, or in other words the energy released by that organ, is the basic answer to both the behavioristic and electrical activities. The causal order of events in a hypoglycemic coma may therefore be outlined as follows:

1. Low blood sugar
2. Decreasing of the metabolism in the brain
3. Manifestations of waning cerebral function
   a. Electrical activity
   b. Clinical symptoms

B. *Oxygen consumption and the EEG during anoxia*

In Chapter 9 a detailed description was given of the changes in cerebral AVO_2 difference wrought by the substitution of some other gas for the oxygen of the inspired air. It is true that when nitrous oxide was substituted for the oxygen, the effects were not those of anoxia alone because this gas possesses a specific pharmacologic action. However, when carbon monoxide was used, or nitrogen, in place of the oxygen, the results as far as the central nervous system was concerned were to the greatest extent produced by lack of oxygen. No matter which of these gases is used, however, the cerebral AVO_2 difference falls into the same general pattern, namely a depression. The oxygen removed from the cerebral blood becomes so small as to be within the experimental error of the method so that irrespective of any acceleration of cerebral blood flow, the oxygen intake of the brain is profoundly cut down. Thus, the neurologic symptoms of acute anoxia may be ascribed to the same underlying cause as the symptoms of hypoglycemia: the brain is struggling under an energy deficit.

Since with anoxia and hypoglycemia cerebral metabolic rate is depressed, it would be surprising if the behavioristic changes were not the same, or nearly the same, in both conditions. And our review of their respective symptoms also revealed a striking similarity both in the precipitation of the condition and in the recovery therefrom. Indeed, if we could graduate the progressive diminution of brain metabolism in anoxia as finely as we do in hypoglycemia, we would expect to find similar clinical pictures in both conditions.

The EEG. The congruity between hypoglycemia and acute anoxia is not limited to clinical manifestations of cerebral activity, but also extends to the EEG. It has been well established that when the oxygen supply to the brain is shut off, the electrical activity suddenly slows, the faster waves

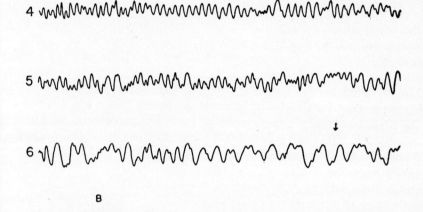

FIG. 42. Brain waves of patient under low oxygen tension, breathing from the closed system with carbon dioxide absorbed. Record No. 4 shows $10\frac{1}{2}$ per second activity though patient has been gradually depleting the oxygen supply. In No. 5 the dominating frequency is 7 per second. In No. 6 all activity has slowed down to 2 to 4 per second. At the arrow the patient became unconscious. Shortly thereafter the nose clamp was removed and the patient began to breathe room air. Strip 7 shows that for 3 seconds the slow waves persist, and directly afterwards, the patient regains consciousness. Remainder of strip 7 pictures the $10\frac{1}{2}$ per second activity.

(Partial record taken from Atlas of Encephalography, Gibbs and Gibbs, Lew A. Cummings, Co., Cambridge, Mass., 1941, page 141).

giving way to the slower ones, as in hypoglycemia (396). Anoxia is more difficult to manage from a technical point of view and for that reason the electrical activity may cease entirely, whereas such a contingency is easily avoided in hypoglycemia if the signs of the fourth and fifth phases are heeded. Just before the record is extinguished in anoxia, there may be seizure-like disturbances foretelling the possibility of a convulsion (9, 836). When the normal oxygen supply is reestablished, first the slow waves reappear and eventually the alpha ones take over until a normal record is obtained. As described in Chapter 6, the work of Gibbs *et al* (397) has demonstrated that the slow potentials arising in anoxia are probably conditioned by the elimination of carbon dioxide due to overbreathing. When 5 per cent carbon dioxide is added to an anoxic mixture containing but 2 per cent oxygen, slow waves do not appear on the EEG. The slow waves exerted in hypoglycemia, however, are probably unassociated with the elimination of carbon dioxide.

VIII. Differential sensitivity of cerebral regions to hypoglycemia and acute anoxia

As discussed in Chapter 1 the central nervous system is so organized that the new portions contain delicate analyzers of sensation and centers for fine co-ordination of neural activities. This high degree of integration is permitted to express itself because of the cortical impulses which either inhibit or reinforce the activities of the older portions of the brain. We have referred to this conception as Hughlings Jackson's theory (558). Strong support for the clinical observation that inhibition is a function of the brain has been afforded by the physiological experiments of Marion Hines (528a). Her work revealed that stimulation of a strip of cortex in the foreward zone of the motor area (area 4s) resulted in inhibition of maintained extension of a limb. Thus stimulation of this part of the cerebral cortex stops activity supported by other portions of the CNS. Moreover extirpation of 4s produces spasticity, exaggerated extensor tone and brisk reflexes. This spasticity however is short-lived and effects chiefly the proximal joints. With the removal of additional extrapyramidal injections by extirpation of areas 4 and 6[12] the spasticity becomes enduring and involves all the joints of the limb. This power of inhibition is not limited to the highest phyletic layer but is exhibited by subcortical structures and therefore applies to the lower levels as well. As will be described below not only inhibitory areas but also facilitory ones are found in the brain (see Fig. 43) and both types bring their influence to bear and modulate that of the motor cortex, executed through the pyramidal tracts upon the anterior horn cells. Starting with the cortex McCulloch, Graf and Magoun (721) have traced impulses down the brainstem to the medulla oblongata and suggest that bulbar centers constitute a relay in the inhibitory extrapyramidal system. The bulbar areas (703) in turn send projections, in the ventral part of the cord, which transmit inhibitory influences on a wide variety of motor performance. Suppressor fibres arising in the cerebellar cortex, like those of the cerebral hemispheres, form synapses in the bulbar reticular formation, thus bringing two groups of inhibitory influences to bear on the anterior horn cells (889). See Fig. 43 (4).

With decortication the entire subcortex is freed from the most cephalad suppressor constraint. But the clinical picture as in insulin hypoglycemia

---

[12] The part played by other suppressor areas (262) is being re-examined (1042).

emphasizes the release of the highest parts remaining in function. The mechanism by which these portions of the brain assume a regulatory role over the rest of the neuraxis during the stages of hypoglycemia and acute anoxia is not entirely understood. But suggestions arising from clinico-pathologic studies emanating from the Vogts' laboratory (457) as well as from physiologic experiments (261) indicate that in addition to suppressor areas in the cerebral hemispheres, the cerebellum, and the medulla, other subcortical regions may exert inhibitory powers and thus in turn regulate lower structures. As an example Mettler and his co-workers (732) have demonstrated that excitation of the caudate nucleus or of the putamen inhibits movement induced by cortical stimulation. In Fig. 43 the series of suppressor (−) centers influencing the phenomenon of spasticity is presented.

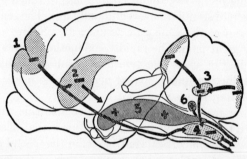

FIG. 43. Reconstruction of the cat's brain showing the suppressor (−) and facili-tatory (+) systems concerned in spasticity. Suppressor pathways are (1) cortico-bulbo-reticular, (2) caudato—spinal, (3) cerebello-reticular and (4) reticulo-spinal serving as a final common path for cortical and cerebellar suppressor areas. Facilitatory pathways are (5) reticulo-spinal and (6) vestibulo-spinal (667).

This figure has been included because it illustrates a portion of the chain of suppressor areas. Thus, after midbrain transection, the loss of the in-hibitory function, caused by a cessation of the impulses from the suprabul-bar suppressor areas to the bulbar suppressor region, is expressed in the phenomena of decerebrate rigidity (974). Another factor to be considered in the production of this type of rigidity is the continued function of facilitatory sites (820, 667) which receive afferent impulses from the cranial nerves and cord. See Fig. 43 (5) and (6). If this viewpoint is ac-cepted normal cortically induced movements are subjected to two opposing groups of influences: inhibitory and facilitatory. But in any case the point to be emphasized is that suppressor modifications exerted continuously, though of varying intensities, emanate from different levels of the neuraxis to control and regulate bodily movements. This phenomenon may be closely allied with that named by Cannon as the "Law of Denervation" (147). He states that when one unit in a series of neurones is inactivated, the subsequent neurone becomes more sensitive to stimulation. In Cannon's observations the stimuli are limited to those of a chemical nature. Another aspect of this phenomenon is observed in the cord. Van Harreveld and Marmont (445) present evidence for the existence of a mechanism which normally depresses the reflex excitability of the isolated cord of a spinal animal. Increased reflex excitability ensues in cats after recovery of the spinal cord from periods of asphyxia. These investigators conclude that the hyperactivity after asphyxia is due to the release of these spinal reflexes from a mechanism normally depressing them and that the neurones responsible for this inhibiting mechanism are more sensitive to asphyxia than are the other reflexes. A similar hierarchy is observed in peripheral nerves (173). Following the application of a tourniquet to a limb, asphyxiating its nerves, the usual response to touch—awareness of a localized and discrete stimulation—is gradually lost. The sensation becomes more indefinite, but at the same time assumes an affective character, being accompanied by great pain. The rapidly conducting nerves responsible for the fine discrimination cease function as a result of asphyxia before the older, slower-conducting unmyelinated nerves which mediate the affective impulses. The latter fibers are more resistant to asphyxia presumably because of a lower metabolic rate. Very much like this transition from a highly specialized to a primitive type of sensation is that observed when the thalamus is released from cortical control, i.e. in the second phase of insulin hypoglycemia. The resemblance between asphyxia of the leg and release of the thalamus becomes clear when we recall that the lateral spino-thalamic fibers carrying primitive, or protopathic pain terminate in the midline nuclei of the thalamus, while those fibers mediating epicritic, or finer sensory discriminations travel on to the cerebral hemispheres, using the thalamus only as a relay station. In both instances one and the same mechanism is affected. Both depress the epicritic pathways, but each does so in a different place of action. The tourniquet interferes with the carrying of these impulses in the nerves of the lower extremity, while hypoglycemia depresses the centers for accurate localization in the cerebral hemispheres. To what basic factor can we attribute this loss of the highly specialized, phyletically newer elements at a time when the older and less highly specialized parts are still carrying on?

It would seem that the symptoms observed in the various stages of hypoglycemia can best be explained by the depression of these phyletic layers, starting from the cerebral hemispheres and working down to the medulla oblongata. This subject of localizing each symptom to a specific area of the brain has been treated by Dr. Frostig in his forthcoming book on *The Insulin Treatment of Mental Disorders* (350). He admits that this "phyletic interpretation of the synchronous and successive syndromes is, of course, subject to serious challenge". Dr. Frostig is conscious, himself, of many weaknesses in the theory, but nevertheless, "the more one ponders the evidence the more the conviction grows that the most economical and adequate theory to account for the findings to date is expressed in the formula of phyletic regression, even if all facts do not fit perfectly into the scheme." From this point of view, then, we may conclude for the present that the five stages in the picture of insulin hypoglycemia, or any

TABLE 32

Glycogen content (mg.%) of parts of the central nervous system of hypoglycemic dogs

NO. OF EXPER.	CAUDATE	CORPORA QUADRI-GEMMINA	CEREBRAL GREY	THALA-MUS	CERE-BELLUM	MEDULLA	CORD
Hypoglycemia							
1.	8	26	56	45	40	35	46
2.	12	28	33	40	32	26	14
3.	8	32	21	27	33	24	14
4.	1	8	16	8	30	49	122
5.	20	0	11	18	18	36	45
6.	12	13	19	20	8	19	16
7.	6	15	10	8	1	31	43
8.	0	0	2	0	1	31	32
9.	0	2	6	0	6	13	26
Normal							
Aver.	58	50	73	62	35	37	29
Range	44–71	37–60	45–108	41–68	23–46	21–47	15–31

The observations of nine experiments are presented in the table. A heavy line has been drawn to separate the glycogen contents of the animals into two divisions. The values to the left of the heavy line are significantly lower than the lowest values for the normal range for that same part, while those to the right are not significantly lower than the normal (166). In general the upper parts of the brain lose their glycogen deposits before the lower areas are depleted.

other kind of hypoglycemia or acute anoxia, represent the dominant activities of five phyletic cerebral layers.

In hypoglycemia when the brain is deprived of its carbohydrate supply from the blood, it must draw upon its own glycogen stores to support cerebral energy. It is therefore significant that in dogs subjected to insulin hypoglycemia the various parts of the brain are depleted of their glycogen in accordance with a pattern which in general proceeds from the newer to the older parts of the brain (166) (Table 32). If a similar phenomenon occurs in man, we can see how the exhaustion of this only remaining source of cerebral energy may produce the step-wise regression in the clinical picture.

Even if phyletic regression does reveal the design of symptomatology, it is still another matter to determine *why* the symptoms obey such a strict routine of action. If the youngest and most recent additions to the brain should possess the highest metabolic rate, then we would expect to observe just such an order as we have described throughout this chapter, since the regions most active metabolically would naturally fall out first should their energy be withdrawn. The next step in our evaluation must therefore be an examination of the metabolic rate in each section of the brain in an effort to determine whether or not they do fall into an orderly fashion.

Remembering that metabolic activities may be probed either *in vivo* or *in vitro*, we will investigate our problem by both of these methods. To study the metabolic activities of the brain *in vitro* involves the *intrinsic* rate of the tissues deprived of their normal physiologic functions, while observation of the intact human or animal has the advantage of combining the *intrinsic* energy demands with the additional energy required for carrying out nervous functions. If the various divisions of the brain possess diverse energy requirements, it may be expected that they would not suffer equally during hypoglycemia. The regions with the highest oxygen consumption, and therefore, greatest demand for carbohydrate, should be most sensitive.

A. *Studies on excised tissues*

The earliest study of metabolic rates in the brain was done in 1917 by MacArthur and Jones (698) who reported that the cerebral components of various species respire at different rates and in the following order: cerebral hemispheres, cerebellum, midbrain, medulla, corpus callosum, spinal cord, and nerve. These early findings have since then been confirmed in principle, if not in detail, as a result of the great impetus given to the study of excised tissues by the improved methods of Warburg. A similar order of respiration was noted by Dixon and Meyer (244) for the grey matter of ox brain, except that the cerebellum exhibited the greatest oxygen utilization. (The largest portion of the cerebellum, functionally connected with the cerebral hemispheres, develops late in phylogeny which is in keeping with the high metabolic rate). Following the cerebellum and in decreasing magnitude, Dixon and Meyer listed the caudate nucleus, cerebral cortex, thalamus, hypothalamus, and globus pallidus.

The adult rat has also been subjected to numerous metabolic studies which may be compared with those of the ox. In the observations of ox brain, white matter was discarded, and the metabolic rates were reported as representative of grey matter only, though some contamination with white cannot be ruled out entirely. In the investigation of rat brain, however, Himwich, Sykowski and Fazekas (523) used entire areas consisting of white and grey matter. The data presented in Table 14 of Chapter 7 reveal that the cerebral cortex possesses the highest oxygen intake (column 3). Brain stem, cerebellum, and medulla follow in the order given. The differences in the metabolic rates are significant. One factor which influences the metabolic activity of any region in the brain is its relative amounts of grey and white matter, the white having a much lower metabolic rate. Therefore, when we remember that the medulla has the largest ratio of white matter, it is not surprising that this section also metabolizes the slowest. It is interesting that despite this difference in experimental materials (the grey in the ox brain, as against the grey and white in the rat) the results on ox brain, in the main, agree with those of the rat, with the exception of the cerebellar cortex.

In all determinations on dogs (495) an effort was made to eliminate white matter in the hope of determining the metabolism of grey matter alone. Among the various parts of the adult brain, the caudate nucleus exhibits the highest oxygen consumption and the medulla, the lowest (see Fig. 22 of Chapter 7). Intermediate and with descending values are the cerebral cortex, cerebellum, thalamus, and midbrain.

The different cerebral areas possess characteristic distributions of metabolic rates, not only for oxidations but also for glycolysis. Observations on adult dogs and cats showed that the caudate nucleus and cerebral grey form lactic acid most rapidly, and with descending rates come the thalamus, midbrain, cerebellum, medulla and cord (168). In experiments of Craig and Beecher (201) the cerebral cortex, medulla and cord were compared and the rates of aerobic and anaerobic metabolism were found to decrease from the higher to the lower levels of the central nervous system. In general, the order in the ability to put out lactic acid is similar to that in utilizing oxygen. Summarizing these *in vitro* results, we may conclude that in general, with the exception of the cerebral hemispheres, there is a decrease of metabolic rate as the neuraxis is descended.

B. Studies on the intact human and animal

Evidence that the cerebral cortex in the human being demands more fuel than the subcortical portions was obtained in a hypoglycemic patient who on two occasions was given different amounts of intravenous glucose (495). Before the first injection the patient displayed the signs of sympathetic hyperactivity and violent motor phenomena which we have seen in the second stage. The myoclonic twitchings became generalized and a convulsive seizure developed. Four grams of glucose were then injected intravenously, much less than the amount used as a routine procedure to avoid further convulsions. All the neurological symptoms disappeared except that the patient failed to regain environmental contact, which in this case, could not be accomplished by merely 4 grams of glucose. One hour later, as the insulin continued to work, the patient again sank deep into the second stage as evidenced by perspiration, salivation and stereotyped movements. As soon as the tonic spasms of the third stage became evident, 8 grams of glucose were injected, an amount double the first dose. With this larger dose, recovery was complete, environmental contact was maintained for one-quarter of an hour, the slow waves were replaced by the faster ones on the EEG, and the oxygen consumption rose to the lower border of normal. Thus, a greater amount of glucose *is* needed to support cortical functions than subcortical. A parallelism was again noted between the three variables—the oxygen intake, electrical activity and clinical symptoms—as the patient shuttled back and forth, losing and regaining contact with his environment. The blood sugar level, true to our first observations, had little bearing on these variables and remained low throughout the entire observation.

There seems to be a discrepancy between the *in vitro* and *in vivo* observations as to the cerebral portion which occupies the highest metabolic position. We have just seen how the energy demands of the cerebral hemispheres exceed all others in man whereas the caudate nucleus was most active in the dog. A suggestion immediately arises in one's mind to explain this incongruity: the studies on human beings were made on the intact brain which was still functioning instead of on excised tissue, and the energy for operation adds an additional quota to that which is needed for maintenance. Support for this explanation is found in observations of dog brain made *in situ* (538). Blood drawn from the superior longitudinal sinus and therefore representing in a preponderating manner the cerebral hemispheres shows a C.M.R. greater than any hitherto recorded either for the entire brain *in situ* or for any excised cerebral region. The discrepancy between the results obtained from excised tissues and on the intact animal is therefore ascribed to a difference in the experimental conditions and resolved in favor of the *in vivo* observations. The cerebral hemispheres occupy the cardinal position for integrative centers and their metabolic requirements including both components for rest and for work appear to be highest.

Electrical activity. Further evidence that the cerebral cortex works at a higher rate of activity and therefore has greater energetic demands than does the subcortex, may be obtained by an examination of the brain waves in each of these two regions during hypoglycemia.

Dogs were used for these experiments since they lend themselves more readily to this type of observation than do human beings (529). In the first place, we found that the effects of hypoglycemia in the dog are similar to those of man as far as *cortical* activity is concerned. The rapid rhythm disappears and the slow waves increase in prominence; and in the more prolonged hypoglycemia, the alpha cortical responses fail completely and are restored only an hour or so after injection of glucose (protracted shock). When, however, electrodes are placed on *both* the cerebral cortex and the hypothalamus of the dog, it is observed that the hypothalamus shows more stability than the cortex, the fast cortical rhythms vanishing long before those of the hypothalamus. Conversely, the injection of glucose during

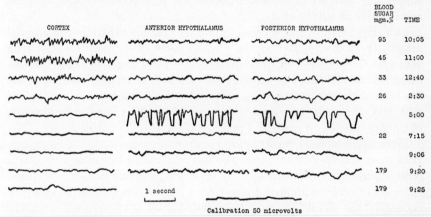

Fig. 44. Records from cortex, posterior hypothalamus, and anterior hypothalamus during insulin hypoglycemia and recovery. At each recorded time successive records were made from the three regions about one minute apart. Note augmentation of cortical slow waves at 2:30 and flattening of record by 7:15. 37 gm. of glucose were given from 9:04 to 9:16. Note slowness of return of cortical activity after administering sugar. The hypothalamic responses are much less depressed and return more rapidly after sugar injection as seen in records taken at 9:06 and 9:20. Note the violent responses of the hypothalamus at 5:00, producing amplifier block. These surges were not accompanied by convulsions nor were they associated with pulse or respiration (529).

profound hypoglycemia restores the hypothalamic waves before those of the cortex. Also submitting evidence of this type on hypoglycemic cats are Bartley and Heinbecker, stating that the cortex may be depressed at a time when the basal ganglia and the medullary centers still show integrated activity. The peripheral nerves are unaffected by hypoglycemia even just prior to the death of the animal (63).[13] This differential sensitivity of cortical and subcortical tissues is in agreement with the above observations on

[13] But by excising the nerves and applying anoxia it can be shown that those with the lower oxygen consumption rate possess the longer survival period (1030) as indicated by ability to conduct the nervous impulse, a relationship between deprivation of energy and loss of function which corresponds to that observed in the brain.

oxygen intake, as well as with work cited in Chapter 7 that metabolic activity in the lower parts of the brain does not keep pace with that of the higher parts.

Until now we have been comparing the sensitivity of the cortex with the subcortex, but have not distinguished between the many areas of the subcortex itself. In the next experiments to be described, not only was the ability to survive anoxia and hypoglycemia used as an indicator, but also the capacity for restoring normal function after the glucose or oxygen supply has been reestablished. In other words, revivability was as much an objective as survivability.

As early as 1858, Brown-Séquard (121) demonstrated the differential sensitivity to oxygen lack of the various parts of the nervous system in animals. He studied decapitated dogs by perfusing the head through cannulas inserted into the carotid and vertebral arteries. He watched for the revival time of each section of the central nervous system and noted that the cerebrum was least able to withstand anemia. The medulla oblongata, the spinal cord, and peripheral nerves followed in order.

More recent work of this type are the dramatic experiments of Heymans, Bouckaert and co-workers (466) who used the isolated head of a dog, or a head connected to the trunk only by the vagus, and this head was perfused either by blood from another dog or from a perfusion pump. By temporarily cutting off the circulation from the isolated head, they were able to study the time allowance which insured recovery for each section of the brain. After cerebral circulation had been occluded from 4 to 5 minutes, the functions of the isolated head were apparently suspended. But if perfusion was again resumed before the end of the five minutes, the activities of all parts of the brain including the cerebral hemispheres could be restored. Under the same experimental conditions the midbrain may regain function after 10 to 15 minutes, as indicated by active palpebral and pupillary reflexes, both of which have motor nuclei in the midbrain. The medulla was still able to recover after a half-hour or longer of occluded circulation as confirmed by the fact that respiratory, cardio-regulatory and vasomotor reflexes were reestablished. Experiments like these prove the sensitivity of the cerebral hemispheres over any other part of the brain, and also differentiate between the resistance of the midbrain and the medulla oblongata.

Sugar and Gerard (926) were able to make an even finer discrimination than Heymans and Bouckaert by using several electrodes, each one placed on a different part of the brain. The records thus obtained were witness to the exact time each portion of the brain could survive without oxygen, and could revive after oxygen had been restored. In their experiments, abrupt and functionally complete anemia of the brain of cats was produced by temporary occlusion of one carotid artery after ligation of all other vascular channels to the brain. Sugar and Gerard, according to their table (Table 33) observed that the electrical potentials of the cerebellar and cerebral grey disappeared earliest, the medulla latest, and the other parts, among which were subcortical white, caudate nucleus and the thalamus, were intermediate in that order. The recovery of normal waves after release of the occlusion occurred in the reverse order. For example, the dorsal nucleus of the thalamus recovered quickly while the cerebral cortex and cerebellar grey required the longest time before the normal waves recurred.

Weinberger, Gibbon and Gibbon (986) made a distinct contribution to this type of experiment by determining the relationship between the exact

TABLE 33

Survival times for particular regions of the brain following complete cerebral anemia

CEPHALIC REGION	TIME FOR DISAPPEARANCE OF POTENTIALS (SECONDS)
Cerebellar grey	10–12
Ammon's horn	10–12
Cerebral grey (cortex)	14–15
Subcortical white matter	20–22
Corona radiata	20–25
Caudate nucleus	25–27
Ventrolateral nucleus of thalamus	28–33
Lateral geniculate body	32–37
Medulla:	
Reticular formation near n. vagus	30–40
Tuberculum cuneatum	over 2 mins.
Spinal V tract	over 2 mins.

Times given are for representative occlusions performed at the beginning of experimentation: successive occlusions lower these values from 1 to 5 seconds.

duration of cerebral anemia and the consequent neurologic changes. These workers using a series of cats, abruptly stopped the circulation by clamping the pulmonary artery. In this way, for the first time, a combination of three experimental advantages was achieved: (1) arrest of the circulation to the *entire* central nervous system in the intact animal, (2) a definite period of time was calculated in minutes and seconds, and (3) the results were strengthened with histologic check-ups. The cats were arranged in order of increased length of circulatory arrest. The main objective was to study the relationship between the duration of circulatory arrest and the extent of ultimate loss in neurologic function of the cats. The animals were operated on under sterile precautions with the thought in mind of studying their recovery after release of the pulmonary clamp. These authors write that arrest of the circulation for 3 minutes and 10 seconds or less was tolerated by all parts of the brain without any obvious neurological disturbances. But, at 3 minutes and 25 seconds or more, permanent alterations in behavior were manifest. The animals lost all spontaneity and appeared disinterested in their environment, signifying (and upon later examination proving) lesions in the cerebral hemispheres. As the brain was exposed for longer intervals to anemia, the cerebral damage became more profound. Vision and sensation suffered permanent injury after 6 minutes of occlusion. After 7 minutes and 36 seconds of circulatory blocking cerebral damage was evidenced by visual, sensory and auditory defects, motor, postural and reflex abnormalities, and dementia. When the circulation was interrupted for as long as 8 minutes and 45 seconds, life could not be restored for more than a few hours. The minute histologic check-up of these animals on the effects of anoxia on the brain will be dealt with in the next section.

Morphologic evidence. By examining the actual site of lesions which have been wrought by want of cerebral energy, whether due to hypoglycemia or other causes, we can encourage still further our belief that there is an intimate alliance between the vulnerability of each part of the brain and its respective metabolism.

Weinberger, Gibbon and Gibbon (987) continued their work on the same cats which they had previously studied neurologically. Sacrificing the animals, they looked for lesions throughout the brain of each cat. Disregarding those animals subjected to anemia for less than 3 minutes and 10 seconds since their brains showed no injury, these writers report the first lesions in animals who had undergone anemia for 3 minutes and 25 seconds. Frank necrosis was found in small and limited areas of the cerebral cortex. In other cats where circulation was arrested for periods of $7\frac{1}{2}$ minutes, the cerebral cortex was destroyed completely. According to these experiments, laminas III and IV[14] were the most vulnerable of the cortex while the Purkinje cells of the cerebellum rank next to the nerve cells of the cerebral cortex in susceptibility. The basal ganglia were more resistant to cerebral anemia than the higher cortical centers, and the lower parts of the brain stem and spinal cord were uninjured even by the longest period of circulatory arrest compatible with continued survival of the animal.

The results of Weinberger and his co-workers confirmed and extended those previously gathered by Gomez and Pike (410) who ligated the carotid and subclavian arteries of the cat, and observed the following order of decreasing sensitivity: small pyramidal cells of the cerebral cortex, Purkinje cells of the cerebellum, the cells of the medulla oblongata, the cervical portion of the spinal cord and the spinal ganglia. Gildea and Cobb (401) also occluded the cerebral vessels of cats and found the most severe

---

[14] The cells of the cerebral cortex are divided into 6 layers, called laminas and numbered from I to VI, the first lamina being most external.

lesions in the cortex, consisting of focal areas of necrosis. The lesions in their animals were usually diffuse, but the most marked changes took place in laminas III and V of cortical grey. Large and small pyramidal cells appear more susceptible than other cerebral cells.

Morrison (753) who exposed monkeys and dogs to simulated high altitudes observed all the lesions previously reported for anoxia irrespective of the method of production though he noted that the pathologic changes varied in some ways according to the type of anoxia. In general, the damage grew with the number and severity of the exposures. The cells of the cortical grey matter were the first to suffer and then those of the other parts of the brain yielded to the deprivation of energy. In order of decreasing frequency of involvement, the frontal lobes came first and then the parietal occipital and temporal followed in turn by the cerebellum and basal ganglia. In further agreement with previous workers the medulla and spinal cord remained unchanged so long as the animal was capable of survival. The white matter was affected only after repeated exposures to a more severe anoxia than was required to injure the grey. Disease of the myelin moreover did not localize itself in accordance with that of the cellular grey, for example, the lesions were profuse in the frontal grey matter but the myelin of that region was involved only in a minority of the animals.

The work of Finley and Brenner (325) is especially notable. By subjecting monkeys to hypoglycemia rather than anoxia, they had the advantage of studying cerebral metabolic depression, but on a much slower time-scale. They found that the acute swelling and vacuolation of the nerve cells seen in comas of $3\frac{1}{2}$ to $4\frac{1}{2}$ hours' duration are readily reversible, but that permanent damage is certain when comas last for $9\frac{1}{2}$ hours or longer. At $14\frac{1}{2}$ hours the entire cytoplasm of the cells disappears so that only nuclei remain. It should be noted that the earliest injury is to the cells of the cortex. According to Finley and Brenner, the lesions were more abundant in the frontal poles and anterior part of the hemispheres than in other regions. Only after prolonged or repeated insulin comas do the basal structures become involved. Lesions in the phyletically older portions of the brain, the basal nuclei and the brain stem, are minimal. An acute reaction consisting of a multiplication of the glial supporting cells (in both grey and white matter) is seen in brain tissue exposed to coma for more than 14 hours. The white matter also showed striking and widespread pathologic changes in the cerebral and cerebellar hemispheres. Many authors concur with Finley and Brenner (33, 857, 935, 984, 1012), in that small doses of insulin, and consequently coma of short duration, inflict no demonstrable changes, but that under the impact of large doses which lengthen the coma, the damage is severe.

When cells are deprived of their energy by hypoglycemia, brain tissue may degenerate. For example, in Chapter 8 on Human Cerebral Metabolism it was found that at least $\frac{1}{4}$ of the normal cerebral metabolic rate is necessary to maintain the structure of the whole brain and to insure the functions of the lower brain stem. If metabolism is depressed beyond this minimum of cerebral integrity, the energy supplies are not sufficient to save the structure of the brain nor the functions remaining in the medulla oblongata. Chaikoff and co-workers (848) provide an opportunity to examine the relationship between energy and cerebral structure. They studied the phospholipids, the building stones of nervous tissue, and found that the brain absorbs from the blood both phosphoric acid and lipid molecules, synthesizing them into phospholipids. According to their work, this synthesis can take place only with the energy afforded by respiratory metabolism. In hypoglycemia the energy is not available for this phosphorylation, and those lipids which are continually being broken down in the wear and tear of life cannot be replaced. Hence cerebral tissue finally disintegrates. Not all parts of the brain, however, are deprived of their energy to the same extent. For example, observations of hypoglycemic dogs reveal that the rostral portions of the adult brain are depleted of glycogen first (166). These cerebral areas are therefore the earliest to suffer from lack of energy and show destructive changes before the more caudad cerebral regions.

Most important of all are the results obtained on human beings.[15] At this point we do not intend to enter into the vexing controversy of whether or not the insulin hypoglycemia treatment of schizophrenia destroys cerebral tissue (659). Some report no irreversible changes; most indicate some cerebral damage (33, 857, 935, 984, 1012). The human brains that have been studied are those of patients whose hypoglycemia was so severe that they died, and the results are therefore not typical of the treatment. Clinically, one is but rarely able to find any irreversible neurological changes in patients who have been properly treated.

Earlier in this chapter we have discussed the phenomena of protracted shock. We have shown that recovery is impeded and even impossible if the fifth phase of insulin hypoglycemia is permitted to last for more than 15 minutes to one-half hour, but that the administration of carbohydrate before this time produces rapid and complete recovery. The only way to determine whether patients receiving the hypoglycemic treatment for schizophrenia suffer permanent brain injury would be to study morphologically the brains of patients subjected to hypoglycemia with termination early enough to prevent protracted shock, which of course, could be done only on patients who have died of an intercurrent cause, or experimentally on animals. The brains of human beings and animals so treated should give

[15] See Chapter 11 for correlation between antemortem clinical symptoms and cerebral neuropathologic alterations.

the answer to this question. But until experiments are done which take into consideration the clinical border of complete reversibility, the final word on this question cannot be given.

In the meantime we can examine cerebral lesions in persons who have died in hypoglycemia, in order to study the sequence in which the parts of the brain succumb to lack of foodstuff. Some observers emphasized the gross vascular lesions, but most workers were more impressed with changes in the grey matter leading to necrosis in the cortex and other nerve centers. A degeneration of the white matter and an increase of glial cells were also observed. The conclusions of Lawrence, Meyer and Nevin (640) are based on a review of the literature and six cases of their own. They found that the degeneration and disappearance of nerve cells were most widespread in the cerebral cortex, somewhat less so in the caudate nucleus and putamen, and still less in the cerebellum, while the lesions in the remaining centers of the brain stem were slight. In general Stief and Tokay (913), Bodechtel (96), Leppien and Peters (657), Cammermeyer (143), Ferraro and Jervis (315), Malamud and Grosh (704) all report a similar distribution of lesions, agreeing with the conclusions of Lawrence, Meyer and Nevin (640). Thus, the human material, like that of animals, shows more widespread destruction in the newer phyletic layers in proportion to their intense metabolic activity.

Patients who have died from lack of oxygen present another opportunity to study the morphology of brain tissues. Courville (199) in reporting his patients who died under nitrous oxide anesthesia comes to the conclusion that their death was asphyxial. Of interest to us at this point were his discoveries on the cerebral lesions of these patients, that the order of devastation begins first with the highest parts of the brain, the cerebral hemispheres and the lenticular nucleus. Lowenberg, Waggoner and Zbinden (692) in general agree with the results of Courville, for they too find that their patients who died from nitrous oxide poisoning showed widespread destruction in the hemispheres and the basal ganglia. They write, "the changes in the brain stem and cerebellum were in all cases much less than those of the cortex and basal ganglia". They also point out that destruction is distributed in this same manner with pantapon, morphine and ergoapiol poisoning. Gebauer and Coleman (369) have reported irregular degeneration of the cortex, the greatest cell defects being apparent in the laminas III, IV and V, of a patient who died 7 days after cyclopropane anesthesia. Cellular degeneration was also present in the globus pallidus, but no sign of assault to any other part of the brain was detected.

In all cases of anoxia this same order of the disintegration in the brain is observed. The lenticular nucleus however is especially vulnerable and not only so when the effects of nitrous oxide are superimposed on those of anoxia, as mentioned above, but also when the deprivation of oxygen is caused by carbon monoxide poisoning. These lenticular reactions exemplify the specific susceptibility of various cerebral regions to toxic agents. One factor that must be considered is the high rate of metabolism of the striatum (caudate nucleus, 495) making it susceptible to the anoxic deprivation of energy. In addition, its vulnerability to substances injected via the carotid artery (289) suggest that the relatively short unbranched arrangement of the striate arteries affords a higher concentration of the injected substances, to this region than areas fed by other cerebral arteries. The Vogts (959) term this selectivity pathoclisis, and suggest a physiocochemical basis as an explanation of the affinity displayed by an injurious substance for a given structure, rendering the latter a site of least resistance. In a conversation with these neurologists they pointed out to the author that the phyletic regression observed in hypoglycemia and acute anoxia whether expressed in terms of damaged cerebral areas or clinical signs may be regarded as an instance of specific susceptibility with however a known mechanism. Regression and specificity are not mutually exclusive but may operate simultaneously and in Chapter 12 the analysis of the phenomena of thiopental anesthesia reveals the progressive advance of the metabolic depression as well as the specific affinity of various masses for that depressant drug.

A specific affinity exhibited by neural structures for agents is only one of the factors competing with the descending order of susceptibility, for that broad generalization does not necessarily apply equally to every type of cell within a given layer. As Grenell (420) points out the sensory cells of the pontine and medullary regions are more susceptible than the motor groups. In a similar fashion areas with associative functions are vulnerable to anoxia. Whether or not the exceptions to the general rule can be traced to the respective metabolic rates of the cell groups involved, is a problem of the future.

IX. RESISTANCE OF THE NEWBORN TO HYPOGLYCEMIA AND ACUTE ANOXIA

It is a remarkable fact that infants sustain hypoglycemia much better than do adults. A paper by Kettringham and Austin (592) shows that newborn babies have a normal level of blood sugar at birth, but that it drops immediately to hypoglycemic levels and remains so for at least the first three days of postnatal life. Allweiss[16] obtained average values of 57 mg. per cent at birth and 45 mg. per cent four hours thereafter. This latter value rose gradually so that the average for all his infants was 67 mg. per cent after the 10th day. Despite their low blood sugar, newborn babies are usually free of hypoglycemic symptoms. Priscilla White (568)

---

[16] Personal communication from Dr. M. D. Allweiss.

reports a large number of subnormal blood sugars on 19 babies, yet she notes only one instance of a hypoglycemic reaction. Contrary to the general belief, she finds that the low level of blood sugar in babies of diabetic mothers is not, as a rule, much more severe than that in the newborn from normal mothers. Before discussing the reason for the relative insensitivity of the newborn to hypoglycemia, data on the comparative susceptibility of the newborn infant and the adult to anoxia are in order.

There has been some question as to the period that an adult can survive without respiration. Evidence has been carefully evaluated in a review published in the *Journal of the American Medical Association* (807) on the greatest length of time of submersion under water compatible with revival. At the end of this review is quoted the conclusion of Taylor in his *Principles and Practice of Medical Jurisprudence* (936) in which he sets the longest time at 7 to 8 minutes, and this figure may be considered as the outside limit for adults. Babies, however, may survive beyond this limit. For instance, Smith and Kaplan (884) report a baby who had a perfect recovery after a period of apnea of a full 14 minutes. The resistance of the human infant is in keeping with the wealth of information assembled in Chapter 7 that the newborn of several mammalian species was able to withstand anoxia and hypoglycemia much longer than the adult of the same species. We have suggested that the tolerance of newborn animals both to hypoglycemia and anoxia may be associated with their low cerebral metabolic needs (953, 523, 495); and continuing with this thought in Chapter 8, found that the same may be applicable to the human newborn, as well (497). But, the question must be asked: why do lower energy requirements render the human newborn better able to withstand any deprivation of energy?

Reverting back to Figure 23 in Chapter 7, we find that the infant brain of an animal obtains a large proportion of its energy from glycolysis, much larger than an adult (165). The infant brain, therefore, creates an energy deficit much more slowly than an adult, since this deficit is in fact the difference between the total cerebral demand and the amount of energy which can be contributed through glycolysis (that is, without oxidation). It follows then that if the infant brain does not sink into energy debt as quickly as an adult, survival will be that much longer when the child is exposed to insufficient glucose or oxygen in the blood.

If such is true of an animal brain, can we assume that the brain of a human babe has extra time for accumulating its energy debt? Before this question can be resolved, we must first ask ourselves: do human beings have the same resources of anaerobic energy through glycolysis as an animal? We know that all tissues glycolyze to some extent in the absence of oxygen (973), and in most cases this glycolysis no longer continues when the oxygen is restored to carry on oxidations. But there are certain tissues which, even in the presence of oxygen, persist in glycolyzing and in fact never cease putting out lactic acid. Among these singular tissues is the brain (22, 238). We have shown that more glucose is utilized by the brain than can be accounted for by oxidative processes, and the excess glucose is glycolyzed at least in part, leaving the brain in the form of lactic acid (770) and pyruvic acid (524). The energy so obtained comes to about 1.7 per cent of the total energy requirement of the brain. If we are sure that the human brain does glycolyze even in the presence of a full complement of oxygen, certainly we would expect to see glycolysis, but much more abundantly, in the brain which is suffering from oxygen lack.

Energy made available by glycolysis would naturally go a longer way in the event of anoxia if the total cerebral energy requirement were very small, as it is in the infant brain. However, the anaerobic supply of energy finally exhausts itself even in the newborn child, if oxygen is delayed for too long. In this case, the brain of the newborn child will also suffer destruction, but the process is prolonged over a period of time far beyond that in which the adult succumbs. We would not expect, however, that the order in which the areas of the brain are destroyed would follow the same sequence in both infant and adult, because the distribution of metabolic activity is not the same in both. The resistance of a cerebral district varies inversely with its metabolic activity; that is to say, the less energy a tissue demands, the stronger will be its resistance. In the newborn animal the medullary regions are the most active (953) (see Chapter 7, Table 17), while the reverse is true of the adult, in whom the rostral portions of the brain have the fastest energy metabolism. The prime position of the medulla oblongata during early development is not only supported by oxidations (495) but also by glycolysis, (168) cholinesterase activity (757) and acetylcholine content (990).

We have already seen how the newest phyletic parts of adult human brain are the first to be hit by hypoglycemia or anoxia (325, 640, 986, 987). In the infant, on the contrary, the older areas become involved earlier as is the case with the glycogen content in the caudad regions during hypoglycemia (319; see Fig. 31, Chapter 7). We might therefore expect that their cerebral hemispheres would be damaged only after the lower portions had been injured. An observation of Steiner quoted by Schreiber (860) supporting this suggestion was made on a newborn babe who suffered from apneic periods and died from convulsions after three days, and whose medulla was the only portion of the brain to show necrosis. An additional bit of evidence is obtained from Racker's observation on a human fetal brain in which the medulla oblongata exhibited an oxygen intake 38 per cent higher than that of the cerebral hemispheres (812).

Minkowski's study (746) of the response to stimulation of the foot of the human fetus revealed that the cerebral hemispheres are not active at birth

He reported that the spinal mechanisms regulating this response come in succession under the influence of the bulb, midbrain, and basal ganglia (pallidum), but not the cerebral hemispheres until after birth. A step-wise expansion of fetal behavior was also observed by Hooker (539). Youngstrom (1035) found a similar sequence in the increased concentration of cholinesterase, appearing first in the spinal cord and then, by turn, in a pooled sample including midbrain and medulla, the diencephalon, basal ganglia, and finally in the cerebral hemispheres. Youngstrom's observations agree with those of Minkowski and Hooker, for as might be expected the metabolic foundation precedes the development of behavior in each part of the brain. It would seem that quantitative differences between the brain of the newborn and the adult may be the basis for their contrasting reactions.

The importance of apnea at birth has been emphasized as one of the outstanding causes for cerebral injury during childhood (860). Though this concept probably applies in a certain number of cases, one wonders how widely it can be effective in view of the tolerance of the newborn to anoxia. Almost any birth involves a period of asphyxia, but according to Yannet (1031) only in a very small percentage of cases can birth injury be assigned to cerebral anoxia. His data do not indicate that birth trauma is the most prominent causative factor and he concludes that in most instances there are antenatal factors to be blamed for cerebral palsy. The dietary of the mother before the birth of the child may be one of these factors (978).

X. Summary

In the present chapter we have started to apply our knowledge on the energy metabolism of the brain to an analysis of how the central nervous system operates. By the use of insulin treatment for schizophrenia as a method for study, it was found that the complex activities of the central nervous system may be resolved into a series of five patterns allocated to different layers of the neuraxis.

When the brain is deprived of its foodstuff, the symptom-groups come into view and replace each other one by one in the order of their relation to the cortex, subcortico-diencephalon, midbrain, upper and lower medulla respectively. As we witness first the phyletic regression of the central nervous system, and the recovery therefrom, it is important to note that the latter is the recapitulation of the phyletic development of the brain. In other words, we are following by means of symptomatic and biochemical studies the embryologic formation of the central nervous system. According to this working hypothesis, the brain in perfect working order depends upon the co-ordination of 5 separate layers, each capable of mediating a distinct pattern of response, and all integrated with the cerebral cortex.

Studies of blood sugar, brain waves, and oxygen utilization of the brain were all made on the same schizophrenic patients in order to shed more light on the question at hand, that is, to what factor can the arrangement of these symptom-complexes be attributed? Barring the first phase of hypoglycemia blood sugar had no bearing on the clinical picture, but a direct association was detected between the electrical activity and the symptoms. Cortical rhythm finds its expression in the alpha waves of 10 per second frequency; displacing these at approximately the time when the cortex loses its hold are the slower undulations signalling that the patient has slipped from his environmental contact.

Most informative were the studies of the oxygen intake during hypoglycemia. Blood samples drawn at stated intervals throughout the treatment proved beyond a doubt that the brain uses less and less oxygen. If the answer to the symptoms and electrical activity could be compressed into one underlying cause, it might be this progressive dampening of brain oxidations.

Parallel to the results obtained with hypoglycemia are those of acute anoxia. A striking resemblance between the two was disclosed when the anoxia was produced by inhalation of nitrogen and this resemblance held true throughout recovery from the anoxia. In the light of this likeness between hypoglycemia and anoxia, it was concluded that the common denominator for cerebral reactions in both conditions would be that brain metabolism suffers.

Upon investigating the oxygen demands of each part of the brain, it was found that the higher phyletic layers of the brain need greater metabolic support, and therefore succumb earlier to lack of foodstuff or oxygen. From these studies, the principle was evolved that the newest phyletic layers in the brain metabolize most vigorously, and are therefore most vulnerable to injury. This principle which has been used to explain the succession of hypoglycemic symptom-complexes as well as the electrical record on the EEG, is also useful in accounting for the order of injury inflicted on the brain under the rigors of hypoglycemia or anoxia. Thus, a whole wealth of morphologic material, both experimental and clinical, when analyzed in accordance with this principle, reveals that a relatively mild deprivation of energy affects only the newest parts of the brain, and as energy is severely curtailed more and more of the lower structures become involved.

What looks to be an exception to this generalization, that is, the fact that the newborn possesses extraordinary resistance to hypoglycemia and anoxia, is in truth only an apparent discrepancy, and also finds its answer in metabolic terms. The metabolic activity of the infant brain is slow and therefore less sensitive to a blocking of its energy supplies.

CHAPTER 11

THE AUTONOMIC DIVISION OF THE CENTRAL NERVOUS SYSTEM

Patterns of Activity in the Five Phyletic Layers

I. PURPOSE OF THE CHAPTER

So far our analysis of the symptoms of hypoglycemia and acute anoxia has been limited to the somatic activities, or the relation of the central nervous system to posture and movement of the skeletal muscle. The purpose of this chapter is to study and analyse the autonomic division of the central nervous system, as we have done with the somatic, by using the step-like process of hypoglycemia or anoxia, as well as examining areas of destruction in human fatalities, to disentangle the contributions of each layer of the brain and to demonstrate the total integration of the autonomic nervous system.

II. SITES OF AUTONOMIC CONTROL IN THE BRAIN

Each and every motor activity of the body must necessarily be supported by appropriate changes in metabolism. These, in their turn, are the result of accommodations in respiration, circulation and glandular activity. It is the function of the autonomic nervous system to innervate the organs which are responsible for all the mechanisms supporting the motor activities of the body. In a word, the autonomic nervous system controls visceral activity: the heart rate, the secretory action of the glands, and the contraction of smooth muscle, whether in blood vessels or in organs. The fact that we have separated the somatic from the visceral division of the central nervous system and treated them in two different chapters does not imply that each acts independently of the other. On the contrary, they form two component parts accounting for the reaction of the body to one and the same stimulation, mutually assisting each other in adapting us to our environment. Nevertheless, for clarity of exposition, the visceral is singled out from the somatic and thereby each is studied more accurately. Such a separation is helpful because the autonomic alone acts in behalf of the internal environment of the body.

In Chapter 3 we have treated the anatomy of the autonomic nervous system as a whole, and traced the nerve fibers of both the sympathetic and parasympathetic branches from their origin in the brain and cord to their respective viscera.[1] Like the somatic division, the autonomic probably

[1] As indicated in footnote on page 317 the functional classification of cholinergic

303

has offices in each phyletic layer. The representation of the autonomics in the cortex is found in several regions including the frontal lobes (585, 842) and an area on the medial surface of the hemispheres, the cingular gyrus (886, 976). In the cerebral hemispheres, the operating nuclei for autonomic regulation are situated, in general, close to those for the corresponding somatic functions (357). In the subcortico-diencephalic layer, there too is a separation of the somatic from the visceral centers. The hypothalamus is the main harbor for visceral regulation in the second layer, and there is some clinical evidence that the striatum should also be included (995). The nuclear masses of the hypothalamus may be divided into four groups: the anterior and midline (parasympathetic), and posterior and lateral (sympathetic) (357). As for the third and fourth layers, the anatomic stations are still undisclosed, except for the group of mesencephalic cells (Edinger-Westphal nucleus) which give rise to the autonomic fibers causing constriction of the pupils. At any rate, we do know that there must be some nervous connections between the hypothalamus and the medulla. The fifth, or lower medullary layer, is a leading site for parasympathetic activity, containing nuclei whose outflow go to the salivary glands, the viscera of the thorax—heart and lungs—and those of the gastro-intestinal tract down to the transverse colon, as well as to the islands of Langerhans. The medulla oblongata also houses important sympathetic centers whose functions are to constrict blood vessels, accelerate heart rate and bring on sweating. As mentioned above, these centers will be examined from the viewpoint of hypoglycemia, but not included in the study are nerve cells as far down as the spinal cord and in the organs of the body themselves, cells which are functioning even in the fifth stage of hypoglycemia. Some of these cells belong to one branch and some to the other. The parasympathetic nuclei located in the lumbar cord control the rectum, the bladder, and the blood vessels of the generative organs. The sympathetic nerves arising in the grey cells of the lateral horn of the cord innervate blood vessels and most of the viscera. From this brief description we see that there is a continued path of autonomic connections starting from the cerebral hemispheres, passing down through each successive layer of the brain, and ending in the visceral effectors. We can therefore understand how the stimulation or release of any cerebral component except for the proprioceptive ganglion, the cerebellum may make itself known in terms of visceral manifestations.

The smooth integration between the somatic and visceral components of the central nervous system constantly manifests itself in bodily activity.

and adrenergic fibers, which depends upon the particular neurohormone released by the terminations of the autonomic nerves, agrees in general with the anatomic classification.

Moreover, the two branches of the autonomic division, parasympathetic and sympathetic, are also working in a harmonious balance. Under what may be called the state of the body in calm life, i.e. when the environment is free from threats to the organism, the balance of these two components encounters only moderate fluctuations. Not by any means static, this balance is a result of a dynamic equilibrium which may be upset in one direction or another in accordance with the environment and constitution of the individual. If something happens to excite him or to arouse his emotions for any reason whatsoever, there is an immediate somatic response assuming the attitude of defense or attack, and allied with this is a visceral adaptation which mobilizes the body for the emergency. No matter what the stimulus may be, so long as the emotions are aroused, the balance between these two branches is always upset by a sympathetic preponderance. And this occurs regardless of whether the parasympathetic is simultaneously stimulated or inhibited, a topic which will be considered later in this chapter. Blood pressure rises, heart rate accelerates, respiration increases, and pupils dilate while the skin becomes flushed, viscid sweat covers the body and metabolism mounts. In the reverse condition, when the rapport with the environment recedes temporarily, as in sleep, the parasympathetic branch outweighs the sympathetic and the phenomena of the former are spread over the individual. His blood pressure falls, heart rate slackens, respiration becomes shallow, the pupils are constricted, his face turns pale, and this time his perspiration is watery while the metabolic rate decreases. So we see that the equilibrium between parasympathetic and sympathetic is seldom at rest, but continually vacillating. Sometimes the shift is tremendous as when a soldier plunges into battle, or for that matter when any threat is made to one's life. Other examples of such extreme unbalance will be seen in the next section when we study the autonomic nervous system and its visceral symptoms in human cases in which hypoglycemia and different forms of anoxia were instrumental in producing these symptoms.

III. Autonomic activity studied on human cases

In Table 34 we have reviewed the shift in balance between sympathetic and parasympathetic during insulin hypoglycemia. A similar order of autonomic symptoms may be seen in anoxia, starting with a marked release of the sympathetic and if the acute anoxia is maintained for some time (say, up to 2 minutes) a parasympathetic slowing of the heart rate will finally be observed. A major difference in the neurologic symptoms of hypoglycemia and acute anoxia, therefore, is the fact that in anoxia the symptoms are unfolded faster than in hypoglycemia (Chapter 10). Thus, for the autonomic, as for the somatic, the effects of acute anoxia are similar to those of hypoglycemia.

TABLE 34

Autonomic symptoms according to phasic progress in insulin hypoglycemia

PHASE	SYMPTOMS	DOMINANT AUTONOMIC SYNDROME
Cortical	a. when patient is settled and undisturbed: 1. slow heart rate 2. constricted pupils 3. water salivation and perspiration b. if the patient is stimulated by any approach, as from the examiner: 1. quickening of heart rate 2. moderate dilatation of pupils 3. salivation and perspiration becomes viscid	a. Parasympathetic b. Transitory sympathetic
Subcortico-diencephalic	1. characteristically, the pupils dilate, but may be intensified upon any stimulation 2. pulse follows the trend of the pupils: faster with dilatation; less fast with constriction 3. flushed face and free sweating after any violent motor activity 4. eyeballs bulge	Basic sympathetic predominance with waves of intensified activity
Mesencephalic & Upper Medullary	a. between tonic or extensor spasms: 1. face is pale 2. heart rate drops to normal or below 3. pupils contract b. during spasms: 1. very fast pulse 2. pupils widen but do not react to light 3. face is flushed 4. spasms of pulmonary and intestinal musculature	a. Parasympathetic b. Sympathetic
Lower Medullary	1. face deathly pale, almost grey 2. pulse slow and hammer-like 3. eyeballs deeply sunken, pupils pinpoint, and do not react to light 4. respiration slow and silent 5. extremities cold	Maximal Parasympathetic

The changes in autonomic dominance come on in two rising swells. Throughout the first phase there is an oscillation of sympathetic and parasympathetic gradually working up to a maximal sympathetic in the second phase; in the third and fourth phases there is again a varying of the two tones which finally resolves into a maximal parasympathetic in the fifth phase.

In the patients receiving the insulin treatment for schizophrenia (Chapter 10), it was possible, by an ever-deepening depression of brain metabolism, to make an analysis of cerebral functions and to allocate them to five phyletic layers (473). In no way, in these studies, however, could we show experimentally that as a certain layer was depressed, its respective symptoms appeared. In other words, all our reasoning was necessarily by analogy, since in all these patients the metabolic depression had only a fleeting effect upon the brain. For the most part we relied on animal experiments both for our data on relative rates of metabolism in the various cerebral areas and also for the results of a series of transections proceeding caudally down the neuraxis. These facts, then, together with our neurologic observations on human patients, gave us a general idea of where the anatomic locus might be. Only when a human fatality resulted from a deprivation of cerebral energy was it possible for us to show that the newest parts of the brain were destroyed first, thus allowing us to conclude that the rostral parts of the brain metabolize more intensely and therefore suffer the first destruction. It would bring strong confirmation to our phyletic point of view if it were possible to obtain the brain for autopsy and thus correlate the antemortem syndromes directly with actual examination of the brain postmortem. This, of course, means that the patients were injured so fundamentally that they could not survive. Heretofore, we have studied some of these patients who either recovered from or succumbed to overdoses of insulin, carbon monoxide poisoning, or faulty nitrous oxide anesthesia. Our object then was to compare their behavior with their cerebral metabolic rates to see what bearing one had on the other. In none of those cases was an autopsy performed. The literature does provide several instances of this same type of death where the study of the patient was completed by an autopsy, and these patients supply us with the necessary link in our reasoning.

Two such patients have been reported by Wortis and Maurer (1023).

Case 1. A woman who accidentally received an overdose of insulin failed to recover and was sent to Bellevue Hospital in New York City. She presented a bizarre picture; except for the vocalization of one or two meaningless words buried in a stream of unintelligible jabber, she gave practically no evidence of contact with her environment. When stimulated painfully or by loud noises, or more usually when there was no external stimulus, she showed signs of diffuse sympathetic discharge. The reactions were stereotyped and lasted from 30 seconds to 2 minutes. During these attacks, her eyelids widened, exophthalmos occurred and the pupils dilated so widely that the iris was no longer visible. The pulse rate rose from 100 to 140 and the blood pressure from 120 to 170. She would strike out blindly and usually not in the direction of the stimulus, and would literally snarl and spit. Respirations were forced and rapid, sweating was generalized. She never made any attempt to avoid the stimulation and there was never any evidence of aggression directed against the examiners. These reactions were observed in almost unchanged fashion for 30 days occurring on the average of 100 times a day. She eventually died of pneumonia and autopsy revealed a generalized cerebral softening. Histologic sections unfortunately were not made.

Case 2. The second case concerns a woman with a practically identical clinical picture which was the result of exposure to an illuminating gas. In this case an autopsy revealed gross congestion and hemorrhage both of the cortex and of the subcortical white matter, and necrosis of the globus pallidus. There were no gross nor microscopic changes in the cerebellum or medulla other than hemorrhage. The authors, referring to both patients, point out: (1) there was no continuation of the "sham rage" syndrome (51) once the stimulation was removed, thus indicating that the patients did not experience true rage or fear, and (2) despite the fact that the physicians induced several hundred attacks, their approach to the bedside was never a source of anxiety to the patient. (3) The rage was never purposeful. At no time did either patient attempt to untie her restraints, strike the examiner, or escape painful stimulus.

Here, then we see two patients who on autopsy disclosed destructive changes in the cerebral hemispheres, and who exhibited phenomena similar to those observed in the second stage of hypoglycemia.

Case 3. Courville (199) writes of another instance where the brain was injured to the extent of reproducing the symptoms of the second phase of hypoglycemia. The patient, a young Mexican primipara, was delivered uneventfully of a normal male child. A nitrous oxide-oxygen ether mixture was administered for repair of her perineum. Towards the close of the operation, respiration had become shallow and slow. After this, several short periods of apnea were noted. Pure oxygen was administered and respirations improved though they continued much slower than normal. Instead of regaining consciousness, the patient remained deeply comatose and developed generalized convulsions. Two days later she still presented a picture of coma punctuated by periods of involuntary laughing and crying. An examination on the third day revealed that she was covered with perspiration, had lost contact with the environment except for outbursts of crying when she was disturbed in any way. No formed words or sentences were uttered, voluntary movements were absent or extremely limited, and all four extremities were held in a position of slight flexion. The Babinski sign was present. The patient grew progressively worse and after surviving for $6\frac{1}{2}$ days, succumbed.

On autopsy various sections of the brain were taken for histologic study. The cerebral cortex showed various degrees of necrosis in the numerous sections. The cells of the corpus striatum and thalamus were devoid of any gross changes and areas of necrosis were not found. The nerve cells of the midbrain and pons showed no appreciable change. This patient, then, who showed symptoms which closely resembled those in the second phase of hypoglycemia had suffered widespread destruction of the cerebral hemispheres, but the subcortex had been spared, a picture which is the morphologic counterpart of that obtained through a metabolic depression of the cerebral hemispheres. Unlike a temporary metabolic depression from which recovery was assured, these patients could not survive the permanent damage and so succumbed.

The next four cases have been chosen because they illustrate release of symptoms as far down as the fourth layer. The authors do not mention the autonomic balance, but the reader will recall from Table 36 that this fourth phase features a parasympathetic superiority, which gives way to the sympathetic whenever the patient is seized by muscular spasms.

Case 4. Another of Courville's interesting case histories concerns a second Mexican woman also giving birth to her first baby, and to whom nitrous oxide-oxygen and ether were administered for perineal repair (199). About $\frac{1}{2}$ hour after anesthesia, she suddenly ceased to breathe. Artificial respiration and carbon dioxide-oxygen mixture were promptly given, and then for over a period of 6 minutes, the patient would alternately take a deep breath between periods of apnea lasting about a minute. After that, spontaneous deep respiration was resumed. Shortly thereafter generalized convulsions made their appearance. These were finally controlled with sedatives though muscular twitchings still persisted after the major convulsions had ceased. The muscles were spastic and the Magnus-deKleyn phenomena were observed (see Chapter 10 for Magnus-deKleyn reflex). Apparently the woman had reached the symptoms characteristic of the fourth phase with freeing of the upper medulla from supramedullary control. The patient went downhill rapidly, and died 46 hours after the induction of anesthesia.

In the autopsy blocks of tissue for histologic study were taken from parts of the cerebral cortex, basal ganglia (lenticular nucleus), cerebellar cortex and medulla oblongata. Examination revealed that the cells of the superficial layers of the cortex were destroyed. The deeper layers of the cortex adjacent to the white matter were found to be seriously injured universally. The lenticular nucleus had suffered softening of the grey matter and early necrosis. The nerve cells showed the same type of change as those of the cerebral cortex. The cortex of the cerebellum also was affected and the cells of Purkinje were its most seriously damaged elements. The author does not report on the medulla oblongata, possibly because it showed no change. In this observation we have excellent evidence that the second phyletic layer was involved in the destructive process. It is too bad that midbrain sections were not taken in this case, because if this layer had also been damaged (as was actually shown in cases 6 and 7), then we would have the last evidence needed in favor of premyencephalic release. However, the areas of cerebral injury observed by Courville do agree with the clinical symptoms of the patient just before her antemortem sinking: extensor spasms, and the Magnus-de Kleyn postural reflexes.

Case 5. The symptoms which Courville characterizes as decerebrate rigidity appeared in a colored boy, aged 6 (199). They were observed after an operation was performed under nitrous oxide anesthesia to drain an abscess. At the time the operation was completed the child suddenly stopped breathing and his pulse was imperceptible. Stimulants were given and artificial respiration had to be continued for $\frac{1}{2}$ hour before automatic breathing was resumed. Within a few hours generalized hypertonicity of the body musculature developed associated with repeated convulsive seizures. Four hours later the child was found to be comatose, vomiting and perspiring freely. The deep reflexes were hyperactive. "The state of decerebrate rigidity became progressively more marked," and death ensued a little after four days following the episode of respiratory failure. Courville examined blocks of tissue from the cerebral hemispheres, the corpus striatum and the cerebellum. The cerebral cortex revealed areas of extensive alterations. These lesions were also common in the lenticular nuclei. The Purkinje cells in the cerebellum were devoid of any trace of chromatic material. In this brain, too then, the three parts examined all showed extensive changes, in accordance with symptoms allocated to a lower portion of the brain stem.

Cases 6 and 7. Lowenberg, Waggoner and Zbinden (692) report two patients with a minute histologic study of all cerebral parts. Both patients, like those of Courville, were comatose and exhibited opisthotonic convulsions. These symptoms can best be explained by their neuropathology, which was practically identical in both cases. In the cerebral hemispheres severe disturbances of the laminar type were seen, which upon closer examination showed that all of the 6 cerebral lamina were involved, but that the 3rd, 5th and 6th were completely destroyed. The second phyletic layer was as severely affected as the cortex. The parenchyma of the caudate nucleus, putamen, globus pallidus, thalamus and hypothalamus, all received insult. The destruction was somewhat less marked in the midbrain, but nevertheless there was moderate degeneration of the neurones of the grey masses in this layer. The cerebellum was destroyed in many areas, in fact even in the medulla the neurones were somewhat shrunken. As a result of faulty nitrous oxide anesthesia, these patients clearly display the destructive processes in all supramedullary portions of the brain, and with it the development of the extensor spasms characteristic of liberation of the fourth phyletic layer

On such an important subject as this, additional data would be welcome. Perhaps with such histologic data and careful neurologic study over a period of time we might be able to accumulate enough cases to illustrate amply how each layer possesses its characteristic neurologic integration.

Discussion. These seven case histories together with the work on patients receiving shock therapies for schizophrenia, have yielded much additional information on the sympathetic-parasympathetic balance. The oscillations in balance during the first, third and fourth phases are fairly clear, that is, the visceral symptoms which we have described above in human subjects are readily understandable on the basis of functional co-ordination of the autonomic and somatic divisions of the central nervous system. In the first phase we have found a parasympathetic predominance which is over-turned whenever the organism is mobilized by any sensory stimulation. For example, Parker (782) notes that during this parasympathetic stage, even though pupils are constricted, they are very unstable and the slightest stimulus, say the approach of the physician to the bedside, will cause their dilatation. Analogous sensitivity occurs in the pulse rate during this phase. Pupil dilatation is accompanied by an increase in pulse rate from 6 to 15 beats faster per minute. "Evidently," Parker adds, "the effect of a disturbance which would normally produce little change is greatly increased in patients with insulin hypoglycemia."

Both branches of the autonomic system are represented in the cerebral hemispheres (150, 533), and the autonomic symptoms of the first phase are referable to both sympathetic and parasympathetic. In the third and fourth phases we also saw a parasympathetic overactivity except when the third-phase tonic spasms and the fourth-phase extensor spasms appear (Chapter 10), at which times the co-ordination of the autonomic division presses mobilization of the sympathetic in order to support the energy demands of muscular activity. To explain this co-ordination two suggestions are offered: either the sympathetic and parasympathetic symptoms can be attributed to undiscovered nuclear masses in these layers, or sympathetic and parasympathetic centers in the medulla oblongata are active in the autonomic integrations. The second suggestion takes into account that the first and second phyletic layers are depressed while the third, fourth and fifth are still left functioning. The medulla oblongata therefore may be responsible for mediating the visceral adaptations of the third and fourth phases.

The analysis of the sympathetic hegemony in the second phase and of the parasympathetic in the fifth phase requires further clarification. Here the tendency of the autonomic predominance is contradictory to what we would expect to see. Our human cases all demonstrated a release of the visceral patterns mediated by the hypothalamus, manifested in pupil dilatation, rapid heart rate, viscid perspiration and saliva, all increasing in intensity periodically and accompanied by a bulging of the eyeballs, rise in blood pressure and deep, fast respiration. We know that anatomically both branches have governing nuclei in the hypothalamus, suggesting that the second layer expresses itself in a balanced relationship between the two branches, the autonomic integration of a normal quietly resting individual. And, if there were any unbalance, one would anticipate a parasympathetic rule in the second phase, because we know that parasympathetic centers are located in front of the sympathetic ones in the hypothalamus.

The question then is: why do we actually observe a sympathetic reign in the second phase? The answer must involve one of the following alternatives:

(a) that the parasympathetic is completely inactive, or
(b) that the parasympathetic is working at its normal rate and the sympathetic is hyperactive, or
(c) that both sympathetic and parasympathetic are actually stepped up, but sympathetic more so than the parasympathetic.

The apparent parasympathetic predominance of the fifth phase may be subjected to the same type of questioning. We know that there are sympathetic posts in the medulla which are responsible for raising blood sugar and blood pressure and accelerating heart rate. We also are aware that the medulla possesses nuclei of parasympathetic activity acting in the reverse direction.

The question regarding the medullary phase, therefore, is: why do we see only parasympathetic signs in the fifth phase? Again the answer lies in one of the following:

(a) because the sympathetic has been rendered inactive, or
(b) because sympathetic remains unchanged while parasympathetic moves ahead, or
(c) that the function of both sets of nuclei have undergone an acceleration, but the parasympathetic more than the sympathetic.

The answer to these questions can only be resolved by resorting to work on animals, the subject of the next section, since by various operative and other experimental procedures on animals, we can separate one autonomic tone from the other and thus evaluate each independently from the other.

IV. ANIMAL EXPERIMENTS TO STUDY THE AUTONOMIC BALANCE

A. *Hypothalamic and medullary patterns in hypoglycemia*

Since the activity of the heart responds with delicate sensitivity to either sympathetic or parasympathetic stimulation, this organ has been used with considerable convenience to test the autonomic balance during hypoglycemia (518). Dogs and cats were used in these observations. Some dogs were studied without any operative interference with their autonomic system, while others were subjected to section of their vagus nerves to the heart in order to remove parasympathetic influence, and thereby better determine the effects of the unopposed sympathetic. Still other experiments, not in this same series, but performed considerably earlier by Dworkin (264) were done on cats whose sympathetic chains were extirpated in order to reveal the unopposed parasympathetic. In the dogs the ECG was employed to follow cardiac activity but in the cats the heart rate was counted by means of a stethoscope attached to the chest wall.

Intact autonomic system. Taking first the animals whose autonomic nervous system was left intact, we permitted the hypoglycemia to proceed until the definite sympathetic preponderance became apparent through the electrocardiographic record. Until this point the record showed only hazy and transitory deviations from the normal. A most reliable sign of the sympathetic predominance in the second phase is the noticeable acceleration of the heart rate, which occurred at this time (Table 36). The sympathetic syndrome has been studied in great detail by Cannon and his school (146). They find that the sympathetic sway may be initiated after blood sugar has fallen below 70 mg. per cent, thereby disclosing the hypothalamic integration. In the observations made in the author's laboratory, (518) however, the hypoglycemia was allowed to continue until the blood sugar fell to values as low as 13 to 25 mg. per cent, assuring a depth of blood sugar far below the superficial stage, in order to study the medullary reaction. Under these conditions, the ECG tells an entirely different story. The abnormally fast heart rate which we had seen in the second phase now has given way to one which is abnormally slow—true to the symptoms in the final stage of hypoglycemia. In the earlier literature, the emphasis has been laid upon the sympathetic tone represented here by a fast heart rate as an important sign of hypoglycemia, but more recent studies reveal that the parasympathetic response indicated by a retarded heart rate is of equal importance in the later phases of hypoglycemia. Further proof for this conclusion will be adduced in the experiments where operative interference was employed to inactivate either one or the other branch of the autonomic division.

Extirpation of the sympathetic chains. In Dworkin's experiments (264) particular care was taken that no peripheral portion of the sympathetic was active. The complete sympathectomy removed accelerator nerves to the heart, the splanchnic nerves to the adrenal medulla, and all other peripheral nerves which might give rise to sympathin. When such a cat was placed under hypoglycemia, the only cardiac sign was a retarded heart rate. The hastened heart rate which is characteristic of early hypoglycemia did not occur. This work proves once more that:

(1) a fast heart rate is dependent upon sympathetic control, and in addition, establishes that:

(2) the parasympathetic branch is active even in early hypoglycemia in spite of a prevalence of the sympathetic.

Section of the vagus (518). In the experiments to be described all parasympathetic influence on the heart was eliminated by section of the vagus nerves. Here, instead of the initial sympathetic rule which is later overcome by a parasympathetic predominance, the dog displayed a continuous sympathetic hyperactivity throughout the entire experiment. This points to two conclusions: (1) that the slow heart in the animal whose autonomic system was left intact is the consequence of parasympathetic action, which could not manifest itself when the vagus nerve was severed, and (2) that the retarded heart seen in the first group of experiments on intact animals did not mean that the sympathetic tone had died out, but that the overflow of parasympathetic activity has inundated and submerged the sympathetic.

These experiments indicate the correct choice from among the three alternatives proposed at the end of the preceding section: whereas it might appear to the examiner that the second phase of hypoglycemia is solely sympathetic activity, and the fifth entirely parasympathetic, our analysis clearly shows that neither branch is quiescent, for in fact, both may be increased, but one side is overridden by the other.

B. *Further analysis of hypothalamic integration: anoxia, fright, and direct stimulation*

Blood sugar level as indicator. The nature of the hypothalamic integration is disclosed not only in the second phase of hypoglycemia but also in a number of other conditions and some of these—anoxia, fright, struggle, and direct stimulation of the hypothalamus—are reviewed by Gellhorn in his book "Autonomic Regulations" (374). We will only briefly summarize his experiments. Using the level of blood sugar as an indicator, he observed: rabbits respiring oxygen in low concentrations (313); cats either confronted by their hereditary enemies, dogs, or subjected to direct stimulation of the hypothalamus (376). Rats, in some observations were frightened by the noise of fire crackers, or by being tied down to a board (376), while in others the rodents were injected with metrazol (313), cocaine, or bulbocapnine (312). The methods used to disclose the activity of each branch of the autonomic were similar in all these experiments in so far that the animals were studied in three conditions: either the entire autonomic division intact or the peripheral portion of the sympathetic inactivated, or with the latter in addition to vagotomy. We shall review the experiments of Feldman, Cortell and Gellhorn (313) on rabbits respiring only 7 per cent oxygen, since these results are typical of all the others. The usual response to anoxia was observed in the rabbits whose autonomic nerves were unchanged. This reaction in terms of blood sugar, was made evident by an increase from 71 to 84 mg. per cent. In those rabbits whose adrenal glands had been dener-

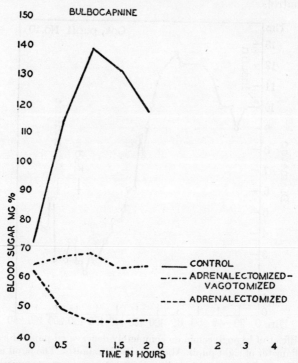

FIG. 45. Influence of bulbocapnine phosphate on blood sugar of rats. Bulbocapnine (50 mg/kg) was injected immediately after the first blood sample was taken.

vated prior to the experiment, instead of a rise in blood sugar, a mild hypoglycemia was effected. Confirming their work on the rabbits, they also found that the blood sugar of adrenalectomized rats in partial anoxia fell from 63 to 42 mg. per cent. In the rabbit and the rat, when the sympathetic influence was removed, the parasympathetic component of the hypothalamus was permitted to express its supernormal activity, causing the secretion of insulin and consequently, a fall in blood sugar.

When all autonomic control of blood sugar was eliminated by section of the vagus and removal of the adrenal glands, there was no significant change in the blood sugar level despite the partial anoxia. The instruments for both lowering and raising the blood sugar had been removed. Essentially the same results were seen when bulbocapnine was injected. In intact rats blood sugar rose; on the other hand, in adrenalectomized animals hypoglycemia ensued. Again when the animals were both adrenalectomized and vagotomized, blood sugar did not change significantly (Fig. 45). These experiments like those of anoxia reveal the two elements of hypothalamic control.

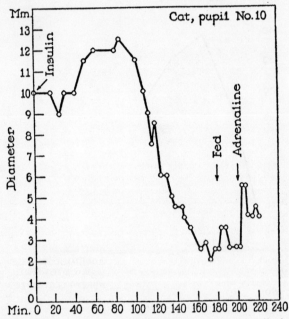

FIG. 46. Effect of hypoglycemia on completely denervated pupil of cat. Ordinate: horizontal diameter of right pupil. Abcissa: time in minutes. The pupil is found to be sensitive both to adrenergic and cholinergic substances, first constricting and then dilating

Adrenergic and cholinergic substances as indicators. Another method of studying the hypothalamic pattern is to observe the effects of sympathetic and parasympathetic substances in the blood stream. By means of these indicators, Bender and co-workers were able to demonstrate the swing from sympathetic to parasympathetic hegemony during progressive hypoglycemia as well as to bring into view the two opposing tones of autonomic pull in the hypothalamus. Bender and Siegal (77) used the pupil of the totally denervated eye as an objective indicator. Deprived of all its nervous innervations, any fluctuations in the diameter of the pupils must be due either to a sympathetic-dilator (adrenergic) substance or to a parasympathetic-constrictor (cholinergic) substance. A cat with pupils so prepared received a large dose of insulin. As can be seen from Figure 46, the diameter of the pupils measured 10 mm. before insulin injection. About 70 minutes after the injection, their diameter had widened to 12.5 mm. Subsequent to this maximal dilatation, there was a progressive narrowing, returning at 110 minutes to the original measurement, then constricting to practically a line, 2 mm., at 170 minutes of insulin action. According to these data, early hypoglycemia is characterized by an adrenergic phenomenon, which is later replaced by a cholinergic reaction.

Bender (75) also used adrenergic and cholinergic substances to examine the hypothalamic pattern, and his method was to cause voluntary muscle to become hypersensitive to acetylcholine,[2] the chemical (cholinergic) media-

[2] Within comparatively recent times we have learned that nerves secrete chemical substances which are released at the nerve-ends and may excite effector organs. The proof first came from Loewi (676) who showed that a vagus substance was liberated in the heart on vagal stimulation, and another substance on stimulation of the sympathetic fibers. The vagus substance later proved to be acetylcholine and another acetyl compound (760) and the sympathetic secretion, adrenaline and nor-adrenaline (149, 295, 708). Dale (218) proposed the words cholinergic and adrenergic to distinguish between the two fibers: the cholinergic secreting the acetyl compounds and the adrenergic, adrenaline, and nor-adrenaline. The components of the parasympathetic system are mostly cholinergic. The motor nerves to the muscles (120) also liberate acetylcholine. On the other hand, most post-ganglionic sympathetic nerve fivers are adrenergic. Because denervated skeletal muscle reacts sensitively to acetylcholine it was possible for Bender to use muscular contraction to indicate the activity of parasympathetic nerves and their neurohormones.

Proponents of two viewpoints support either an electrical or a chemical mechanism for the carriage of the nerve impulse. According to one group of observers, influenced by the data reviewed above the transmission of the impulse depends upon the formation of chemical intermediaries (127, 128, 129, 744). Another group stresses the electrical potential which accompanies the nerve impulse and concludes that the process is an electrical one. Nachmansohn incorporates the chemical concept into the electrical theory and regards acetylcholine as playing an essential role, but a role evoked by the electrical variations (758). Acetylcholine is formed all along the nerve fiber and is rapidly destroyed by cholinesterase or more specifically acetylcholine-esterase (26a) in order to permit further activity (99). The same process occurs not only along the nerve but also across the synapse (360). The acetylcholine associated with neuronal function is probably split off from a precursor (1) and following the activity may either be reconverted to the acetylcholine precursor or hydrolyzed with the aid of the enzyme acetylcholine-esterase. The choline thus freed is reacetylated at the expense of energy from phosphate bonds (763) which in turn is made possible by oxidations and glycolysis (772, 180) (see Chapter 5, p. 72, ft.). Thus the process of neuronal recovery includes, among other restorative phenomena, acetylation of choline and reconversion of acetylcholine to the precursor form. The latter, like the former, is an endothermic action requiring energy (1).

Today the participation of the electrical phenomena in the passage of the nerve impulse is firmly established both for the nerve cell and the synapse (285, 365), but the position of acetylcholine as a chemical mediator in either situation has been questioned (384, 209).

tor between motor nerves and the muscles they innervate. The device he used to render these muscles hypersensitive was to denervate them, cutting their motor nerves. In this way, muscles can be made to reveal slow involuntary contractions as acetylcholine increases in concentration in the blood. That these contractions actually are responses to cholinergic substances in the blood and not to adrenaline, is substantiated still further by the fact that the contractions could be reproduced by injection of acetylcholine, while adrenaline in small doses did not create such responses. Bender used monkeys prepared by cutting the left facial nerve (Fig. 47). These animals were then permitted to scamper about in their cages as they were threatened with a catching net. The usual sympathetic mobilization took place, but about 2 or 3 seconds after the threatening had ceased, slow contractions on the left half of the face appeared, thus disclosing the increased parasympathetic effects occurring at the same time as the usual sympathetic.[3]

Bender and Kennard (76) showed that this response to acetylcholine in the blood did not result from its local liberation since resection of combinations of the third to the twelfth cranial nerves, simultaneous with extirpation of the cervical sympathetic did not change the "fright reaction". The authors conclude that the effect is probably due to a general secretion of acetylcholine-like substances with secondary diffusion through the blood stream to the denervated muscles.

These experiments enlarge our interpretation of bodily integration in an emergency. Cannon (146) emphasized the importance of the mobilization of the sympathetic branch in the attack and defense mechanism of the animal. Bender amplifies Cannon's conception and suggests that during fright there occurs a general discharge of autonomic action with secretions

According to Loewi (677) transmission in ganglia, post-ganglionic cholinergic autonomic nerves and neuromyal junctions is a function of acetylcholine. He also takes into consideration post-ganglionic adrenergic fibers and concludes that the chemical mechanism applies to all peripheral synapses. Despite suggestive evidence for the participation of acetylcholine in transmission in the central nervous system and along nerve trunks we do not possess conclusive proof that stimulation releases acetylcholine in central synapses, nor that sensory nerves are cholinergic. Except then for peripheral synapses the manner in which acetylcholine and cholinesterase affect nerve function is not clear (110, 157). We know however that anticholinesterase drugs, which presumably cause accumulation of acetylcholine, can induce increased cerebral function, as indicated by changes in the brain waves (425), to the point of convulsive electrical patterns (342). Acetylcholine moreover has been found in the cerebrospinal fluid of patients with grand mal epilepsy (948). An excellent review of the recent work on the pharmacology of the nervous system with special reference to the functions of acetylcholine and adrenaline is presented by Marrazzi (708).

[3] An important experiment would be to prepare monkeys by cutting the motor nerves to the facial muscles, and then study the relationship of the parasympathetic to the sympathetic phenomena in the second stage of insulin hypoglycemia.

not only of sympathetic-adrenergic hormones, but also of a parasympathetic-cholinergic substances, both groups entering into the role of bodily defense in times of emergency. The responses to an emergency however are even

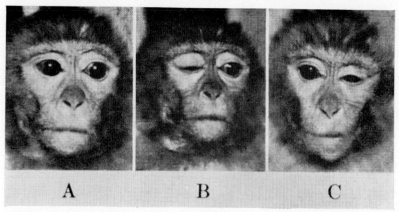

FIG. 47

A shows picture of facial expression of a monkey at rest following sectioning of the left facial nerve. Note that the left eyelids on the paralyzed side are somewhat further apart than on the right.

B shows the effect of voluntary activity on the part of the monkey. The right eyelid closes; the left remains open because of paralysis.

C reveals the "fright reaction." The otherwise paralyzed denervated muscles of the left side are now involuntarily contracted. The contraction of the eyelids and wrinkling of the left side of the face are evident.

TABLE 35

Heart rate as an indicator of autonomic activity in anoxia

BLOOD SUGAR MG. %	AVO₂ DIFF. VOL. %	HEART RATE PER MINUTE ACCORDING TO THE ECG	REMARKS
61	5.5	158	Dog under pentobarbital but before nitrous oxide inhalation
62	0.2	33	$2\frac{1}{4}$ minutes of nitrous oxide
		91	Respiring oxygen
93	0.3	188	Vagi sectioned and ECG taken again after $3\frac{1}{4}$ minutes of nitrous oxide
		160	Respiring oxygen again

more widespread for adrenaline stimulates the activities of the anterior pituitary. That gland therefore secretes its trophic hormones and thus increases the production of thyroxin and of the adrenal cortical steroids, glandular products which are probably utilized more rapidly in conditions of stress (684a). Thus not only the sympathetic and parasympathetic branches but also the anterior pituitary and its dependent glands are mobilized when the safety of the organism is threatened.

C. Medullary autonomic responses in anoxia

In anoxia as in hypoglycemia the heart rate and the electrocardiogram were used to obtain objective evidence on the autonomic integration of the medullary or fifth phyletic layer. A series of dogs was studied before and after vagotomy, and we are submitting a table with the results of a typical experiment (518). In this particular dog anoxia was induced by the inhalation of pure nitrous oxide. The cerebral AVO_2 difference before breathing the gas was 5.5 vol. per cent and heart rate 158 beats per minute. During $2\frac{1}{4}$ minutes of inhalation, the heart rate decreased sharply to 33 beats per minute, and the AVO_2 difference fell to a value within the experimental error, 0.2 vol. per cent. Blood sugar was unchanged. Upon reinhalation of oxygen, the heart rate rose to 91 beats per minute.

As soon as the dog had recovered, both vagi were sectioned and the animal was again subjected to nitrous oxide anoxia for $3\frac{1}{4}$ minutes. Heart readings were again taken. This time, instead of falling, the heart rate increased to 188 beats per minute, and the blood sugar rose from 62 to 93 mg. per cent, both signs to be expected considering that the sympathetic syndrome was in undisputed hegemony. At the same time the cerebral metabolic depression was evidenced by an AVO_2 difference down to 0.3 vol. per cent. Upon restoration of oxygen the heart rate fell to the original beat. From this experiment and the accompanying table we see that by means of vagotomy we could unmask the sympathetic tone when the animal was in the medullary phase.

D. Relationship of autonomic and metabolic findings

Because brain metabolism decreases as the phases of hypoglycemia are traversed (Chapter 10), it would seem possible to determine at what values of the cerebral metabolic rate, first the sympathetic and then the parasympathetic take over. Such a correlation was made for the parasympathetic by sampling blood from the brain, drawn at specific times when the ECG, or clinical symptoms, revealed a distinct deviation from autonomic equilibrium. By this process, we found that when the cerebral oxygen difference of dogs diminished from the normal values of 9.3 vol. per cent to to 4.3 vol. per cent, the heart slowed (518). If cerebral blood flow (and we remember that this factor must be considered) remains constant, then a fall in metabolism to 46 per cent (4.3/9.3) is accompanied by a release of the lower medulla from rostral influences and discloses the signs of the fifth phyletic phase in the dog. The finer analysis of the signs possible in human beings under insulin hypoglycemia invites a correlative study of cerebral metabolic rate both when the second phase features the sympathetic, and the fifth phase, the parasympathetic.

V. Discussion

We have been studying the sympathetic and parasympathetic under a variety of conditions and found that their interactions may follow one of two general patterns (636, 911). They may either bear a reciprocal relationship to each other, or they may increase and decrease together. The first of these patterns is seen in the reaction of the heart when the subject is startled (101). The heart is speeded up, not only because the sympathetic is stimulated but because the parasympathetic is, at the same time, inhibited. In accordance with this pattern the sympathetic has been described as mobilizing the body for emergency, as in strenuous muscular activity, and the parasympathetic as correlating the reconstruction of bodily reserves, characteristic of digestion and sleep. This type of integration has been compared by Eppinger and Hess (284) to a balance on a fulcrum. When one arm of the balance rises, the other falls. But, autonomic activities may follow the second pattern in which both branches act together in the same direction, though not necessarily to the same degree of intensity. Because this direct relationship has not been stressed adequately and especially because it appears, under certain circumstances, to be the more significant of the two, we have assembled the data throughout this chapter using hypoglycemia, anoxia, or hypothalamic stimulation as a basis for examining the parallel or direct action of the two branches.

It must be clear that if the sympathetic were allowed to reign unchecked, the organism would be aroused to an emergency, but the tremendous burst of activity could not be maintained for any protracted duration unless moderated and supported by the parasympathetic. Apparently in some cases, it is more to the biologic advantage of the individual for the parasympathetic to check the sympathetic, than for the former to diminish its own activity. A most striking example showing the benefit of this dual mobilization can be seen in the second phase of hypoglycemia. A patient in the subcortico-diencephalic phase exhibits a picture involving most of the emergency adaptations innervated by the sympathetic branch. But, at no time is the parasympathetic dormant. Instead, a constant watch is kept over the sympathetic, checking any uneconomic bursts of activity. The heart rate has been known to increase during this phase from its normal frequency to one of 110 beats, and concomitant with each wave of further sympathetic release, to a temporary acceleration as fast as 140 beats. Fast as this may seem, it is not, by far, the upper limit of cardiac rate, so we may assume that the parasympathetic has worked its effect to restrain the heart.

In addition to heart rate, blood pressure and size of pupils, as well, do not reach their maxima because of parasympathetic activity.

Whereas the sympathetic dominance of the heart rate is impeded by the parasympathetic in the second phase of hypoglycemia, preventing an excessively fast heart rate, the reverse happens in the fifth phase where the sympathetic moderates the action of the parasympathetic thus keeping the heart from beating too slowly. We know that during the fifth phase the heart rate becomes ever slower, and yet we find that sympathetic activity is also present to prevent an uninhibited parasympathetic sway. These deductions made from observations on human beings receive strong support from animal experimentation, in which excision of the sympathetics prevents the early rise in heart rate (264), and severence of the vagi (518), the late slowing seen in hypoglycemia. This kind of interaction may be compared to a tug-of-war. Neither the sympathetic nor the parasympathetic is permitted to run away with the control, and extremes either to one side or the other are prevented (662).

While the parasympathetic checks the sympathetic in some parts of the body, in others it seems to act independently of the sympathetic. In such cases, the simultaneous mobilization of both branches integrates diverse bodily activities. Bulatao and Carlson (126) showed that hunger contractions gave evidence of parasympathetic activity as soon as blood sugar began to fall in hypoglycemia. Their work, though done on dogs, is in agreement with observations on human beings where the secretory activity of the gastro-intestinal tract, a parasympathetic function, is found to be increased during the second phase of hypoglycemia, even though sympathetic activity is prepotent in other parts of the body. Thus, any food ingested before or during hypoglycemia is rapidly digested and counteracts the hypoglycemia.

Another instance when the sympathetic and parasympathetic are both active on different parts of the body is seen again during the fifth phase where the vasomotor tone and the circulation are maintained by the sympathetic. This phase is most dangerous to the patient because all functions are slackening from a prevailing parasympathetic influence which diminishes heat formation and promotes its dissipation. At this time, more than any other, the continuation of the thin thread of life depends upon the sympathetic centers. In spite of the slow heart, blood pressure is limited in its fall by the vascular adaptation governed through the medullary centers of sympathetic origin. If the parasympathetic were permitted free dominance, and all supporting reactions of the sympathetic withdrawn, vasomotor tone would collapse and survival become precarious. The loss of these sustaining sympathetic activities is best seen where hypoglycemia has been unduly prolonged and in the resulting protracted shock, the vital medullary centers are temporarily in abeyance. (See protracted shock in Chapter 10.)

Not only in hypoglycemia but also in "startle" and in extremely cold temperatures is a biologically useful integration of the body observed under the combined stimulation of the sympathetic and parasympathetic. We have seen that when a subject is startled or frightened, the heart rate is increased because of sympathetic stimulation as well as removal of vagal inhibition. But in other parts of the body a simultaneous mobilization of both branches is observed. As Gellhorn showed (376), blood sugar rises, a sympathetic effect, and at the same time insulin is liberated, a parasympathetic influence. The sympathetic release of hepatic glucose and the parasympathetic liberation of insulin work together to facilitate the oxidation of carbohydrate and thereby furnish an abundance of energy to maintain the startled individual.

Intense cold, too, calls forth the simultaneous actions of both autonomic branches, which interact to speed up carbohydrate metabolism, and in this way aid the organism in withstanding the environmental hardship (377). This action of the autonomic nervous division may be likened to that of a team of surgeons. The chief surgeon performs manipulations distinctive from those of his assistant, but both surgeons are nevertheless working toward a common objective.

Still remaining to be solved are the physiologic mechanisms subserving the different types of autonomic integration. These integrations, reciprocal and direct, must be laid down either in the central or peripheral portions of the autonomic division.

Any attempt at analysis must include the responses in two different kinds of integrations: one affecting the entire area of the brain and the other more discrete in application. The first occurs characteristically when a region is released from cephalad control and involves the simultaneous mobilization of all its components. The second is the result of the receptor stimulation and the immediate response may be either sympathetic or parasympathetic, in which case the other autonomic branch may be inhibited, a reciprocal relationship,[4] or may be activated secondarily so that both autonomic elements are aroused. One suggestion (134) as to the mechanisms underlying the varying interdependence of the sympathetic (946, 962) and the parasympathetic is afforded by evidence which indi-

---

[4] The reciprocal relationship recalls Sherrington's (875) "reciprocal innervation of voluntary muscle" in which for example, the nerves evoking the flexor muscles are stepped up as the nerves to the extensors are inhibited. Perhaps the same stimulus that excites sympathetic centers inhibits those of the parasympathetic, and vice versa. The direct relationship may be compared with the simultaneous neural activation of agonistic and antagonistic muscles, an intergration taking place during standing.

cates that a small dose of adrenaline increases the response to acetylcholine (252, 130) while a large dose reduces the response (708). Another suggestion (709) stresses the importance of the temporal element in determining the nature of the ganglionic actions exerted by adrenaline: a primary inhibition of transmission is followed by a secondary facilitation and a biphasic reaction is disclosed. But until the position of acetylcholine is better understood it would not be rewarding to pursue this analysis further. In the meantime, however, certain facts may be taken into consideration, for example, in the second phase of hypoglycemia when both the sympathetic and parasympathetic hypothalamic centers are hyperactive the sympathetic dominance may be accounted for in part by the presence of the chief centers for the secretion of adrenaline which are housed in the hypothalamus. The situation is different in the medulla oblongata where the parasympathetic hegemony may be ascribed to the fact that its representation is quantitatively greater than the sympathetic. Though we do not fully understand the mechanisms for the different reaction patterns we have begun to correlate them with the character of the nervous stimuli and the physiological status of the body.

The phyletic evolution of the central nervous system is well exemplified in its autonomic division. The lower phyletic layers representing the nervous integration of our earliest vertebrate ancestors is chiefly parasympathetic in character. It is representative of cold-blooded animals, the fish, amphibia, and reptiles, who except for special occasions, were relatively inactive and in whom it was not necessary to maintain a fixed body temperature higher than that of their environment. Their nervous organization, therefore, permitted the ready loss of heat and did not call for a high metabolic rate. For a higher and more complex achievement, centers present in the lower phyla undergo further development and take on additional functions for the appropriate bodily co-ordinations. Thus, we find that the hypothalamus, one of these centers, contains the sympathetic offices necessary for survival in a faster and more complicated way of life. This explanation which is confessedly teleologic nevertheless does more than merely recapitulate the evidence. It shows how the evolution of the nervous system was an essential preliminary step in the adaptation of warm-blooded animals to their environment.

VI. SUMMARY

Applying methodically the results of hypoglycemia and of anoxia as well as of other conditions destructive of cerebral tissues, we have been able to separate the functional levels and analyse the patterns of autonomic control in each. Thus, it has been shown that the concept of "levels of function" can be employed in the analysis of the autonomic nervous division, as well as of the somatic division.

Cited first were human cases which when studied after death revealed distinct lesions in various cerebral areas, the degree and extent of which was in close alliance with the antemortem neurologic symptoms. It was also found that the autonomic control, which is normally balanced, is upset in two great waves during any progressing hypoglycemic coma. The symptoms of the patients conformed to this finding, the first wave climaxing with a sympathetic predominance in the second phase, and the second wave reaching its maximum with a parasympathetic control in the fifth phase.

Further experimentation on animals in which one or another branch of their autonomic nervous system was inactivated, showed that in neither of these two swells of predominance was the other side dormant, but both branches of the autonomic were accelerated, one more so than the other. Therefore, in the second level or phase where the sympathetic is seen to be in command, the parasympathetic is also working, and even at an increased speed. And likewise, where parasympathetic assumed superiority in the fifth phase, the sympathetic is merely cloaked from view, but still active. Considering the second and fifth phases, as well as the first, third and fourth in which there are less conspicuous oscillations, we may conclude that the symptoms observed throughout indicate that both branches of the autonomic nervous system are active in all five phases.

The analysis of the autonomic division throughout this chapter reveals that integration between both its branches may vary in accordance with the kind of stimulation and with the organ which reacts to the stimulus. Either one branch increases while the other is inhibited, the reciprocal integration of strenuous physical exertion, or as in hypoglycemia both are stimulated simultaneously, the direct relationship. With "startle" both the reciprocal and direct reactions are observed: the first on the heart rate, and the second on the level of blood sugar. The chief function of the direct co-ordination is to prevent an extreme response either sympathetic or parasympathetic; and though in general, the reaction of the body may be preponderantly sympathetic or parasympathetic, yet this relationship does not hold in all parts of the body, and in the second stage of hypoglycemia the parasympathetic achieves control of the gastro-intestinal tract despite the general sympathetic predominance.

CHAPTER 12

THE BARBITURATES AND SOME OTHER
DEPRESSANT DRUGS

A Classification of Clinical Signs and a Theory of Narcosis

I. INTRODUCTION

To enter the debated field of narcosis is an adventure for few signposts are available to guide the traveler toward the goal of understanding the underlying mechanisms. A new avenue of approach, however, has been opened by the development of a method for the determination of cerebral metabolic rate *in vivo*. Though this method has been employed in this field for the first time, it has made substantial advances possible, advances, however, that have been prepared for by the work of earlier investigators and particularly Quastel (803) on the action of narcotic drugs.

The term narcosis has been construed in many ways, but it is always referable to a depression of some sort. The particular meaning in this chapter is a depression of nervous function. This involves a diminished sensitivity of all types, a loss of motor responses, and in a word, a condition in which there is a temporary and reversible decrease or abolition of pain and normal automatic activity, usually accompanied by deep sleep.

A good narcotic depresses the newer phyletic portions of the brain while the medulla is left relatively free so that the vital vegetative functions, such as respiration and blood pressure, are maintained. This depression of the higher centers brings on unconsciousness, or prevents the perception of pain, and indeed depresses most reflex excitability so that the patient lies quietly on the operating table despite incisions and other operative manipulations. Notwithstanding the recent advances on the nature of anesthesia, it would seem too early to single out one conception which would apply to all members of such a heterogeneous group of drugs as the narcotics. Nevertheless, there are some suggestions which seem to help us across the first hurdles.

The observations of Meyer and Overton (734) on the lipid solubility of most narcotics, the conclusion of Traube (949) that narcotics lower surface tension, and that of Hoeber (531) to the effect that they diminish cellular permeability, all indicate the method by which narcotics leave the blood and pass through the cellular membranes into the brain proper. But, they do not expound the influence of these drugs once they are within the cell. Quastel (803) has accumulated much evidence from the *in vitro*

326

point of view showing that barbiturates and some other narcotics depress brain metabolism. An analysis of patients subjected to anesthesia in the operating room is necessary, however, in order to obtain a decision as to whether inhibition of brain metabolism is the important factor or whether some action on nerve function is the root of a narcotic condition. The foremost purpose, therefore, of our discussion is to examine brain metabolism following the use of various narcotics, in the hope of determining: (1) whether there is a depression in brain metabolism, and (2) if there is a depression, to evaluate its role in creating narcosis.

II. BARBITURATES

The barbiturates have received a vast amount of attention, the principal incentive being their extensive therapeutic use. By choosing an appropriate member of the barbiturate group any desired degree of depression can be produced, from shallow sedation to deeper sleep and profound surgical anesthesia. Those which act over a long period of time must necessarily be employed for the lighter degrees of depression while the shorter-acting barbiturates may be given intravenously for a brief period of operative anesthesia. Our discussion of the barbiturates is divided into four sections: (A) the effect of barbiturates on brain metabolism, (B) the question of a special influence of this group of drugs on the hypothalamus, (C) a description of the clinical signs during thiopental anesthesia, and (D) using the data assembled in the first three sections as a working basis, we shall discuss the relation of cerebral metabolic depression to the narcotic effect of the barbiturates.

A. *Barbiturates and brain metabolism*

The study of barbiturates and brain metabolism was pioneered by Quastel and his school (803) who have brought forth much reliable evidence to show that barbiturates depress metabolism of excised cerebral tissues. They showed that these drugs do not act as cell poisons which might exert a progressive decrease on the oxygen intake; on the contrary, with a given concentration of a barbiturate, they found that the metabolism did not fall progressively in a steady decline, but was depressed to a constant degree throughout the period of observation. Furthermore, washing the tissues free of the barbiturate reverses its influence so that the oxygen consumption rises towards the original value. Quastel continued his work, finding that the metabolism of the brain was depressed more than that of other tissues that he studied, and even more important, that the barbiturates interfere with the oxidations of carbohydrate and carbohydrate-split products, but not with non-carbohydrates, such as succinic acids.[1] The weight of this discovery is appreciated when we remember that the brain oxidizes chiefly carbohydrate. Of prime significance for the use of barbiturates is an understanding of the order in which the different parts of the brain succumb to their influence (523). By turning to Table 15 of Chapter 7, we see that pentobarbital in 0.012 per cent solution exerts the most profound absolute depression on the cerebral cortex (Col. 5). The percentage inhibition of the brain stem is less than that of the other parts of the brain (Col. 6). This pattern of action with its chief accent upon the cortex furnishes the pharmalogic basis for this entire group of drugs because it applies not only to excised cerebral tissues but, as shall be presented later in this section, also to the intact brain of the living body. The concentrations of barbiturates used in the *in vitro* experiments, however, are much greater even than those employed to produce profound surgical anesthesia. The work of Quastel and others demonstrating that barbiturates depress the metabolism of excised cerebral tissues cannot, therefore, be applied directly to the intact organism until it is verified on living animals and human beings.

The work on our problem, the determination of the *in vivo* effects of barbiturates on brain metabolism, may be divided into two parts: the earlier, concerned only with the cerebral AVO₂ difference and the latter, including not only the oxygen difference but also cerebral blood flow. The earlier results are presented because they add strength to the conclusion that barbiturates interfere with cerebral oxidations *in vivo*. First, then, we shall discuss briefly the investigations on the cerebral AVO₂ difference, beginning with those of Damcshek, Myerson and Loman (219), whose group of patients, comprised of 17 schizophrenics, received intravenously a dose of sodium amytal, sufficient to put them in sound sleep but not in surgical anesthesia. The average cerebral AVO₂ difference before injection was 6.4 vol. per cent, and afterwards, 5.7 vol. per cent. Confirming this small diminution are the results of Dr. F. A. Hale and the author who, in some unpublished observations, found that 5 psychotic patients, narcotized by intravenous injection of sodium amytal, possessed an average oxygen difference of 5.8 vol. per cent, a lower value than the average arterio-venous oxygen difference of normal man, 6.7 vol. per cent (497). These decreases in arterio-venous oxygen difference are less than those reported subse-

---

[1] The value of sodium succinate as an antidote for barbiturate poisoning has been both affirmed (898) and denied (637). Pyruvate has also been suggested as an analeptic for barbiturates (994).

Contradictory results have been reported by Lamson, Greig and Robbins (635a). They found that glucose and some products of glucose metabolism including succinic and pyruvic acids exert potentiating effects on barbiturate anesthesia in certain species of animals. This potentiation is marked in the guinea pig definite in the hamster and rabbit, variable in the dog and not present in the rat.

quently (293) because consideration was not taken of the anatomic arrangement in the cerebral venous return nor of the resulting discrepancies between the right and left arterio-venous oxygen differences during light

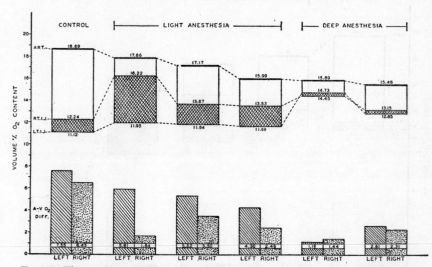

FIG. 48. The results on patient ♯1 are illustrative of the group in which the right arterio-venous differences are reduced more than the left in all observations made during light depression. In deep anesthesia both differences are of lowest value and in agreement with each other. The same data are presented in two ways: the columns in the lower part of the figure depict the right and left arterio-venous oxygen difference in terms of volumes per cent, while in the upper portion of the figure are the actual values for arterial and venous oxygen content. The cross-hatched area shows the difference between the oxygen content of the right and left internal jugular venous blood. The gradual decrease of arterial oxygen is evident as the anesthesia becomes deeper.

Erratum: The arterial content of the control should be 18.22 volumes per cent and the left and right control arterio-venous oxygen differences, 7.10 and 5.98 vols. per cent respectively.

anesthesia (Stages 1 and 2, see Section C). The determination of both arterio-venous oxygen differences in 12 subjects revealed that before thiopental all but one pair of differences were equal within the experimental error. Inequalities appeared however during light thiopental anesthesia. The subjects may be divided into two groups: a larger one of 9 patients, in which one AVO₂ difference was more depressed than its fellow, with averages of 2.8 vol. per cent and 5.9 vol. per cent respectively, and a smaller group of 3 patients, in which both arterio-venous oxygen differences were equally reduced. One example of the first group is patient No. 1

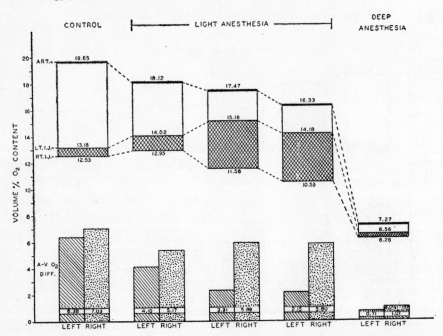

INTRAVENOUS PENTOTHAL SODIUM - PATIENT NO. 5

PREDOMINANT CORTICAL COMPONENT - LEFT INT. JUG. VEIN

FIG. 49. The data of patient #5 are characteristic of the group in which the left arterio-venous oxygen difference is consistently smaller than the right during light anesthesia. In deep depression both right and left arterio-venous oxygen differences are equal and within the experimental error. The data are shown in two ways: the right and left arterio-venous oxygen differences are presented in the columns of the lower part of the figure and in the upper portion are the values for the oxygen content. The cross-hatched area shows the difference between the oxygen content of the right and left jugular veins. The prolonged depression of respiration in deep anesthesia is exhibited in the low oxygen content of the arterial blood.

Erratum: The control values in the right internal jugular venous oxygen content should be 12.53 volumes per cent, and the left and right arterio-venous oxygen differences 6.47 and 7.31 volumes per cent respectively.

(Figure 48), whose right arterio-venous oxygen differences were smaller than the left in each experiment made with sufficient thiopental to secure light depression. In another instance of group I, patient No. 5 (Fig. 49), the left arterio-venous oxygen difference was the lesser and remained so throughout light narcosis. In deep thiopental anesthesia, however, both patients exhibited right and left arterio-venous oxygen differences which were low and equal within the experimental error, irrespective of the pattern displayed when the patient was lightly anesthetized. The smaller

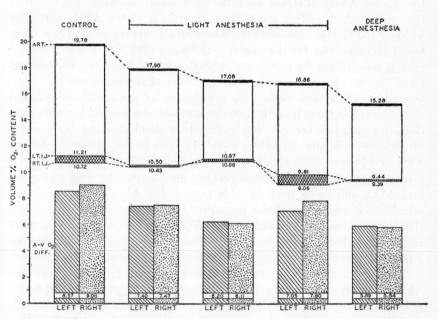

FIG. 50. Patient #10 is representative of the group in which the right and left arterio-venous oxygen differences changed together. The data is presented twice, once in the lower columns showing the paired right and left arterio-venous oxygen differences, which vary within the error of the method, and again in the upper portion of the figure with the value for oxygen content. The cross-hatched portion shows the differences between the oxygen content of the right and left internal jugular blood, none of which, however, is significant. The comparatively large arterio-venous oxygen difference in deep anesthesia is associated with a profound fall in blood pressure.

group, typified by patient No. 10 (Fig. 50), revealed only insignificant differences between the right and left side both in light and deep anesthesia.

It must be emphasized that repeated observations yielded consistent patterns for each group, i.e., if in the *lighter stages* the right arterio-venous oxygen difference was smaller than the left in the first observation, it was smaller in all succeeding ones. This difference between the two sides is not the usual occurrence. Despite the dissimilar sources of blood in the two internal jugular veins the AVO_2 differences are the same, in most instances, due in part to the mixing of the venous blood in cortical-subcortical anastomoses. When discrepancies are observed they may be imputed to differences in oxygen metabolism too great to be entirely overcome by the venous anastomoses. Light thiopental anesthesia imposes an additional strain on venous mixture so that individuals with bilateral equality of AVO_2 at rest exhibit disparities under anesthesia. The suggestion is that the smaller AVO_2 difference is caused by a lower metabolic rate and that the region which suffers the greater depression of the AVO_2 difference includes the cerebral hemispheres. These results appear to supply a functional corroboration for the anatomical finding (389, 64) of asymmetrical venous return from the cortex and subcortex and to indicate a biochemical basis for the well known decorticating action of the barbiturates.

A more satisfactory method for the solution of this metabolic problem was achieved in three investigations on monkey, dog and man, which were definitive in nature because they included the simultaneous measurements of both determinants of cerebral metabolic rate. In the monkey, Schmidt, Kety and Pennes (856) noted that cerebral metabolism was impaired to a greater degree in deep than in superficial anesthesia. The results on cerebral AVO_2 differences were variable but cerebral blood flow was always retarded. A similar metabolic impairment was noted in the dog (538), though in contrast to the monkey the AVO_2 difference was decreased more consistently than blood flow. Finally observations of man (528) demonstrated that cerebral oxidations were depressed in thiopental anesthesia.

In order to prepare for the simultaneous drawing of blood samples, which was necessary in the observations on this group of patients with cerebral disease, needles with stylets were inserted into the femoral artery and the two internal jugular veins after the areas had been numbed by novocaine. The stylets were removed from the needles for the collection of blood samples before and during anesthesia which was produced by the intravenous injection of thiopental in 1% solution. In all observations the depth of anesthesia was evaluated by means of clinical signs (see Section C) and cerebral blood flow was measured according to the method of Kety and Schmidt (596, 598), in which the subject breathes a gas mixture containing 15% nitrous oxide, 21% oxygen and 64% nitrogen, with soda lime being used to remove the expired carbon dioxide. The samples of blood were analyzed for oxygen in order to determine AVO_2 difference and for nitrous oxide to measure cerebral blood flow. Cerebral metabolic rate was calculated from these two factors and expressed in terms of cc. oxygen/100 gm. tissue/minute. (In the remainder of this discussion only the number of cubic centimeters of oxygen will be presented and the rest of the designation, cc. oxygen/100 gm. tissue/minute, is to be understood). The average cerebral metabolic rate for all observations made during anesthesia was found to be 1.6, a reduction of approximately 35% from the average control value of 2.5. Both AVO_2 difference and blood flow may be lowered to produce this result, for in 18 observations made during anesthesia, AVO_2 difference decreased 12 times and cerebral blood flow 13.

It should be pointed out however that the results which were used to obtain these average values differed on both sides in the same patient. Such differences are not usual in resting individuals unencumbered by brain pathology. Kety and co-workers (598) in observations of ten unanesthetized subjects did not find a significant difference between the cerebral metabolic rates as calculated from the right and left internal jugular blood. The mixing of the venous blood by means of cortical-subcortical anastomoses on which this equality largely depends is not always adequate so that in some instances, even in individuals without brain pathology, the bilateral metabolic rates are not the same (1032). This discrepancy moreover occurs more frequently in patients with organic changes of the brain (399) (see p. 94, Chapter 6 for discussion of relation between cerebral vasculature and metabolic observation on these patients). But whether the right and left values are averaged together or whether they are taken separately a decrease of CMR is observed in thiopental anesthesia. Such a decrease however does not occur while the patient still retains some degree of environmental contact as in narcoanalysis (600).

The information gained from the experiments on monkey (856), dog (538), and man (528), proves beyond a doubt that thiopental induces a fall in cerebral metabolism *in vivo*, a conclusion which is corroborated by the *in vitro* observations on the rat (523). This decrease in metabolism places the barbiturates among the group of drugs which can produce histotoxic anoxia, which, as will be discussed at the close of the chapter, is created by blocking the transfer of hydrogen atoms, at some stage, from substrate to oxygen.

B. *Barbiturates and the hypothalamus*

A relationship between the barbiturates and the hypothalamus has been claimed on the grounds that barbiturates bring on sleep, and it is well known that sleep mechanisms are closely bound up with the hypothalamic region, regardless of whether the hypothalamus contains a center for sleep, or as is now more generally held, a center for wakefulness (452, 863, 230, 612, 816). In the latter event, sleep is brought about by a decreased rather than an increased activity of such a center, an explanation in accord with the influence of barbiturates upon the hypothalamus. The experimental basis for this linkage between the hypothalamus and the action of the barbiturates has been probed by many authors. An example of the specificity of barbiturates for the hypothalamus has been disclosed by Pick

(792) and Feitelberg and Lampl (311) who studied temperature changes with the aid of thermocouples in cortical and subcortical loci; and using phenobarbital, they found that though the brain takes part in the general fall of body temperature, not all the cerebral areas react simultaneously. The temperature of the brain stem falls earlier than that of the cortex. Further evidence for the selectivity of the barbiturates for subcortical centers is obtained in the observations of Leiter and Grinker (648) who noted that vasomotor and respiratory responses to electrical stimulation of the hypothalamus were more readily elicitable during ether anesthesia than during that of dial, a barbiturate. Masserman (714) observes that amytal anesthesia diminishes or completely abolishes the sympathetic and emotional mimetic reactions to electrical stimulation of the hypothalamus, leaving the neuromuscular responses to excitation of the motor cortex apparently unaffected.

An opportunity to observe the quieting influence of barbiturates on man is afforded by the use of thiopental for surgical anesthesia. Not only are the early rise of blood pressure, quickening of the heart rate, and widening of the pupils absent but the succeeding stage of wild excitement, characteristic of the hypothalamic release immediately following loss of environmental contact due to ether or other volatile depressants, is not evident with thiopental. Such widespread nervous manifestations of sympathetic hyperactivity are greatly reduced by the hypothalamic depression of barbiturate origin, but are sometimes seen in individuals in the lighter stages of anesthesia who suffer pain or exhibit idiosyncrasies to barbiturates. The work of Keeser and Keeser (579, 580) who found barbiturates in greatest concentration in the hypothalamus has been questioned by Koppanyi and co-workers (620) who obtained an equal distribution of barbiturates in all parts of the brain. Vogt's results (958) are in essential agreement with Koppanyi's. An equal distribution however does not rule out an enhanced action upon the hypothalamus. On the grounds of all this work, it would be difficult to deny that the functions of the hypothalamus are selectively influenced by the barbiturates.

In view of this special barbituric action on the hypothalamus it would be interesting to determine whether the respiratory metabolism of the hypothalamus is preferentially depressed by studying the effects of barbiturates on various regions of the human brain and of the rat brain. In excised rat brain the inhibition of the cerebral hemispheres is greater than that of the brain stem (see Chapter 7, Table 15, Cols. 5 & 6). Our respiratory observations were, however, not limited to the hypothalamus alone which was only a small part of the structures examined. But if our results do represent the hypothalamic metabolic effect, we are, aware of a discrepancy between metabolism and function. In any case, we here see the first example of a point that will be made again later on, that the depression of the brain metabolism is not adequate by itself to explain the changes in behavior wrought by the barbiturates.

C. *Clinical signs of thiopental anesthesia*

The full gamut of the signs of thiopental anesthesia are best seen when this drug is given intravenously in a dilute, usually 1 per cent solution. The anesthetist, whose purpose it is to bring the patient to the operating table expeditiously, injects a stronger concentration of thiopental as fast as compatible with the patient's safety and so is apt to miss the early stages of thiopental anesthesia, which are telescoped by the rapid administration of the drug. But when the thiopental is administered slowly, the full spectrum of the signs is gradually displayed. However, irrespective of the concentration and injection rate of the drug, the clinical signs remain consistent for any given stage.

Although some of the pharmacological actions of thiopental may not be influenced by the depression of cerebral oxidations, as for example, the transitory apnea occurring in the earlier phases, in most instances, the clinical changes are related to a diminution of oxygen utilization and may be segregated into four groups conforming, in general, to a definite pattern (291, 488). Such a pattern is compatible with a metabolic inhibition, which involves the entire brain at all times, but in the beginning is most intense in the cerebral hemispheres, an intensity that spreads, like a wave, in turn over the subcortico-diencephalon, the midbrain, the pons and medulla. The reader should turn to Chapter 10, Fig. 39 on the "transverse section of the brain revealing the five phyletic layers to which the symptoms of hypoglycemia have been allocated," because a similar neuroanatomic localization may be applied to the clinical signs of thiopental narcosis. Except in rare instances, the spontaneous motor phenomena, which are of such importance in elucidating the phyletic stages of hypoglycemia, are entirely blotted out by thiopental. It is, therefore, necessary to seek recourse to stimulation in order to determine the depth of narcotic depression, and by this method the various centers of pain proved to be the keys required to unlock the diagnostic secrets. The difference between the cortical type of discrete and finely coordinated response to pain in the unanesthetized individual, and the less appropriate, broader, and excessive, reaction places the patient in the second phyletic layer, while an even earlier link in the chain of centers for noxious stimuli turns out to be useful in determining the mesencephalic stage of narcosis. Though the following classification is based upon a phyletic plan, its prime principle is to be a guide to the anesthetist. The patient's operability is, therefore, made the chief criterion and the third, surgical, stage of anesthesia cuts across the evolutionary concept to include in its three planes both the subcortico-diencephalic and midbrain phases. The succeeding fourth, or pontine, stage is considered too close to that of medullary failure to be desirable

STAGE	ANESTHESIA	CHARACTERISTICS	SITE of DEPRESSION	BRAIN
I	CLOUDING	EUPHORIA LOSS of DISCRIMINATION *TO* IMPAIRMENT of ENVIRONMENTAL CONTACT	SLIGHT DEPRESSION of CORTEX *TO* MODERATE DEPRESSION of CORTEX	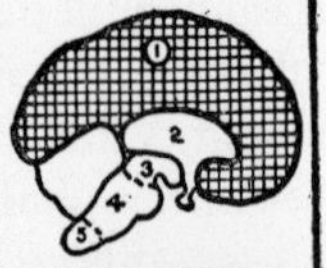 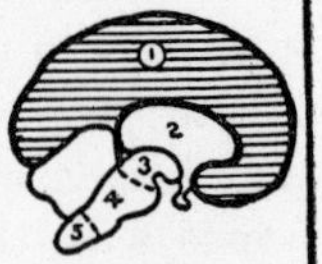
II	DELIRIUM	LOSS of CONSCIOUSNESS	PREDOMINANT CONTROL by SUBCORTEX	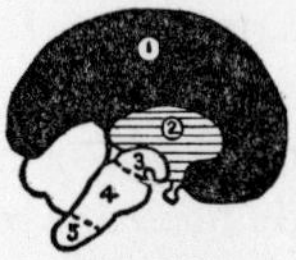
III Plane I	LIGHT SURGICAL	HYPOACTIVITY to PAINFUL STIMULUS	MODERATE DEPRESSION of SUBCORTEX	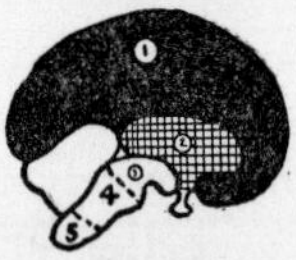
Plane II	MODERATE SURGICAL	LOSS of SOMATIC RESPONSE to PAIN	PREDOMINANT CONTROL by MIDBRAIN	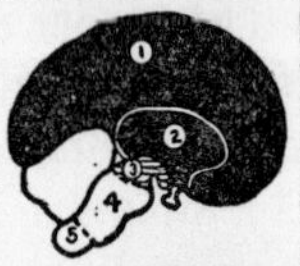
Plane III	DEEP SURGICAL	LOSS of VISCERAL RESPONSE to PAIN	MODERATE DEPRESSION of MIDBRAIN	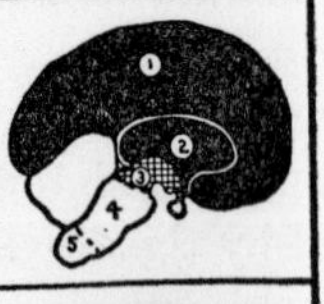
IV	IMPENDING FAILURE	FALL in PULSE PRESSURE	MODERATE DEPRESSION of PONS	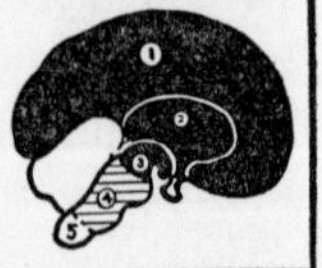

FIG. 51. The neuroanatomic allocation of the stage of anesthesia is correlated with the predominant clinical sign. In the representations of the cerebral transverse sections horizontal lines indicate slight depression, cross-hatching, moderate depression and completely black area, suppression of function.

for practical use, and this admonition applies, though with less emphasis, to the third plane of surgical anesthesia.

The first stage of anesthesia, clouding of consciousness, is associated with depression of the cerebral hemispheres. The second, of delirium, includes suppression of cortical function and slight obtundation of the subcortico-diencephalon. Somewhat greater inhibition of the same layer produces the first plane of the third stage, surgical anesthesia. With the suppression of the first two layers and slight inhibition of the midbrain, the second plane of the third stage appears. Further impairment of the midbrain brings on the third plane of surgical anesthesia. The fourth stage, of impending failure, involves the practical elimination of the activities in the three top phyletic layers and some depression of pons and medulla. It must be realized, however, that the changes do not take place in an abrupt step-wise manner but develop gradually from one stage to the next. Infrequent variations are not included in the following clinical description which represents the usual picture in the nonpremedicated and nonoperative subject. The reader is referred to Figure 51 for the correlation of the anesthetic stages and their neuroanatomic allocations.

Stage I. Clouding of consciousness. The functions ascribed to the highest phyletic layer undergo deepening depression throughout this stage. First among the alterations observed after the injection of several cubic centimeters of thiopental solution is that of personality, as the patient becomes euphoric. If he has previously had a worried, preoccupied expression, it disappears and instead a smile is apt to spread over his countenance. Taciturn individuals become talkative and, in general, freedom from the usual constraints is observed. Euphoria begins the clouding of consciousness, which is the chief characteristic of the first stage. The clouding is made evident by an impairment of environmental contact both as to time and place while specific performance in response to command becomes inept. The patient can still answer questions, but the character of the reply both in content and in physical execution reveals depression of cortical control. Fine discrimination is impeded early and the patient's reaction to pain is altered as it becomes less compelling of attention. But the reverse reaction, increased response to touch and pain, indicates the lower portion of the first stage and this susceptibility, in regard to pain, becomes intensified in the next one. Finally it should be pointed out that this stage of thiopental narcosis, though of little aid in surgery, is effective for narcoanalysis and narcosynthesis (424, 631).

Stage II. Delirium.[2] The stage of delirium begins with the loss of con-

[2] The term delirium is chosen for the second stage of thiopental anesthesia because the term has been used to describe the condition of individuals exhibiting depression of their customary mental activities and reintegration of behavior at a lower function-

sciousness when the patient is no longer aware of his environment. If the patient has been counting aloud, on the command of the anesthetist, the numbers gradually are articulated less clearly. Perhaps the final one the patient is capable of uttering is repeated several times before he stops counting, no longer able either to execute or to receive commands of any kind. The functions of the cerebral cortex seem to be suppressed and those remaining appear to be integrated chiefly by the second phyletic layer, the subcortico-diencephalon, which, however, is itself under limited, though definite depression. The comparatively inept and crude activities of this layer are manifested by the patient's behavior following a painful stimulus. Though the thalamus is deprived of most of its modalities, sensitivity to pain is retained, and to an exaggerated degree, because of the release from the higher centers. A noxious stimulus elicites a hyperactive response exemplified by excessive and inappropriate movements of the arms and legs. The application of various types of pain: pin prick, pressure exerted either on the tendo Achilles or on the superorbital nerve, pinching of the skin with covered or uncovered clamp, all give rise to violent movements of the four extremities. These somatic reactions are supported by visceral adaptations: faster heart rate, raised blood pressure, increased respiration, and widened pupils. Another distinguishing characteristic of this reaction to pain is that it recedes rapidly when the stimulus is withdrawn.

Though a noxious stimulus may evoke hyperactivity, most frequently the second stage of thiopental anesthesia is differentiated from that of ether anesthesia and hypoglycemic coma by the absence of motor excitement. In fact, thiopental anesthesia is characterized by paucity of motor phenomena and specific depression of hypothalamic mechanisms. Though the hypothalamus contains both sympathetic and parasympathetic centers, the sympathetic pattern is predominant. Thiopental, therefore, depresses sympathetic activities in a more obvious manner than those of the parasympathetic. For that reason the emotional mimetic responses are less dramatic than those seen either with other central nervous system

---

al level (829). Though the third and fourth stages of thiopental narcosis might be included within the borders of this definition, it is usually reserved for a more superficial depression and for that reason is also employed in naming the second stage of ether anesthesia (411, 428). With equal justice the term is applied to reversible psychotic episodes characterized by impaired awareness and release of apparently purposeless emotional and motor activities. These episodes are associated with drug intoxications, toxic-infectious exhaustion states and may also occur spontaneously (829).

In the original description, stage II was designated as hypersensitivity because of the exaggerated response to painful stimuli. That term however is incorrect because the threshold for afferent stimulation is not lowered and may be raised. The term dysesthesia is more appropriate because the sensation appears to change character and assume a painful affective tone.

depressants or with hypoglycemia and the patient when free from pain, remains quiet even in this anesthetic stage.

Stage III. Surgical anesthesia. The stage of surgical anesthesia is divided into three planes which are characterized by alterations in responses to pain whether muscular, pupillary or respiratory as well as by changes of eyeball movements.

Plane 1. Light surgical anesthesia. With the beginning of the first plane, the response to a painful stimulus becomes diminished. Even the application of a clamp to the skin can evoke only a slight movement of the arm or leg, and for this reason it is felt that minor surgical procedures may be performed here. At this time, not only are the cerebral hemispheres suppressed but the second phyletic layer, though still active, is depressed more deeply than in the second stage.

Plane 2. Moderate surgical anesthesia. In the second plane, muscular response to a painful stimulus is abolished but pupillary dilatation and respiratory changes are still evoked on the application of a clamp to the skin. The suppression of the second phyletic layer, which accounts for the failure of somatic or muscular reactions to a noxious stimulus, leaves the midbrain, though somewhat depressed, the highest remaining active level. The persistence of pupillary and respiratory responses may be attributed to a mesencephalic pain center (966). From this center inhibitory impulses emanate to the Edinger-Westphal (third) nucleus, temporarily preventing its tonic constrictor effects upon the pupil (379).[3] When the patient is not stimulated, however, the pupils in most instances are constricted and no longer react to light.

Plane 3. Deep surgical anesthesia. As muscular responses to pain have ceased in the previous plane, the distinguishing signs of this one are the loss of pupillary and respiratory reactions to a noxious stimuli as the lowest pain center becomes increasingly depressed with the other mesencephalic mechanisms.

Stage IV. Impending failure. All visible responses to pain have previously disappeared, but the diagnosis of this stage is aided by an evaluation of pulmonary and cardiovascular function. The predominant signs of the fourth stage are extreme depression of respiration and diminution of pulse pressure. The onset of pupillary dilatation frequently observed may be ascribed in part, at least, to anoxia. Though the signs of the fourth stage

---

[3] Harris, Hodes and Magoun (446) conclude that the perception of pain and pupillodilation possess afferent pathways which are distinct throughout their courses. Their conclusion, however, does not exclude the inhibitory relationship between the pain and the pupillary centers presented above. Kuntz and Richins (633), however, note that anesthesia induced by pentobarbital, a member of the barbiturate group of drugs, lowers the threshold for pupillodilation which they believe is caused by activation of the third nerve center rather than by its inhibition.

disclose that the pons and medulla are not free of sensible metabolic inhibition, they are the highest cerebral regions which are still in activity. This stage must be regarded as a warning sign that further progression in the depth of anesthesia would suppress the vital centers and lead to the dangerous fifth stage of medullary failure.[4]

Signs of Anesthesia. The series of progressive changes in the clinical signs throughout the entire course of anesthesia are briefly commented upon in the order of their appearance in the following table.

Pupil size: The size of the pupil gradually becomes smaller with increasing depth of anesthesia and constriction is the rule in the second and third planes of the third stage. The absence of earlier dilatation of the pupil may be attributed to depression of the hypothalamic mechanisms (714) though the pupil may become enlarged when anoxia supervenes.

Pupillary reactions to light and to pain: The pupillary reaction to light disappears in the second plane of the third stage when the Edinger-Westphal nucleus is obtunded. The dilatation with pain fails to occur in the third plane of the third stage, probably due to depression of the midbrain pain center.

Eyeball activity: Eyeball movements become involuntary in the second stage and even in the first plane of the third stage some slight activity is present. Then, in the lower part of the second plane and in the third plane the eyeballs become fixed and centrally placed. The loss of movement can be explained by a depression of the median longitudinal bundle and the nuclei of the third and fourth cranial nerves.

Eyelid tone: The eyelid tone gradually recedes in conformity with skeletal muscle tone throughout the body.

Corneal reflex: The corneal reflex exhibits a greater inconsistency than any of the other signs, perhaps because of its association with pain centers situated in three different phyletic layers. Thus, this reflex may disappear in the second stage or in the first and the second planes of the third stage. But it is not invariably absent until the third plane is attained, when the three top phyletic layers are obtunded.

Muscular reaction to pain: The muscular responses to all kinds of pain are unchanged in most of the first stage but are hyperactive in the second when the second phyletic layer is dominant. All reflex movements become minimized in the first plane of surgical anesthesia with depression of the second layer. When the functions of this cerebral area are entirely suppressed skeletal muscular reactions fail completely.

[4] Swank and Foley (931) did not confirm this series of signs. These investigators however, employed another species, dog, and other conditions: for example, the control observations were not made before the barbiturate was injected but afterwards.

TABLE 36
Signs of thiopental anesthesia

STAGES OF ANESTHESIA	PUPIL SIZE	PUPIL REACT. TO LIGHT	PUPIL REACT. TO PAIN	EYE BALL ACTIVITY	EYELID TONE	CORNEAL REFLEX	MUSCLE REACT. TO PAIN	PULSE	B.P.	RESP.
Stage I	4+	4+	4+	voluntary	4+	4+	+4	N	N	N
Stage II	4+ to 3+	4+	4+	roving	4+ to 2+	4+ to 0	6+	N	N	N
Stage III Plane I	3+ to 2+	3+ to 1+	3+	slight	2+ to 0	4+ to 0	1+	N	slight fall	diminished
Plane 2	2+ to 1+	0	2+	deviate then central	2+ to 0	4+ to 0	0	Inc.	varies	depressed
Plane 3	1+	0	0	central	0	0	0	Inc.	varies	depressed to apnea
Stage IV	dilate with anoxia	0	0	central	0	0	0	Inc.	fall in pulse press	apnea

The preanesthetic state is expressed as 4+ and deviations therefrom by corresponding changes in the number of pluses (+), increasing to 6+ and diminishing to zero (0). In the last three columns N stands for preanesthetic values.

Pulse: The pulse rate is altered by thiopental only when anoxia or CO_2 accumulation supervenes and at such times the rate increases.

Blood pressure: The blood pressure will fall frequently in the lighter stages of anesthesia and especially during a rapid induction. This phenomenon, however, is usually transient. There are often slight variations in the systolic and diastolic pressure but a fall in pulse pressure is characteristic of the fourth stage.

Deep tendon reflexes. Tendon reflexes are not included in Table 36 because of their inconsistencies. Not only are there discrepancies between the responses on both sides of the body but little positive correlation is found in regard to the depth of anesthesia: for example, reflexes are occa-

TABLE 37

Arterial hemoglobin oxygen saturation in thiopental anesthesia

CONDITION	HB. PER CENT
Preanesthesia	95
Stage I	94
Stage II	94
Stage III	
Plane 1	92
Plane 2	82
Plane 3	39

A correlation of arterial hemoglobin saturation with stages of thiopental anesthesia is presented. The results are the averages obtained on a series of 12 patients (528). The dangerously impaired saturation of arterial hemoglobin when the patient's spontaneous respiration is deeply depressed by thiopental reveals a need for the anesthetist's aid in improving the oxygenation of the patient's blood (292).

sionally hyperactive even in the fourth stage in some patients and yet are absent in the third stage in others.

Effect of thiopental on respiration. Respiratory activity must be considered separately throughout the four stages, for respiratory arrest may take place at any of the last three stages and in that case is out of proportion to the other narcotic effects. Depression of respiration may be brought about by a rapid injection of even a relatively small amount of this drug. This type of apnea is temporary and respiration is resumed quickly or is easily reinvoked, by painful stimulation and other analeptic measures, except in deepest anesthetic stages. If, however, this transient type of apnea is avoided by a slow and gradual administration of thiopental, a respiratory pattern, more consistent with the degree of cerebral metabolic inhibition, is observed. An apparently normal rate and rhythm persist until the second plane of the third stage when a diminution of amplitude and an increase of rate are observed. Breathing, which becomes increasingly shallow and rapid in the third plane, occasionally gives way to apnea which, however, is the frequent occurrence in the fourth stage.

In Table 37 will be observed the oxygen saturation of the arterial hemoglobin during the various stages of thiopental anesthesia (292). The dangerous arterial depression, mirroring the inadequate pulmonary exchange, is observed beginning in the second plane of surgical anesthesia and becoming extreme in the third plane. This brings to a brain already laboring under the disadvantages of depression of nerve function and impairment of cellular respiration the added impediment of a deficiency in arterial oxygen (292, 814) which unfortunately is a handicap shared by all the organs of the body. The depression of respiration results not only in anoxemia but also in acidoses as CO_2 is retained and pH falls (814). If it is necessary to continue a profound stage of anesthesia, the patient should be aided. Instead of air he should be given oxygen. Instead of depending on his own inadequate respiratory movements, the anesthetist should enlarge the thoracic excursions by alternately compressing and releasing the rubber rebreathing bag filled with oxygen, parts of the anesthetist's apparatus. The benefits derived throughout the body from the improvement of the arterial oxygen do not, however, extend to the barbiturate inhibition of cerebral cellular respiration which ceases only with the detoxication of the drug.

Though metabolism is depressed to such an extent, in thiopental narcosis, as to be insufficient to support function in the upper portions of the brain, it must not be thought that their energy exchanges are entirely eliminated. On the contrary, their metabolic rates even in deep surgical anesthesia are adequate to maintain cerebral structural integrity. It would require a much greater dose of thiopental than the amount used for surgical anesthesia to cause cellular destruction. Such a lethal dose may be compared with the concentration of barbiturates employed to impede the oxidation of cerebral tissues which are excised and therefore functionless. Large concentrations are necessary before the basal respiration of excised tissues can be inhibited, while in vivo we have not only to deal with the basal respiration for the maintenance of structures but also built upon and beyond it the metabolism to support function. The latter may be checked by a comparatively small dose of drug. And that is why even after the spontaneous activities of the respiratory centers fail, so long as the patient is aerated by the anesthetist and the complicating factor of an anoxic anoxia is avoided, recovery is assured. Since structural maintenance is not interfered with by the dose of thiopental used in patients, it is not surprising that after the intervenous injections of thiopental have ceased and the barbiturate is detoxified, cerebral metabolism rises and function is restored.

Another sign of the continued metabolism of the brain even in deep anesthesia is the presence of brain waves. When clouding begins the undulations become higher and faster than before anesthesia and these alterations which appear first in the frontal lobes and then gradually extend to occipital area grow more pronounced as the first stage progresses. The onset of the second stage is signalled by the disappearance of the fast waves and the presence of large slow ones. But beyond the inception of the stage of delirium the EEG no longer correlates with the depth of anesthesia for the delta waves remain predominant during the entire period of profound narcosis (322, 108). The change in character of brain waves with loss of environmental contact is therefore similar to that observed in hypoglycemia (508).

Recovery. In recovery, the patient's signs reveal that he advances upward through the various planes and stages of anesthesia, passing through the midbrain, subcortico-diencephalic and cortical stages, before complete recovery is gained. Additional evidence for the retracing of the anesthetic path during recovery is afforded by the electroencephalogram for the slow frequencies which give way to faster ones reappearing first in the occipital region, then in the parital and finally in the frontal, the newest part of the cerebral hemispheres, an order which is the reverse of that observed during the propagation of the narcosis (108). If the course of the anesthesia is brief and superficial, the return is more rapid than if it is prolonged and of greater depth. As a general rule, restitution requires a longer time than is necessitated for the production of anesthesia and this disproportion becomes greater the more profound the narcosis. Neither the EEG changes nor the clinical manifestations are as clearly defined as during induction (322, 108) nor do all signs occur exactly in reverse order during recovery. For example, the restoration of the pupillary size and the reaction to light may be delayed, but in general the course transversed by the patient is the opposite of the one he passed through when he underwent anesthesia.

In this work, we have shown that many of the symptoms observed in thiopental anesthesia may be explained by a phyletic pattern: the depression of cortical functions in the first stage, the release phenomena in responses to pain in the second stage, the loss first of motor and then visceral responses to pain in the midbrain stages, and recovery involving the same path, though in a reverse direction and at a slower rate. We fully recognize, however, the phyletic pattern cannot be applied to all the clinical signs. Examples are the hypothalamic depression, out of proportion to metabolic inhibition, and the variability of the depth at which the corneal reflex is lost and respiratory depression supervenes. As far as the hypothalamus is concerned, a specific affinity of the barbiturates for this region of the brain has been demonstrated. Similarly a special attraction for thiopental has been put forward as an explanation for the inconsistency of the corneal and respiratory reactions. Another complicating factor in the case of the corneal response suggested above is the association of this reflex with pain centers in each of the upper three phyletic layers, while for the respiratory apnea, the exceedingly alkaline titer of the injected thiopental must also be considered. But whatever the exact explanation may be, we can conclude that all the clinical signs do not fall into the phyletic pattern, which must be regarded as a pragmatic aid for further research rather than a completed conception for the neurologist.

The anesthesiologist should remember that the signs were obtained in nonoperative and nonpremedicated patients and that the thiopental was given slowly, in dilute solution. A fast induction renders the differentiation of the various stages more difficult. Furthermore after the drug is given the patient may become lighter and show signs of previous stages. According to Dr. B. Etsten[5] the two signs which are most reliable and fairly constant are the pupillary reactions to light and to pain. The value of these signs should also be considered when other anesthetics are used with thiopental since the specific effects of barbiturates on the respiratory centers make it unsafe to bring the patient beyond the plane of moderate surgical anesthesia by the use of thiopental alone. If nitrous oxide and curare are employed as adjuvants, the pupillary reactions still remain useful as indicators of the planes of surgical anesthesia. Even a mild dose of atropine does not seriously interfere with them. But with cyclopropane and ether to complicate thiopental the pupillary signs are no longer diagnostic. In the operating room it may not be practical to apply the various landmarks presented in the clinical analysis of thiopental anesthesia. Yet from the point of view of understanding the reactions of the central nervous system they yield an insight which is of aid in elucidating the mechanisms involved in barbiturate narcosis.

D. An evaluation of barbiturate depression

Though the data presented so far prove that barbiturates do depress brain metabolism, the role played by this depression in the production of a narcotic state is not its only determinant. Metabolic depression does vary with the depth of narcosis but the extent of the inhibition is inadequate to explain the entire anesthetic effect. This inadequacy is seen on comparing the metabolic deficit observed in hypoglycemic coma with that of thiopental anesthesia (528). If we may take the observations obtained by two different groups, then brain metabolism is decreased from its original value by 40 and 60% (600, 477) during insulin hypoglycemia. On the

[5] Personal communication.

other hand, with thiopental, the average oxygen intake for all observations made in anesthesia, is lowered approximately 35%. The metabolic inhibition of insulin hypoglycemia is, therefore, considerably greater than with thiopental anesthesia. Other reports show that another factor, interference with nerve function, in addition to metabolic impairment, occurs with thiopental anesthesia.

Suggestions as to how barbiturates may act to alter nerve function have been submitted by the work of a number of investigators, one group of which found that certain barbiturates paralyze the vagus nerve (427, 665, 364, 621), preventing its characteristic action to slow the heart. In addition to this autonomic effect, it was found by studying the electrical potentials in the cerebral cortex of the cat (231) and of the dog (529), that pentobarbital greatly increases the amplitude of the slower waves arising spontaneously in the cortex. This seems to suggest an analogy of the action of pentobarbital to sleep. The deepest phases of pentobarbital anesthesia are marked on the EEG by an almost complete cessation of this spontaneous activity of the cortex. Nevertheless, even at this stage, when a sensory nerve is stimulated, it still evokes electrical potentials from the cortex, though any motor response is prevented (231). We can say from the electrical studies that pentobarbital suppresses spontaneous cortical activity, as well as motor response, but does not block the approach through the sensory channels.[6] Despite the relatively weak development of their powers on the sensory side, the barbiturates, in common with other general anesthetics, impair the transmission of the nerve impulse. This impaired transmission may be referred to as an elevation in the threshold of the synapse (460). If a comparison is permissible between central and peripheral synapses then it should be noted that barbiturates and other anesthetics depress synaptic transmission in the excised superior cervical ganglion before a measurable decrease in oxygen consumption is observed (639a), another example of differential depression in function and metabolism.

The action of some barbiturates to inhibit the vagal slowing of the heart is also accomplished by interfering with the propagation of the nerve impulse (427). This interference with neural function is similar, in effect,

---

[6] The failure to evoke motor expression may be ascribed to the absence of afterdischarge or the inability to excite the many additional impulses which normally arrive at the motor neurone as a result of long-circuiting in the central nervous system (69, 711). Usually these additional impulses reinforce, strengthen and prolong the more direct effects of the original stimulus. The depressant effects of the barbiturates are exerted chiefly on the innumerable interneurones rather than on the more direct afferent paths to the cortex (109). The absence of long-circuiting, in turn, is associated with a raised synaptic threshold due in part to an impeded rate in the recovery of the neurone after impulse propagation (712).

to the paralyzing influence of atropine on parasympathetic nerves and curare on motor nerves. It would seem that there are two fundamentally different ways of halting cerebral activity: one involves obstruction of nerve function and the other is a consequence of a diminished metabolic rate. Thiopental occupies an intermediate position, deriving its influence both from inhibiting cerebral metabolism and from obtunding nerve function.

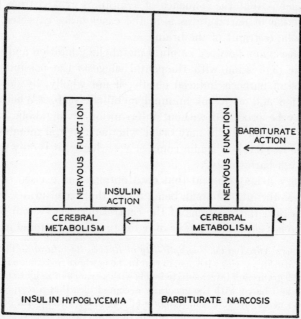

FIG. 52. In insulin hypoglycemia nervous function is affected only indirectly as its metabolic support is withdrawn. In barbiturate narcosis the influence is two-fold: (1) a direct interference with nervous activity, and (2) a depression of cerebral metabolism, though small compared with insulin action.

This bipartite basis of thiopental anesthesia is also revealed by the examination of the clinical signs presented in the preceding section. We do not know whether interference with nerve function takes place in any given sequence, but the phenomena of progressive thiopental anesthesia are best explained by a combination of nerve inhibition superimposed upon the metabolic depression which exhibits a pattern of phyletic regression. According to this viewpoint, the extent to which cerebral metabolism of the individual is lowered is by no means comparable to his loss of nervous activity. For instance, the action of thiopental may narcotize a patient deeply, but his brain metabolism does not fall to a proportional degree. In the case of hypoglycemic coma, however, the brain metabolism and nervous performance fall to equally perilous depths. It is obvious that in insulin hypoglycemia the brain can no longer carry on because the power to perform its work has been turned off. In barbiturate narcosis, part of the energy is still available in spite of the fact that the subject is in deep narcosis. We therefore must admit that the depression of brain metabolism does not tell the whole story of barbiturate narcosis and have indicated that barbiturates interfere directly at some point with nervous activity. The main fact is that the sequence of symptoms evoked from the intravenous injection of barbiturates is in the exact order expected if caused by a metabolic restraint of the brain.

This inconsistency between cerebral metabolic inhibition and the extent of anesthetic depression with thiopental suggests the possibility of still another type of narcosis induced chiefly, if not wholly, by depression of nerve function and with but minimal metabolic factor. Whether or not narcosis may be produced without interruption of metabolic support, it is apparent that anesthesia may occur whether cerebral metabolic rate is forced to the low level of insulin coma or yet whether it is only moderately decreased by a barbiturate.[7]

In summary it may be said that data obtained on excised cerebral tissues as well as the intact human being reveal that barbiturates lower brain metabolism. But, the reactions of the central nervous system to barbiturates seem to have a special power over the functions centered in the hypo-

[7] *Some Factors Affecting the Susceptibility of Rats to Barbiturates.* The resistance of rats to barbiturates varies with age, lowest in the newborn, maximum in rats weighing from 50–200 grams and intermediate levels with advance in weight and age. These results are in agreement with the generally accepted idea that a reciprocal relation exists between metabolic rate and narcotic effect. This relationship, however, may rest for the most part on the metabolic rate of the brain rather than that in the entire body. It is true that in rats the form of the curves for basal metabolic rate and cerebral metabolic rate are similar (602, 165). Both curves are found at their lowest levels for approximately the first three weeks of life before rising rapidly to a maximum at the end of the seventh week and then receding very slowly toward old age. But the early changes of B.M.R. would seen to depend on the entire organism rather than on the metabolism of any organ for the metabolism of kidney and liver slices from newborn rats is found to be approximately the same as in the mature animal (216). Cerebral metabolism on the contrary is much lower in the newborn than in the adult, in accordance with the smaller dose required to anesthetize the neonate. This relationship between C.M.R. and narcosis is to be expected since the primary effect of narcosis is exerted on the brain.

The necessity for the individualization of barbiturate dosage is well known. Observations on rats suggest that in addition to age and weight, sex, strain, and nutritional status are factors. In the first place, mature females are more susceptible to barbiturates than males, a difference evoked by pentobarbital but not by thiopental. Secondly, the LD_{50} dose was found to be quantitatively different in three different strains of rats. Finally, in (537) vitamin B_1 deficiency, resistance to barbiturates is sensibly diminished.

thalamus. Motor activity is also selectively affected. Despite the disagreement caused by a direct influence exerted upon nerve function, the general direction of the symptomatic march, descending the neuraxis, may be ascribed to a metabolic inhibition. The explanation is offered that retardation of cerebral metabolic activities is part of the mechanism by which barbiturates create the condition of narcosis.

It is true that all the barbiturates which were studied for their effect on brain metabolism inhibit energy exchanges, but it is known that though most barbiturates are hypnotic in their action, some in marked contrast are convulsant though they still slow the cerebral metabolic rate *in vitro* (356). This same discrepancy between depression of brain metabolism and stimulation of nervous activity has been observed with the non-barbiturate drug, indole. Hutchinson and Stotz (549) found that the administration of indole to rats in amounts adequate to yield an *in vitro* inhibition of 30% to 50% in brain metabolism led to clonic convulsions instead of narcosis.

To explain the convulsant action of some of the barbiturates it is necessary to examine their metabolic and functional influences in order to determine whether they differ from those exerted by the sedative members of this group of drugs. It must be remembered that the diminution of cerebral oxygen intake does not necessarily prevent motor activity but under certain conditions induces hyperactivity. The excitement and convulsive movements that may occur in the second stages of insulin coma, ether anesthesia as well as during thiopental narcosis in the presence of painful stimuli show that metabolic inhibition of the cerebral hemispheres facilitates the functional release of the subcortico-diencephalic layer. If the convulsant barbiturates lack the specific depressant effects on motor expression possessed by their sedative congeners, the metabolic inhibition will serve only to precipitate hyperactivity. The absence of selective motor restraint in conjunction with the cortical release occurring in the second stage of barbiturate anesthesia provide the conditions required for the precipitation of the convulsive fit.

III. NITROUS OXIDE

The gas nitrous oxide is frequently used to produce anesthesia, either for operations of short duration, or for longer ones in which complete muscular relaxation is not required. A favorable anesthetic concentration is 80 per cent nitrous oxide and 20 per cent oxygen, a mixture containing practically the same amount of oxygen as in the air. But, this mixture is effective only when given to patients who have been properly premedicated with a short-acting barbiturate or a mixture of morphine and scopolamine. Without the necessary premedication, the oxygen percentage must be reduced below 20 per cent to insure surgical anesthesia. Adequate oxygenation during nitrous oxide anesthesia is therefore entirely dependent upon proper premedication (See (411), pages 84–85). In the treatment of schizophrenia undiluted nitrous oxide has been employed (332), in which case the anoxic element must be the predominant one. Nevertheless it should be emphasized that nitrous oxide does possess narcotic properties. For example, if nitrogen were substituted for nitrous oxide in the above named gas mixture, making a combination of 80% nitrogen to 20% oxygen, the anesthesia would abruptly cease (411).

Unfortunately we have no observations on brain metabolism of patients respiring 80% nitrous oxide and 20% oxygen (patients subjected only to the narcotic action of nitrous oxide and no additional anoxic element).

TABLE 38

Effect of undiluted nitrous oxide on arterial oxygen relations

PATIENT	LOSS OF CONTACT			SURGICAL ANESTHESIA		
	Content	Capacity	Hemoglobin Saturation	Content	Capacity	Hemoglobin Saturation
	vol. per cent	*vol. per cent*	*Per cent*	*vol. per cent*	*vol. per cent*	*Per cen*
1	17.6	20.4	86	4.4	21.5	21
2	16.9	18.5	91	7.4	19.9	37
3	15.3	16.3	99	4.4	16.1	28
4	12.7	20.4	62	9.0	20.6	44
Average			83			33

The depression of hemoglobin saturation is slight at the time of loss of environmental contact in comparison with the arterial depletion required for surgical anesthesia.

Nor have we any data on partial anoxia when nitrous oxide is given in a gas mixture containing less than 20% oxygen, i.e. 90% nitrous oxide and 10% oxygen. But we do have observations on 4 patients subjected to undiluted nitrous oxide at two different times—when they first lost contact with the environment, and later in deep surgical anesthesia (Table 38). The average value for the hemoglobin saturation at the time consciousness was lost was 83% and in surgical anesthesia, 35%. In deepest anesthesia the oxygen content was observed to be below 5 vol. per cent (496). This fall in arterial oxygen was reflected in the reduced AVO₂ difference. In an observation not included in the table, a difference of 5.5 vol. per cent before anesthesia was reduced to 0.2 vol. per cent during anesthesia. It is obvious that brain metabolism must have been greatly depressed. It is just such a deep depression of brain metabolism over an extended period of time which can produce irreversible cerebral damage (Chapter 11). Such a devastating sequel is a rare occurrence because nitrous oxide anesthesia can be well controlled and is easily reversible. But, should the anoxic element become overpowering, then the brain will suffer injury, either transitory or of an irreparable nature, the extent of which depends upon the duration and severity of the anoxia. In this connection, the destruction may take the form of permanent neurologic residuals, or if more widespread, may be lethal. Occasionally, death is preceded by a "vegetable" syndrome, so termed because only the vegetative functions of the body remain intact. In this condition the patient may well be described as decerebrate, for only the medulla and cord are functional. (See Chapter 11, Section III, Cases 3–7). Nitrous oxide is not alone in this class, as any other gas which displaces oxygen in the inspired air may produce similar results.

The general conclusion made from clinical observations that the narcotic effect of nitrous oxide cannot be the lethal factor is supported by the work of Bülow and Holmes (131) on excised tissues. According to these authors nitrous oxide left brain metabolism unaffected. On the other hand, reports of patients who succumbed from brain damage after nitrous oxide anesthesia reveal that anoxia was a prominent feature. The damaging effects must therefore be attributed to oxygen deprivation. Courville (199) in his comprehensive monograph concludes that regardless of the immediate cause of the brain damage, the clinical symptoms and pathologic findings are not due to the toxic effect of nitrous oxide but to the insufficiency of oxygen.

IV. Alcohol

Any discussion of the effects of alcohol on metabolism must be considered in at least 2 aspects: alcohol as a food, and alcohol as a narcotic. On general grounds, because it is known that glucose is the chief foodstuff of the brain, we would not expect alcohol to be readily utilized by that organ. In Chapter 2 it was pointed out that patients in hypoglycemic coma who received alcohol either by mouth or intravenously showed no change in the cerebral AVO_2 difference. The clinical symptoms confirmed the metabolic observations because the patients failed to rouse from their hypoglycemic coma after receiving alcohol (408). These experiments point to the conclusion that alcohol does not supply energy in significant amounts for brain metabolism.

Nevertheless there is reliable evidence in literature showing that the brain can oxidize some alcohol (520). Dewan (232, 233) has demonstrated a cerebral enzyme system capable of oxidizing alcohol to acetaldehyde (see footnote page 79). Probably the capacity that the brain possesses to oxidize alcohol is obscured by its narcotic action (520).

The disturbing effect of alcohol on the central nervous system is a common observation. Its action, like that of so many other narcotic drugs, commences on the higher centers of the brain and gradually envelops the lower ones. It is necessary to determine whether the behavioristic changes of the alcoholic individual are associated with a decline of his cerebral metabolic rate, and if so, what the relationship between the two may be. That alcohol does depress brain metabolism was concluded by Goldfarb, Bowman and Wortis (406) who studied the cerebral AVO$_2$ difference in 10 people when they were first admitted to Bellevue Hospital in acute alcoholic coma, and again after they had recovered from their debauch. Their average cerebral AVO$_2$ difference was 5.9 vol. per cent during coma and 7.7 vol. per cent afterwards. These authors quote Thomas (941) to show that alcohol increases the rate of blood flow through the brain, and therefore they might have concluded that the fall in cerebral AVO$_2$ difference was caused by the more rapid flow of cerebral blood. But they did not so conclude because they believed that at the time they made their observations such an acceleration of cerebral blood flow had ceased, and therefore that the low AVO$_2$ difference indicated depression of brain metabolism. Also working on this problem were Loman and Myerson (682) who administered alcohol to human subjects in amounts equivalent to 50–85 cc. of absolute alcohol and found a noteworthy decrease of the oxygen removed from the cerebral blood in two instances. In other words, according to these workers, alcohol along with the barbiturates belongs to the group of agents capable of depressing cellular respiration. A point which may be regarded in favor of the histotoxic action of alcohol may be elicited by means of the EEG. The changes of electrical potential under the influence of alcohol are suggestive of a diminution in cerebral energy (228, 282).

Supporting the conclusion on human subjects are further data obtained *in vitro*. From Keilin's observations (581) we know that alcohol may act against cellular oxidations. He has demonstrated that alcohol does not impair the activation of oxygen by cytochrome-oxidase. In a word, alcohol, like the barbiturates, interferes at some point of the hydrogen transport system.

Such a conclusion receives support from other *in vitro* experiments. We refer to observations on excised tissues where it was necessary to use a 6 per cent concentration of alcohol in order to exert a significant metabolic depression (Table 14, Chapter 7). Six per cent is a value of tremendous strength when we consider that a concentration of only 0.6 per cent in the blood of an intoxicated person may be lethal (277). Perhaps with alcohol as with thiopental the concentration of the drug required to inhibit cellular respiration of excised brain tissue is greater than that necessary to depress the oxygen intake of brain *in situ*. When one observes the profound stupor of an individual in an acute alcoholic poisoning, it is impossible to decide whether his narcosis may be ascribed entirely to cerebral metabolic depression. Until quantitative measurements of cerebral metabolic rate are made in alcoholic individuals, it will be impossible to estimate accurately the importance of the metabolic factor. And so the probability exists that the narcotic effects of alcohol may emanate from other avenues than a depressed metabolism in the brain. This does not exclude, however, the fact that depression of brain metabolism is one factor in the observed effects of alcohol upon the central nervous system. Whatever the narcotic action of alcohol may be, it continues to interfere with normal brain function long after the drug has attained maximum concentration, and even as it is disappearing from the blood. The brain cells of the chronically inebriated individual have been accustomed to function in a certain concentration of alcohol, and when the narcotic effect is first removed, they become hyperactive in a new burst of freedom. This is the explanation offered by Lennox (651) and Kalinowsky (574) for "rum fits" which sometimes appear in the "sobering-up" process.

V. ETHER

Ether is another narcotic drug which has been studied for its influence on the human cerebral AVO_2 difference. Dameshek, Myerson, and Loman (219) have made observations on 12 psychotic patients at Boston State Hospital before and during the administration of ether. Their cerebral AVO_2 differences averaged 6.5 vol. per cent before ether and fell to 1.9 vol. per cent during ether anesthesia, lower than what was observed under either alcohol or barbiturate narcosis. Though the administration of ether may increase cerebral blood flow by its vasodilator action on cerebral vasculature, these writers conclude that the extreme drop in oxygen intake which occurs during ether anesthesia may be due to an almost complete abolition of oxidative processes within the cells. Probably an increase of cerebral blood flow and an inhibitive effect on oxidations are both operative in reducing cerebral AVO_2 difference. We may conclude that brain oxidations are diminished despite the fact that additional evidence obtained by a study of excised cerebral tissues does not yield clear-cut results. With concentrations comparable to those used in operative procedures, ether retards oxygen intake of cerebral tissues only within the experimental error (571, 131). But in the intact organism ether anesthesia induces a 40% decrease in cerebral oxygen utilization even though cerebral blood flow is adequate and arterial blood is well oxygenated (592b). There is therefore no doubt that ether may exert a direct effect on the oxidative process of the brain *in vivo*.

Guedel's classification (428) has rendered the management of ether anesthesia more definite by furnishing the anesthetist with groups of clinical signs indicative of the depth of narcosis. The stages of anesthesia, the first of analgesia, the second of delirium, the third of surgical anesthesia, and the fourth of medullary paralysis are reminiscent of the symptomatic progression ascribed to the metabolic inhibition produced by thiopental. But the consensus of opinion (411) regards the pattern of ether as an irregularly descending one which skips the medulla and goes on to the spinal cord. If ether, like the barbiturates, depresses cerebral metabolism, all suprabulbar areas should be included in the metabolic inhibition before the medulla oblongata is so obtunded. The origin of the clinical differences between thiopental and ether must therefore be sought elsewhere than in their metabolic effects and may be found in the specific actions of these anesthetics upon nerve function. One of the actions of ether is to raise the synaptic threshold and especially so on the sensory side (231). In this regard ether and the barbiturate are opposites. The specific effect of ether to prevent sensory stimulation is a source of its analgesia. The interference with the sensory impulse also blocks reflex action and is part of the mechanism of the relaxation produced by ether. Certainly the similarity between the first stage of thiopental and that of ether is striking except for the analgesia with ether (411). Stage 2 of thiopental and of ether anesthesia likewise show strong similarities. Ether however does not exert a specific effect on the hypothalamus and the hyperactivity may therefore be more marked than with thiopental.

Because of the different special effects of ether and thiopental the signs of their third stages are quite different. The pupils enlarge with ether instead of contracting; the time of the loss of corneal reflex is more consistent, respiration is less depressed and better relaxation is obtained with ether as briefly described above. Nevertheless by careful observation one can find in Plane 2 of surgical anesthesia a relative constriction of the pupil which may be an effect of ether in releasing the Edinger-Wesphal nucleus (411), thus indicating a midbrain rather than a spinal allocation for that plane of surgical anesthesia. The downward metabolic march from cortex in the first stage, subcortico-diencephalon in the second, through the midbrain in the third is carried on to the medulla if medullary paralysis threatens (fourth stage). The observation of reduced cerebral metabolic rate (592b) during ether anesthesia is in agreement with this suggestive possibility and therefore a re-evaluation of the clinical march in terms of cerebral metabolic rate is indicated.

VI. CYCLOPROPANE

Cyclopropane, an anesthetic gas, is usually administered with a high concentration of oxygen. As a result the patient's blood is well oxygenated and his color throughout the anesthesia is good. His healthy color is deceiving, however, and not representative of the oxygen used by the tissues, because as we found in the following experiments, cerebral AVO_2 difference is always greatly reduced in cyclopropane anesthesia (8). For example, the second patient in Table 39 had a cerebral AVO_2 difference as low as 2.8 vol. per cent with light surgical anesthesia and it decreased even further to 1.5 vol. per cent when the narcosis deepened. The other patient had a difference of 3.6 vol. per cent in light anesthesia which fell further to 1.1 vol. per cent when the anesthesia became profound. After the cyclopropane had worn off, the AVO_2 difference rose to 8.0 vol. per cent. In the two observations made on dogs, similar steep reductions in cerebral AVO_2 difference were noted.

An increase in cerebral blood flow during cyclopropane anesthesia is probable. This suggestion arises out of the work of Stormont and his co-workers (919) who observed a rise of systolic and diastolic blood pressure during this anesthesia. When systemic blood pressure mounts, cerebral blood flow is quickened as was explained in Chapter 6. Stormont also finds an acidosis due to the retention of carbon dioxide, which he believes accumulates in the patient's mask when the tidal air is reduced so low that adequate absorption of expired carbon dioxide by the soda lime is no longer possible. A carbon dioxide acidosis is a second factor to hasten cerebral blood flow. This increased flow however does not explain the tremendous falling off of the oxygen difference. It is necessary to invoke an additional histotoxic action to account for an AVO_2 difference which approaches the level of the analytical error. The high oxygen content of the venous blood which probably is responsible for the pink color of the patient is similar to that observed in cyanide poisoning in which the histotoxic effect is well established. Ordinarily this depression of cellular respiration is borne well by the patient, but when an additional handicap in respiration is introduced, such as an impairment of arterial oxygen, perhaps through faulty technic, the double burden may bring the patient to a dangerous pass.[6] Perhaps this double handicap may account for the pathologic changes in the brain of a patient reported by Gebauer and Coleman (369) who succumbed 7 days after cyclopropane anesthesia. The histologic examination revealed irregular degeneration of the cortex. The authors point out that the localization of the degenerated areas was consistent with the order of vulnerability of tissues to anoxia. Though we might desire a larger number of observations, the weight of the evidence is in favor of cyclopropane exerting a histotoxic effect.

There are other substances which have not been studied in the human patient but nevertheless do show a decrease in metabolism of excised cerebral tissues. Among these may be included urethane, magnesium,

TABLE 39

Effect of cyclopropane on cerebral arterio-venous oxygen difference of man and dog

SUBJECT	O₂ CONTENT			O₂ CAPACITY		HbO₂	GLUCOSE		LAC. ACID		COMMENTS
	Art.	Ven.	Diff.	Art.	Ven.		Art.	Ven.	Art.	Ven.	
	vol. per cent			vol. per cent		per cent	mg. per cent				
Man	23.2	20.6	3.6		23.3	99	101	97	26	25	1st plane 3rd stage
	21.6	20.5	1.1		21.7	99	108	108	32	39	4th plane 3rd stage
	20.3	12.3	8.0		20.9	97	120	111	44	49	14 min. after anesthesia stopped.
Man	18.7	15.9	2.8	19.0		98	63		18		light anesthesia
	18.9	17.4	1.5	19.3		98	72		18		deep anesthesia
Dog	21.0	16.3	4.7		21.1	100	101	84	33	24	anesthesia
	19.6	8.7	10.9		21.0	93	101	79	31	29	anesthesia stopped
Dog	15.6	11.5	4.1			96	84	79	25	25	light anesthesia
	14.5	11.7	2.8			102	106	104	31	33	deep anesthesia
	11.6	4.3	7.3			97	134	125	49	52	13 min. after mask was off

Arterio-venous oxygen differences in the fourth column are greatly reduced in cyclopropane anesthesia in comparison with the normal values of 6.7 vol. per cent in man and 10.0 vol. per cent in the dog. The values for arterial oxygen content approximate those for oxygen capacity thus accounting for the high saturation of hemoglobin and indicating the excellent pulmonary arterialization of the blood. The utilization of arterial blood sugar is apparent from the differences between arterial and venous glucose. The lactic acid exchanges suggest a release of that substance from the brain in accordance with the normal pattern.

chloral (803) and the bromides (1029). DuBois, Albaum and Potter suggest that the narcotic effect of magnesium lies in its ability to displace calcium and thus prevent certain energy liberating processes (257).

The point of metabolic action of narcotics. We have concluded that all narcotics mentioned interfere with cellular respiration. Whether or not all these narcotics act upon the same respiratory enzyme is not known, though such a common action is not improbable. At any rate, we are forced to limit our discussion to the barbiturates and chloretone since these were the drugs used to elucidate this question.

We have known for some time that narcotics may inhibit respiration in one of several ways: some, like cyanide, combine with the prosthetic group of one of the respiratory enzymes thus inactivating the enzyme; or, as Quastel (803) proposed, oxidations may be blocked in another way, simply by the preferential absorption of the narcotic to a respiratory enzyme in place of its substrate. Again narcotics may combine with a protein portion of enzymes to produce a temporary denaturation (721a). By any method cerebral cellular respiration may be inhibited in a link of the catalytic chain, including the Embden-Meyerhof (275, 736) breakdown to pyruvic acid, and the oxidation of that intermediary metabolite in the Krebs cycle (626). In either instance the Warburg-Christian (970) transport of hydrogen from substrate to oxygen is involved and the evidence at hand is concerned with this transfer of hydrogen (see Chap. 5).

Quastel and co-workers (803) examined each member of the Warburg-Christian oxidative chain, outlined in Chapter 5, in an attempt to determine the exact point at which such narcotics may act. They found first that the cytochrome-cytochrome oxidase portion of this scheme was little affected, because the oxidation of p-phenylenediamine remains unimpaired in the presence of the barbiturates or of chloretone. Respiratory depression in excised tissues must therefore be exerted upon some other step in the oxidative scheme, associated with the transfer of hydrogen. The earliest suggestion to this problem was that the narcotic effect was exerted upon the dehydrogenase, but later investigation by Michaelis and Quastel (742) revealed that the depression of dehydrogenase activity even in the presence of cozymase was too superficial to account entirely for the inhibition of cellular respiration.

Desirous of defining more closely the point of activity, Michaelis and Quastel used chloretone to seek a highly narcotic-sensitive link in the chain somewhere between the dehydrogenase and the cytochrome-oxidase system. They next examined the influence of chloretone on other members of the enzyme chain of hydrogen transfer. One of the known intermediary enzymes is a flavoprotein, but here again their quest was unsuccessful because the activity of the flavoprotein proved to be but slightly depressed by the narcotic. These same authors were therefore forced to the tentative conclusion from their negative research that chloretone affects some component of the tissues' respiratory system *not* included in their study, but which plays an intermediary role between flavoprotein and cytochrome C. Greig suggests (419) cytochrome b as this highly sensitive link in the enzymatic chain. Another possibility must also be considered because the flavoprotein examined by Michaelis and Quastel (742) was not cytochrome reductase, the form active in the Warburg-Christian-Keilin scheme. It would seem that additional studies, including that of cytochrome b and cytochrome reductase, must be made before the exact locus of action can be discovered. Nevertheless, the general conclusion that narcotics do depress brain metabolism remains unshaken.

VII. Summary

The question of narcotics in relation to brain metabolism has been studied and at least two potent influences have been uncovered. The first is metabolic, a withdrawal of the energy required for the support of the brain, the second is a direct interference with nervous activity characterized by the descriptive phrase, elevation of the synaptic threshold, a property not necessarily developed equally throughout the nervous system. Though both influences are interdependent they may be studied separately.

The metabolic component is proved by a diminution of the oxygen intake of the brain. Like the synaptic depression the metabolic inhibition may not be equally distributed. The entire brain is affected by the barbiturate, yet the inequality of the bilateral arterio-venous oxygen differences in light anesthesia as well as the symptomatic progression observed with deepening anesthesia is compatible with the stepwise advance in the intensity of the metabolic interference beginning with the cortex and spreading down the neuraxis. But some of the phenomena are out of proportion to the metabolic inhibition and can be best explained by an additional factor such as impairment of nerve activity as observed for example in the respiratory center. This bipartite conception has been found useful in the classification of the clinical signs of thiopental anesthesia. The phyletic hypothesis for the functional organization of the central nervous system though incomplete nevertheless proves to be of pragmatic value as it furnishes signposts to aid the management of thiopental anesthesia.

The clinical signs of ether anesthesia as described by Guedel reveal a bipartite arrangement similar to that observed with thiopental: the progressive march down the neuraxis has its basis in the reduction of cerebral metabolic rate and the interference with nerve function, the elevation of the synaptic threshold is especially well developed on the sensory side.

To this and other specific effects are attributed the differences between thiopental and ether.

Barbiturates other than thiopental, as well as nitrous oxide, alcohol, and cyclopropane have been considered in this chapter. Most of these drugs lower the metabolism of excised cerebral tissues though with some of these agents the concentrations required far exceed that necessary to produce surgical anesthesia. The observations of cerebral arterio-venous oxygen differences made on the intact organism are likewise suggestive of a decrease in brain metabolism. None of these depressants, however, has been studied quantitatively for its influence upon cerebral metabolic rate *in vivo*. Thus except for thiopental and ether the energy factor in the production of narcosis has not been measured and differentiated from other such depressions of nerve function. A review of the present knowledge of other narcotics, however, is justified as a beginning for the further elucidation of their obtunding actions. Observations of these narcotics suggest that they too adhere to a similar metabolic pattern. The present task is, therefore, to turn our efforts to estimate the metabolic factor among the others in the creation of narcosis.

CHAPTER 13

PROSPECTS AND PROBLEMS FOR THE FUTURE

In all biological sciences we have repeatedly seen that significant advances in knowledge are made under the impetus of some newly developed method of study. Warburg (973) and his apparatus for determining tissue respiration, Van Slyke (956), and his machine for analyzing blood gases, and Berger (81), the father of electroencephalography, are only a few of the names to which credit goes for contributing these basic instruments which lay the framework for later discoveries. In this book, we have seen many of the advances resulting from the study of internal jugular venous blood in human subjects, a method initiated by Myerson (756). The method gives us access to the blood returning from the brain, and this blood can be compared upon chemical analysis for its sugar and oxygen content with these constituents of the arterial blood. The differences between the concentrations of these constituents indicate the magnitude of the energy turnover. We have not expected that single observations necessarily would lead to consistent results, but averages of a series have proved to be of practical value. We may say, then, that the intensity factor, or the determination of AVO_2 differences in the brain, is fairly well perfected and can be relied upon to furnish undisputed data. But what of the capacity factor, the volume of blood passing through the brain per minute, without which cerebral metabolic rate cannot be quantitatively determined? Throughout this book four methods for measuring human cerebral blood flow have been mentioned, but at least two of them are not entirely satisfactory because of technical inconvenience and quantitative limitations. Inserting into the internal jugular vein an electrode, either heated above or cooled below the temperature of the blood is one of these methods (477, 393). The greater the volume of blood passing this electrode per minute, the more closely does its temperature approach that of the blood. Only relative increases or decreases of blood flow can be registered in this way, unless the diameter of the internal jugular vein is known, in which case absolute values can be obtained (see Chapter 2, page 14, footnote 8). Ferris (316) and his associates have employed a procedure by which cerebral blood flow is estimated on a basis of cerebrospinal fluid pressure, likewise having its quantitative limitations and furthermore involving the use of a lumbar puncture needle. The third method (598) is based upon inhalation of nitrous oxide and requires many hematic analyses.[1] Though

[1] The number of analyses and the volume of blood required for the determination of C.B.F., by the nitrous oxide method, have been reduced by the modifications of

360

it has the merit of checking closely with direct observations in a few instances, more checks are desirable before accepting the values so obtained (see Chap. 8, page 179). The fourth technic requires fewer analyses than the third but depends upon the injection of a dye, Evans Blue, into the internal carotid artery (400). The results so obtained agree within 3% with the cerebral venous return collected through a cannula in the internal jugular vein. To date these last two procedures are, however, the best available for determination of cerebral blood flow. Further advances in this field await the application of these methods or some other one, technically simple and quantitatively accurate, for evidence on cerebral blood flow in man. When these measurements are applied, the many problems discussed and suggested in this book will be placed on a sure basis.

The usefulness of any procedure for determining brain metabolism, far-reaching though it may be, can nevertheless be much more valuable if it is complemented by data gathered from other sources. Sometimes this information can be assembled by simultaneous experiments on the same patient, watching his neurologic symptoms and at the same time employing the EEG. Such an opportunity has been presented to study the brain by the various operations in the field of psychosurgery. For example prefrontal lobotomy, performed on persons suffering from involutional depression, severs the tracts between the frontal lobe and the thalamus. The patient is relieved of his abnormal anxiety and takes on a different outlook (344). The influence of this operation to reduce cerebral metabolic rate is known (596) but other kinds of biochemical studies performed on the brain of these patients would be desirable including those in the field of enzymology. The latter is supplying suggestive leads for the problems of epilepsy and narcosis as discussed below. Supportive evidence for the oxygen analyses can also be gathered by combining these analyses with histologic and physiologic studies, such as the neuropathology of the avitaminoses or the changes wrought by freezing (301a), cerebral anemia (836), electronarcosis (352), and other experiments performed on man. The investigative possibilities of these procedures, like those of the physiologically directed shock therapies for mental diseases, have by no means been exhausted.

Experiments on cerebral metabolism of lower animals and primates are an important source of information because of the insight into human activities afforded by phyletic studies. Not to be discounted is the opportunity to create in animals conditions simulating those in human subjects, thus permitting operations not possible on man. For instance, the excision of cerebral tissues can be performed in animals subjected to hypo-

---

Scheinberg and Stead (848a). Their results for cerebral blood flow are somewhat higher than those reported by Kety and Schmidt (598).

glycemia, anoxia, recurrent convulsions (619), or to a condition resembling that of schizophrenic catatonia by the injection of bulbocapnine (123, 314). The strength, therefore, of any interpretation on cerebral metabolic rate, depends in great part upon the correlative evidence from other disciplines. As soon as the restrictions imposed by the lack of proper methods have receded, the field of immediate objectives is a vast one.

"Functional" and organic psychoses. The work on cerebral metabolic rate in regard to one of the so-called "functional" psychoses (those for which no organic disturbance has been found) is on a firm basis since it has been established that in schizophrenia, the most prevalent of any psychosis, the oxygen consumption of the brain is within the normal range (318, 600). Suggestive evidence indicates that an unchanged C.M.R also holds true for the affective "functional" psychoses as well, one of which is the agitated depression (482) observed most frequently in older persons. But the question can be decided only by the application of quantitative methods to this problem. The determination of C.M.R on patients afflicted with psychoses of proved organic origin may lead to a different conclusion for some of these persons appear to be laboring under subnormal cerebral metabolic conditions. This work adds up to some observations of cardiac decompensation (499, 848d) and pernicious anemia (848c) where the brain is apparently deprived of oxygen and a more substantial number of patients with advanced general paresis (479, 783a, 834) or senile dementia (141, 344a). What of other organic diseases? Will they also comply with this conclusion? The question is an open one in regard to such psychoses as follow trauma, surgical manipulations in the operating room, and childbirth.

Mental deficiencies. We have already noted the rather remarkable fact that the AVO_2 difference in undifferentiated mentally defective persons is normal (497), while those distinguished by physical stigmata of one kind or another as exemplified in mongoloids and cretins (494, 486) exhibit consistently reduced values (498). If the data were extended to include other mentally defective individuals, characterized by stigmata, would this finding still hold? The amount of material yet untouched is enormous; for example, patients whose mental deficiency is associated with congenital anatomic anomalies, i.e. syndactalysm (883) as well as with tuberous sclerosis (835) and other comparatively rare diseases (14, 564). If further experiments, made in order to measure C.M.R., could prove that a deficiency in energy is associated with a deficiency in mentality, it would open a new diagnostic feature for the differentiated mental subjects, and at the same time, suggest a starting point for the therapeutic research. If the underlying cause is partly a faulty metabolic process in the brain, it would at least give us a possible clue for ameliorating the condition. A simple illustration of this is thyroid therapy to raise the brain metabolism of infant cretins.

To the present time, but for a preliminary communication (434), no cases have been reported where cerebral metabolism is above normal, except in fever therapy for general paresis (479) when the metabolism is purposely raised. It would not be surprising to the writer, though, if the future would disclose a higher-than-normal metabolic rate in some hyperactive types of mental deficiency or in some of the hyperkinetic forms of psychoses. In general C.M.R. may be expected to correlate with neuromuscular activity, an extreme example is the excessive C.M.R. associated with convulsions (226, 227, 856). The convulsant hyperactivity is, of course, a peripheral manifestation of a violent central disturbance which continues, apparently unabated, in the organism paralyzed with curare.

Vitamins. The sphere of vitamins is an ever-enlarging one, spurred on by the discovery of new vitamins, as well as fresh theories as to the action of those already known. Work in this field on animals is already far advanced (274, 787). But, as for man, our information in regard to cerebral metabolism is niggardly and goes no further than the pellagrins who have been studied with or without an associated vitamin B_1 deficiency (522). The avitaminoses in human subjects, and preferably those induced by a single deficiency rather than those in groups, is indeed a frontier of tremendous importance. In the same category as the vitamins may be placed the essential amino acids since they may play an important role in cerebral structure and function (832).

Epilepsy. Much work has been done on the biology of epilepsy but the enzymatic approach to the natural history of this group of diseases has not been sufficiently explored. The data available include those on cerebral metabolic rate, within normal limits between attacks (413) and raised in convulsive episodes. This rise however has been determined chiefly by indirect means and in experimental convulsions. Additional quantitative determinations on patients are awaited. Other studies by Gibbs, Lennox and Gibbs (391) indicate that an examination of the cerebral blood gas exchanges not only during the fit but immediately before and after the episode may lead to results of prognostic and therapeutic value. The metabolic consequences of repeated convulsions over a long period of time have not been elucidated, though destructive changes may be feared.

A possible line of attack arises out of the suggestion that epileptic convulsions are associated with abnormalities of acetylcholine metabolism (337, 110). (See Chapter 9, page 251 for acetylcholine and convulsions). Of special interest in this connection are drugs which inhibit cholinesterase activity: prostigmine, eserine, di-isopropyl fluorophosphate (DFP), because their pharmacologic use is linked with the ability to prevent the breakdown of acetylcholine. This reasoning is in line with the observation that such drugs modify the course of petit mal epilepsy (1003). And even more to the point, is the observation that patients with focal epilepsy exhibit an elevated cholinesterase activity in the cortical tissue giving rise to the epileptiform discharges, an elevated activity which may be indicative of an abnormally large acetylcholine turnover (794a).

DFP when injected into the common carotid artery of the curarized rabbit produces brain waves resembling those of long enduring status epilepticus in man (341). These abnormal brain waves are associated with a profound fall in cholinesterase activity and the presumptive accumulation of acetylcholine (442). Trimethadione (tridione) and atropine (487) restore the normal brain wave pattern. Caramiphen (Parpanit) (288) and certain antihistamines Dramamine, Benadryl, Phenergan and Lergigan (286, 564a), drugs with atropine-like actions against acetylcholine, also correct the abnormal brain waves. Atropine (425) while diminishing spiking in the interseizure electroencephalogram of patients with grand mal-type of epilepsy is not effective in preventing seizures.

By using subconvulsant doses of DFP, forced circling movements, away from the injected side, are induced. This compulsive behavior is also probably associated with excessive acetylcholine as it is stopped by injections of atropine or scopolamine (287) and by the antihistamines named above (564a). It would seem therefore that the anticholinesterase and atropine-like agents will repay further study. A comparison of their simultaneous effects on behavior and cerebral metabolic rate should yield new information on the mechanism of this form of experimental convulsions. It would be advantageous to be able to determine the metabolic rates of the various cerebral regions separately as well as that of the brain as a whole. The use of DFP has disclosed that some cerebral structures suffer more severe losses of cholinesterase activity than others and it is not improbable that both forced circling and seizure waves are signs of interactions between subcortical as well as cortical areas.

The resolution of the question set by epilepsy will involve the part played by acetylcholine, or some other acetyl compound (760), in the normal brain. Surely the evidence presented above as well as that reviewed in the footnote on page 318, Chapter 11 show that acetylcholine, somehow, is fundamentally involved in the physiology of the nerve impulse; that acetylcholine plays a part not only in the peripheral outposts of the nervous system but also within the neuraxis. In that case the functional pathology of acetylcholine presents enticing vistas including, to mention one problem, the mechanism of action of atropine and atropine-like drugs in Parkinsonism.

In addition to a possible connection between anticholinesterase substances and convulsions, little is known about the mechanism of convulsant drugs. The observation that picrotoxin (606) and methyl fluoroacetate (272, 125a) interfere with cerebral oxidations is however, suggestive and calls for further metabolic studies. Certainly the convulsions seen in hypoglycemia, anoxia and cyanide poisoning are associated with a deprivation of cerebral energy. Such convulsions are a form of the release phenomena discussed in detail in Chapter 10 of this volume. The opposite effect, namely primary stimulation of the nerve cells instead of metabolic inhibition, may also produce fits and must be considered in convulsions caused by camphor, metrazol, and electroshock. Finally the influence of sensory impulses, not only arising in the carotid body (853) but in any part of the organism, must be considered (375, 938). The determination of the extent to which each of these factors influences the pathogenesis of epilepsy is one of the chief problems in that field, and the solution of the problem should yield a point of direction for research in the anticonvulsant drugs.

Narcosis. The analysis presented in Chapter 12 shows that C.M.R. is reduced in thiopental anesthesia and in addition reveals a point of attack of the barbiturates on cellular respiration, i.e. on hydrogen or electron transfer, but does not afford an explanation for the observation that some of the depressant effects of these drugs are more pronounced than could have been expected from the decrease in cerebral metabolic rate. At present the answer to this question is not at hand. Nevertheless there are certain suggestive trends which base the inhibition of nerve function upon a reduction in the energy available for such function, an action of narcotics against some enzyme reactions supporting function rather than a general effect on all the cellular enzyme systems. It is worthwhile to review some of the evidence which is compatible with this viewpoint despite the absence of complete proof that anesthesia is dependent upon a direct effect of the nacrotic against any enzyme system.

It is doubtful whether the power of a narcotic to inhibit cellular respiration can account entirely for the depression of the conduction and transmission of the nerve impulse. These functional activities would necessarily cease if the energy stored in phosphate bonds, the immediate source of energy for the work of the cell, was no longer available. This possibility should be considered because barbiturates seem to prevent the breakdown of energy-rich phosphate bonds. At any rate LePage's work (656a) indicates that these drugs maintain energy-rich phosphate bonds at a maximum. McElroy (721a) makes the suggestion that the very action of narcotics is to interfere, at some point, with energy-rich phosphate bond metabolism, a process which normally is supported by the transfer of hydrogen atoms or electrons. In more general terms, the coupling between the oxidative and the anabolic activities of the neurone is apparently disrupted by the narcotic: though oxidations do not cease, they are no longer associated with the energy-rich phosphate bonds required to support some of the activities of the nerve cell. This idea appears to be logical in view of the fact that conduction and transmission may be continued for a longer or shorter time in the absence of oxygen and at the expense of the stored energy made possibly by the splitting of energy-rich phosphate bonds and by glycolysis. On the other hand a narcotic acts in such a way as to depress nerve function while oxygen consumption continues.

Experiments with succinate (360a) afford examples of oxidative processes which do not appear to store useful energy. Despite an observed increase in oxygen intake stimulated by succinate, energy-requiring processes like the synthesis of acetylcholine by the brain or the formation of energy-rich phosphate bonds by cardiac muscle were not increased proportionally. In fact these processes occurred at a slower rate than with the normal substrates. In these observations succinate competed successfully with the usual substrates, depressed their oxidation and diminished the useful energy available for energy-rich phosphate bonds. It would seem that the energy liberated during the oxidation of succinate is not necessarily effectual in the anabolic processes of the cell. (The controversial position of the use of succinate in the treatment of barbiturate poisoning is mentioned in the footnote on page 328.)

It is therefore important that barbiturates, in contradistinction to their influence on glucose oxidation, do not depress that of succinate. Thus the oxidations which survive the presence of the barbiturate may have little or no anabolic consequences. Meanwhile it is of interest that another anabolic function, namely the acetylation of choline is inhibited far in excess of the depression in oxygen uptake (725a). A 15% reduction in the oxygen utilization of excised cerebral tissues is associated with a 50% diminution in their ability to synthesize acetylcholine. A crucial experiment in this field would be to determine whether or not energy-rich phosphate bond metabolism is inhibited to a greater extent than are oxidations. To summarize this *ad hoc* argument: during anesthesia the cerebral metabolic rate is slowed but the functional aspects of the nervous system are depressed to a greater extent than might be expected from the inhibition of the oxygen intake. It is suggested by McElroy (721a) that narcotics specifically interfere with the reactions involved in the energy-rich phosphate bond turnover (656a) and therefore remove the immediate support for neuronal activity. At the same time oxidations continue, though at a reduced rate, and maintain the structure of the cell.

Central idea. Many advantages follow the formation of a central idea and not the least of these is a constant stimulus to discovery. The chief point of this volume has been to bring evidence to test Hughlings Jackson's concept (558) of the phyletic organization of the central nervous system. Excised tissues, intact animals, and man as well have all been employed for analyses to examine this conception. Its value as a center of reference has been illustrated throughout this book, but it seems to the writer that the advances to be made by the application of this generalization have only been begun.

A new field for the study of hypnotic and anesthetic drugs has been opened by applying to the pharmacology of these agents the knowledge obtained from anoxia and particularly from hypoglycemia, the clinical progress of which indicates a phyletic regression with loss of nervous activities as metabolic depression grows more profound. With each succeeding loss an adaptive reorganization of the remaining activities takes place but each time at a lower level of function. In the author's laboratory a study of C.M.R. in man, as affected by anesthetic drugs, has been initiated with an examination of thiopental (488, 293). The link between anoxia and hypoglycemia on one side and narcosis on the other is a depression of brain metabolism, for one important element underlying narcosis is histotoxic anoxia. The examination of the phenomena of anesthesia in the light of Hughlings Jackson's ideas may yield a clinical sequence similar in anatomic allocations to those obtained with reversible anoxia and hypoglycemia, or with permanent damage to large cerebral areas, a sequence starting in the cerebral cortex and descending the neuraxis towards the medulla oblongata. If this comparison should prove to be correct, it will bring to the anesthesiologist not only clearer insight into the physiologic basis of narcosis but also disclose signposts for the depths of the patient's cerebral depression at any given moment during the various stages of anesthesia.

These studies of anesthetic drugs have a basis in excised tissues, for it has been demonstrated that many of these agents exert a histotoxic anoxia to depress cellular metabolism. But when applied to the intact animal and man, the picture becomes more complicated because to the effects of metabolic depression are added specific actions which vary with different reagents. An illustration of this incongruity is seen in alcohol which has been observed to depress respiratory metabolism of excised cerebral tissues (523). Nevertheless, its effects on the imbiber are probably much more complicated and not alone produced by depression of brain metabolism (277, 406, 682). The barbiturates are another example. These narcotics depress brain metabolism in the human patient (528) and also inhibit the oxygen intake in bits of cerebral tissue (803, 523). This action accounts for a part of their narcotic power but leaves unexplained some features important in the practical administration of this group of drugs. Those effects of the various anesthetics which do not depend upon an inhibition of a respiratory enzyme may also rest upon an enzymatic basis but of a different kind. Enzymatic interference in the high energy phosphate turnover is suggested as part of anesthesia in the previous section on narcosis. Hypoglycemia, anoxia, and the field of anesthesia do not limit the applicability of the phyletic conception, for it includes some of the avitaminoses, cyanide poisoning and every disorder involving a depression of cerebral metabolic rate. Abnormal metabolic rates are also observed in diseases with anatomic changes; arteriosclerosis, general paresis and some of the mental deficiencies (see Chapter 8). It will be our duty in the future to disentangle the metabolic element from any special complicating effects characteristic of particular chemical reagents, noxious substances, or morphologic alterations before we can comprehend the underlying mechanisms.

In the last analysis, a final objective to be achieved from all the work on brain metabolism is to differentiate whether cerebral disturbance, either of endogenous or exogenous origin, finds its source in (1) deviation from the normal cerebral metabolic rate, or (2) in a malfunctioning whether on a structural or physiologic basis but not dependent upon changes in oxygen utilization, or (3) a combination of both. Practical clinical application in the field of therapeutics, and also the proper channels for research will be unveiled after this preliminary diagnosis can be made.

BIBLIOGRAPHY

1. ABDON, N. O., BJARKE, T. The mechanism of acetylcholine liberation in striped muscles. Acta pharmacol. **1**: 1–17, 1945.
1a. ABREU, B. E., LIDDLE, G. W., BURKS, A. L., SUTHERLAND, V., ELLIOTT, H. W., SIMON, A., MARGOLIS, L. Influence of amphetamine sulfate on cerebral metabolism and blood flow in man. J. Am. Pharmaceut. A., Scientific Edition, **38**: 186–189, 1949.
1b. ADLER, E., EULER, H. v. Über die Komponenten der Dehydrase-systeme., II. Hoppe-Seyler's Ztschr. f. physiol. Chem., **232**: 6–27, 1935.
2. ——, ——, GÜNTHER, G., PLASS, M. *Isocitric* dehydrogenase and glutamic acid synthesis in animal tissues. Biochem. J., **33**: 1028–1045, 1939.
3. ADOLPH, E. F. Tolerance to cold and anoxia in infant rats. Am. J. Physiol., **155**: 366–377, 1948.
4. ALBAUM, H. G., NOVIKOFF, A. B., OGUR, M. The development of the cytochrome oxidase and succinoxidase systems in the chick embryo. J. Biol. Chem., **165**: 125–130, 1946.
5. ——, ——, ——. The relationship between cytochrome oxidase and succinic dehydrogenase in the developing chick embryo. Fed. Proc., **5**: 119, 1946.
6. ——, WORLEY, L. G. The development of cytochrome oxidase in the chick embryo. J. Biol. Chem., **144**: 697–700, 1942.
7. ALDERSBERG, D., DOLGER, H. Medico-legal problems of hypoglycemic reactions in diabetes. Ann. Int. Med., **12**: 1804–1815, 1939.
8. ALEXANDER, F. A. D., FAZEKAS, J. F., HIMWICH, H. E. Unpublished results.
9. ——, HIMWICH, H. E. Nitrogen inhalation therapy for schizophrenia. Am. J. Psychiat., **96**: 643–655, 1939–40.
9a. ALLBUTT, T. C. The electric treatment of the insane. The West Riding Lunatic Asylum Medical Reports, **2**: 203–222, 1872.
10. ALLEN, F. M. Studies concerning glycosuria and diabetes. Boston, W. M. Leonard, 1913.
11. AMES, S. R., ZIEGENHAGEN, A. J., ELVEHJEM, C. A. Studies in the inhibition of enzyme systems involving cytochrome c. J. Biol. Chem., **165**: 81–90, 1946.
12. ANDERSON, E., LONG, J. A. The effect of hyperglycemia on insulin secretion as determined with the isolated rat pancreas in a perfusion apparatus. Endocrinology, **40**: 92–97, 1947.
13. ——, ——. Suppression of insulin secretion by the growth hormone of the anterior pituitary as determined with the isolated rat pancreas in a perfusion apparatus. Endocrinology, **40**: 98–103, 1947.
14. ANDERSON, N. L. The Laurence-Moon-Biedl syndrome. J. Clin. Endocrinol., **1**: 905–911, 1941.
15. ANGYAL, L. v. Über die motorischen und tonischen Erscheinungen des Insulinshocks. Ztschr. f.d.ges. Neurol. u. Psychiat., **157**: 35–80, 1937.
16. ARING, C. D., RYDER, H. W., ROSEMAN, E., ROSENBAUM, M., FERRIS, E. B. Effect of nicotinic acid and related substances on the intracranial blood flow of man. Arch. Neurol. & Psychiat., **46**: 649–653, 1941.
17. ARMSTRONG, H. G. Principles and practice of aviation medicine. Baltimore, The Williams and Wilkins Co., 1939.
18. ARSHAVSKI, I. A. Adaptation to anoxia at different age levels. Am. Rev. Sov. Med., **2**: 508–512, 1945.

19. Ashby, W. Carbonic anhydrase in mammalian tissue. J. Biol. Chem., **151**: 521–527, 1943.

20. ———. A parallelism between the quantitative incidence of carbonic anhydrase and functional levels of the central nervous system. J. Biol. Chem., **152**: 235–240, 1944.

21. Ashford, C. A. Glycolysis in brain tissue. Biochem. J., **28**: 2229–2236, 1934.

22. ———, Dixon, K. C. Effect of potassium on the glucolysis of brain tissue with reference to the Pasteur effect. Biochem. J., **29**: 157–168, 1935.

23. Ashford, C. A., Holmes, E. G. Contributions to the study of brain metabolism. V. Role of phosphates in lactic acid production. Biochem. J., **23**: 748–759, 1929.

24. ———, ———. Further observations on the oxidation of lactic acid by brain tissue. Biochem. J., **25**: 2028–2049, 1931.

25. Ask-Upmark, E. The carotid sinus and the cerebral circulation. Acta psychiat. et neurol., Supp. VI, Copenhagen, p. 1–374, 1935.

26. Aumann, K. W., Youmans, W. B. Differential sensitization of adrenergic neuro-effector systems by thyroid hormone. Am. J. Physiol., **131**: 394–401, 1940–41.

26a. Augustinsson, K. B., Nachmansohn, D. Distinction between acetylcholine-esterase and other choline ester-splitting enzymes. Science, **110**: 98–99, 1949.

27. Avery, R. C., Johlin, J. M. Relative susceptibility of adult and young mice to asphyxiation. Proc. Soc. Exper. Biol. & Med., **29**: 1184–1186, 1931–32.

28. Axelrod, A. E., Madden, R. J., Elvehjem, C. A. The effect of a nicotinic acid deficiency upon the coenzyme I content of animal tissues. J. Biol. Chem., **131**: 85–93, 1939.

29. Babinski, J. Du phénomòne des orteils et de sa valeur sémiologique. Semaine Med., **18**: 321–322, 1898.

29a. Bacon, J. S. D., Bell, D. J. Fructose and Glucose in the blood of the foetal sheep. Biochem. J., **42**: 397–405, 1948.

30. Bainbridge, F. A. The physiology of muscular exercise. New York, London, Toronto, Longmans, Green, and Co., 1931. Rewritten by A. V. Bock and D. B. Dill.

31. Baker, Z. Studies on the inhibition of glycolysis by glyceraldehyde. Biochem. J., **32**: 332–341, 1938.

32. ———, Fazekas, J. F., Himwich, H. E. Carbohydrate oxidation in normal and diabetic cerebral tissues. J. Biol. Chem., **125**: 545–556, 1938.

33. Baker, A. B., Lufkin, N. H. Cerebral lesions in hypoglycemia. Arch. Path., **23**: 190–201, 1937.

34. Ball, E. G. Energy relationships of the oxidative enzymes. Ann. N. Y. Acad. Sc., **45**: 363–375, 1944.

35. Banga, I., Ochoa, S., Peters, R. A. Pyruvate oxidation in brain. VI. The active form of vitamin B_1 and the role of C_4 dicarboxylic acids. Biochem. J., **33**: 1109–1121, 1939.

36. ———, ———, ———. Pyruvate oxidation in brain. VII. Some dialysable components of the pyruvate oxidation system. Biochem. J., **33**: 1980–1996, 1939.

37. Banting, F. G., Best, C. H. The internal secretion of the pancreas. J. Lab. & Clin. Med., **7**: 251–266, 1922.

    ———, ———. Pancreatic extracts. J. Lab. & Clin. Med., **7**: 464–472, 1922.

38. ———, ———, Collip, J. B., Macleod, J. J. R., Noble, E. C. VI. The effect of

insulin on the percentage amounts of fat and glycogen in the liver and other organs of diabetic animals. Tr. Roy. Soc. Canada, **16:** sect. V, 39–41, 1922.

39. ——, ——, MACLEOD, J. J. R. The internal secretion of the pancreas. Am. J. Physiol. Proc., **59:** 479, 1922.

40. BARACH, A. L. The treatment of asphyxia in clinical disease, with especial reference to recent developments in the use of oxygen in heart disease. New York State. J. Med., **34:** 672–681, 1934.

41. BARACH, A. L. The treatment of heart failure by continuous oxygen therapy. Anesth. & Analg., **14:** 79–88, 1935.

42. ——. The effect of low and high oxygen tensions on mental functioning. J. Aviation Med., **12:** 30–38, 1941.

43. ——, Physiologically directed therapy in pneumonia. Ann. Int. Med., **17:** 812–819, 1942.

44. ——. Principles and practices of inhalational therapy. Phila. J. B. Lippincott Company, 1944.

45. ——, ECKMAN, M., MOLOMUT, N. Modification of resistance to anoxia, with especial reference to high altitude flying. Am. J. M. Sc., **202:** 336–341, 1941.

46. BARBOUR, A. D., CHAIKOFF, I. L., MACLEOD, J. J. R., ORR, M. D. Influence of insulin on liver and muscle glycogen in the rat under varying nutritional conditions. Am. J. Physiol., **80:** 243–272, 1927.

47. BARCROFT, J. Presidential address (abridged) on Anoxaemia. Lancet, **Pt. 2:** 485–489, 1920.

48. ——, BARRON, D. H. Observations on the functional development of the foetal brain. J. Comp. Neurol., **77:** 431–452, 1942.

49. ——, ——, COWIE, A. T., FORSHAM, P. H. The oxygen supply of the foetal brain of the sheep and the effect of asphyxia on foetal respiratory movement. J. Physiol., **97:** 338–346, 1939–40.

50. ——, KENNEDY, J. A., MASON, M. F. Oxygen in the blood of the umbilical vessels of the sheep. J. Physiol., **97:** 347–356, 1939–40.

51. BARD, P. A diencephalic mechanism for the expression of rage with special reference to the sympathetic nervous system. Am. J. Physiol., **84:** 490–515, 1928.

52. BARKER, S. B. Effects of increased metabolism on ketosis of depancreatized dogs. J. Physiol., **97:** 394–407, 1940.

53. ——, FAZEKAS, J. F., HIMWICH, H. E. Metabolic aspects of thyroid-adrenal interrelationship. Am. J. Physiol., **115:** 415–418, 1936.

54. ——, SHORR, E., MALAM, M. Studies on the Pasteur reaction: effect of iodoacetic acid on the carbohydrate metabolism of isolated mammalian tissues. J. Biol. Chem., **129:** 33–50, 1939.

55. BARNES, R. H., DRURY, D. R. Utilization of ketone bodies by the tissues in ketosis. Proc. Soc. Exper. Biol. & Med., **36:** 350–352, 1937.

56. BARRERA, S. E., LEWIS, N. D. C., PACELLA, B. L., KALINOWSKY, L. Brain changes associated with electrically induced seizures. Tr. Am. Neurol. A., **68:** 31–35, 1942.

57. BARRON, D. H. The functional development of some mammalian neuromuscular mechanisms. Biol. Rev., **16:** 1–33, 1941.

58. BARRON, E. S. G. Mechanisms of carbohydrate metabolism. An essay on comparative biochemistry. Advances Enzymol., **3:** 149–189, 1943.

59. ——, BARTLETT, G. R., KALNITSKY, G. The oxidative pathway of pyruvate metabolism. Fed. Proc., **5:** 120–121, 1946.

60. BARRON, E. S. G., GOLDINGER, J. M., LIPTON, M. A., LYMAN, C. M. Studies on biological oxidations. XVII. The effect of thiamine on the metabolism of alpha-keto-glutarate. J. Biol. Chem., **141:** 975–979, 1941.

61. ——, SINGER, T. P. Studies of biological oxidations XIX. Sulfphydryl enzymes in carbohydrate metabolism. J. Biol. Chem., **157:** 221–240, 1945.

32. BARTLETT, G. R. BARRON, E. S. G. The effect of fluoroacetate on enzymes and on tissue metabolism. Its use for the study of the oxidative pathway of pyruvate metabolism. J. Biol. Chem., **170:** 67–82, 1947.

63. BARTLEY, S. H. HEINBECKER, P. Effect of insulin on nerve activity. Am. J. Physiol., **131:** 509–520, 1940–41.

64. BATSON, O. V. Anatomical problems concerned in the study of cerebral blood flow. Fed. Proc., **3:** 139–144, 1944.

65. BAUMANN, C. A. STARE, F. J. Coenzymes. Physiol. Rev., **19:** 353–388, 1939.

66. BEAN, J. W. Effects of oxygen at increased pressure. Physiol. Rev., **25:** 1–147, 1945.

67. ——, BOHR, D. F. Anoxic effects of high oxygen pressure on smooth muscle. Am. J. Physiol., **130:** 445–453, 1940.

68. BEATON, L. E., LEININGER, C., McKINLEY, W. A., MAGOUN, H. W., RANSON, S. W. Neurogenic hyperthermia and its treatment with soluble pentobarbital in the monkey. Arch. Neurol. & Psychiat., **49:** 518–536, 1943.

69. BEECHER, H. K., McDONOUGH, F. K., FORBES, A. Similarity of effects of barbiturates anesthesia and spinal transection. J. Neurophysiol., **2:** 81–88, 1939.

70. BEHNKE, A. R. Some physiological considerations of inhalation anesthesia and helium. Anesth. & Analg., **19:** 35–41, 1940.

71. ——, JOHNSON, F. S., POPPEN, J. R., MOTLEY, E. P. The effect of oxygen on man at pressures from 1 to 4 atmospheres. Am. J. Physiol., **110:** 565–572, 1934–35.

72. BELLINGER, C. H., TERRENCE, C. F., LIPETZ, B., HIMWICH, H. E. An evaluatuion of the factor of depression of brain metabolism in the treatment of schizophrenia. Psychiatric Quart., **17:** 164–172, 1943.

73. BENDA, C. E. The central nervous system in mongolism. Am. J. Ment. Def., **45:** 42–47, 1940–41.

74. ——. Microcephaly. Am. J. Psychiat., **97:** 1135–1146, 1941.

75. BENDER, M. B. Fright and drug contractions in denervated facial and ocular muscles of monkeys. Am. J. Physiol., **121:** 609–619, 1938.

76. ——, KENNARD, M. A. The fright reaction after section of the facial, trigeminal and cervical sympathetic nerves. J. Neurophysiol., **1:** 431–435, 1938.

77. ——, SIEGAL, S. Release of autonomic humoral substances in hypoglycemic cats and monkeys. Am. J. Physiol., **128:** 324–331, 1939–40.

78. BENEDICT, F. G., TALBOT, F. B. Metabolism and growth from birth to puberty. Publication 302, Carnegie Institution of Washington, 1921.

79. BENNETT, A. E. Preventing traumatic complications in convulsive shock therapy by curare. J. A. M. A., **114:** 322–324, 1940.

80. BERG, R. L., STOTZ, E., WESTERFELD, W. W. Alcohol metabolism in thiamine deficiency. J. Biol. Chem., **152:** 51–58, 1944.

81. BERGER, H. Über das Elektrenkephalogramm des Menschen. Arch. f. Psychiat., **87:** 527–570, 1929.

82. BERGMAN, H. C., DRURY, D. R. Effect of feeding and fasting on sugar utilization of eviscerated rabbits. Proc. Soc. Exper. Biol. & Med., **37:** 414–417, 1937–38.

83. BERNARD, C. Leçons sur la physiologie et la pathology du système nerveux. J. B. Baillière et fils, Paris, 1858.

84. BERT, P. Leçons sur la physiologie comparée de la respiration, professées au Museum d'histoire naturelle. J. B. Baillière et fils, Paris, 1870.

85. BEST, C. H., CAMPBELL, J., HAIST, R. E. The effect of anterior pituitary extracts on the insulin content of the pancreas. J. Physiol., **97**: 200–206, 1939–40.

86. ——, DALE, H. H., HOET, J. P., MARKS, H. P. Oxidation and storage of glucose under the action of insulin. Proc. Roy. Soc. London, **100B**: 55–71, 1926.

87. ——, HAIST, R. E. The effect of insulin administration on the insulin content of the pancreas. J. Physiol., **100**: 142–146, 1941–42.

88. ——, ——, RIDOUT, J. H. Diet and the insulin content of pancreas. J. Physiol., **97**: 107–119, 1939–40.

89. ——, HOET, J. P., MARKS, H. P. The fate of the sugar disappearing under the action of insulin. Proc. Roy. Soc. London, **100B**: 32–54, 1926.

90. ——, TAYLOR, N. B. The physiological basis of medical practice, fourth edition, Baltimore, The Williams & Wilkins Co., 1945.

91. BIASOTTI, A. Tolérance au glucose chez les chiens recevant des injections d'extrait anté-hypophysaire. Compt. rend. Soc. de biol., **116**: 455–456, 1934.

92. BISSINGER, E., LESSER, E. J. Kohlehydratstoffwechsel der maus nach injektion von zuckerlösungen und von insulin, III. Biochem. Ztschr., **168**: 398–420, 1926.

93. BLACK, P. T., COLLIP, J. B., THOMSON, D. L. The effect of anterior pituitary extracts on acetone body excretion in the rat. J. Physiol., **82**: 385–391, 1934.

94. BLIXENKRONE-MØLLER, N. Kohlenhydrat und Ketonkörperbildung aus Fettsäuren in der künstlich durchströmten Katzenleber. Hoppe-Seyler's Ztschr. f. physiol. Chem., **252**: 137–150, 1938.

95. BODANSKY, M., BODANSKY, O. Biochemistry of disease. New York, Macmillan Company, p. 264., 1940.

96. BODECHTEL, G. Der hypoglykämische Shock und seine Wirkung auf das Zentralnervesystem, zugleich ein Beitrag zu seiner Pathogenese. Duetsches Arch. f. klin. Med., **175**: 188–201, 1933.

97. DE BODO, R. C., BLOCH, H. I., GROSS, I. H. The role of the anterior pituitary in adrenaline hyperglycemia and liver glycogenolysis. Am. J. Physiol., **137**: 124–135, 1942.

98. ——, ——, SLATER, I. The role of the anterior pituitary in the maintenance of normal blood sugar levels and in the physiological mobilization of liver glycogen. Am. J. Physiol., **137**: 671–680, 1942.

99. BOELL, E. J., NACHMANSOHN, D. Localization of choline esterase in nerve fibers. Science, **92**: 513–514, 1940.

100. BOHR, D. F., BEAN, J. W. Dehydrogenase inactivation in oxygen poisoning. Am. J. Physiol., **131**: 388–393, 1940–41.

101. BOND, D. D. Sympathetic and vagal interaction in emotional responses of the heart rate. Am. J. Physiol., **138**: 468–478, 1942–43.

102. BOOTH, V. H. The identity of xanthine oxidase and the Schardinger enzyme. Biochem. J., **29**: 1732–1748, 1935.

103. BOUCKAERT, J. J., JOURDAN, F. Recherches sur la physiologie et la pharmacodynamie des vaisseaux cérébraux. 6. Réactions pharmacologiques des vaisseaux cérébraux. Arch. internat. de pharmacodyn. et de thérap., **53–54**: 168–183, 1936.

104. BOWMAN, K. M. Psychoses with pernicious anaemia. Am. J. Psychiat., **92**: 371–396, 1935.

105. BOYD, E. Outline of physical growth and development. Minneapolis, Burgess Publishing Co., 1942, Plate 39. Taken from Scammon, R. E., and Dunn, H. L., Empirical formulae for the postnatal growth of the human brain and its major divisions. Proc. Soc. Exper. Biol. & Med., **20**: 114–117, 1922–23.

106. BRACELAND, F. J., MEDUNA, L. J., VAICHULIS, J. A. Delayed action of insulin in schizophrenia. Am. J. Psychiat., **102**: 108–110, 1945.

107. BRAZIER, MARY, A. B. Physiological mechanisms underlying the electrical activity of the brain. J. Neurol. Neurosurg. & Psychiat. **11**: 118–133, 1948.

108. ——, FINESINGER, J. E. Action of barbiturates on the cerebral cortex. Electroencephalographic Studies. Arch. Neurol. & Psychiat., **53**: 51–58, 1945.

109. BREMER, F., BONNET, V. Action particuliere des barbituriques sur la transmission synaptique centrale. Arch internet. Physiol., **56**: 100–102, 1948.

110. BRENNER, C., MERRITT, H. H. Effect of certain choline derivatives on electrical activity of the cortex. Arch. Neurol. & Psychiat., **48**: 382–395, 1942.

111. BREUSCH, F. L. The fate of oxaloacetic acid in different organs. Biochem. J., **33**: 1757–1770, 1939.

112. ——. Citric acid cycle; sugar, and fat-breakdown in tissue metabolism. Science, **97**: 490–492, 1943.

113. ——. Ueber Einige Zuckerhydrogenasen in der leber. Enzymologia, **11**: 87–91, 1943.

114. BRITTON, S. W. Studies on the conditions of activity in endocrine glands. XVII. The nervous control of insulin secretion. Am. J. Physiol., **74**: 291–308, 1925.

115. ——. Adrenal insufficiency and related considerations. Physiol. Rev., **10**: 617–682, 1930.

116. ——, KLINE, R. F. Age, sex, carbohydrate, adrenal cortex and other factors in anoxia. Am. J. Physiol., **145**: 190–202, 1945.

117. BRODY, S., KIBLER, H. H. Growth and development. LII. Relations between organ weight and body weight in growing and mature animals. Univ. Missouri Research Bulletin, 328, 1941, p. 18.

118. BRONK, D. W., BRINK, F. Energy requirements for the maintenance of structure and function in nerve. Read at a symposium of the Annual Meeting of the Federation of Am. Societies for Exper. Biol., at Boston, 1942.

119. BROOKS, C. M. A delimitation of the central nervous mechanism involved in reflex hyperglycemia. Am. J. Physiol., **99**: 64–76, 1931–32.

120. BROWN, G. L., DALE, H. H., FELDBERG, W. Reactions of the normal mammalian muscle to acetylcholine and to eserine. J. Physiol., **87**: 394–424, 1936.

121. BROWN-SÉQUARD, E. Recherches expérimentales sur les propriétés physiologiques et les usages du sang rouge et du sang noir. J. de la physiol. de l'homme, **1**: 95–122, 353–367, 1858.

122. BUCHANAN, J. M., SAKAMI, W., GURIN, S., WILSON, D. W. A study of the intermediates of acetoacetate oxidation with isotopic carbon. J. Biol. Chem., **157**: 747–748, 1945.

123. BUCHMAN, E. F., RICHTER, C. P. Abolition of bulbocapnine catatonia by cocaine. Arch. Neurol. & Psychiat., **29**: 499–503, 1933.

124. BUEDING, E., FAZEKAS, J. F., HERRLICH, H., HIMWICH, H. E. Effect of insulin on pyruvic acid formation in depancreatized dogs, J. Biol. Chem., **148**: 97–104, 1943.

125. ——, STEIN, M. H., WORTIS, H. Blood pyruvate curves following glucose ingestion in normal and thiamine-deficient subjects. J. Biol. Chem., **140**: 697–703, 1941.

125a. BUFFA, P., PETERS, R. A. Formation of citrate *in vivo* induced by fluoroacetate poisoning. Nature, **163**: 914, 1949.

126. BULATAO, E., CARLSON, A. J. Contributions to the physiology of the stomach. Am. J. Physiol., **69**: 107–115, 1924.

127. BÜLBRING, E. BURN, J. H. Vascular changes affecting the transmission of nervous impulses. J. Physiol., **97**: 250–264, 1939–40.

128. ——, ——. Observations bearing on synaptic transmission by acetylcholine in the spinal cord. J. Physiol., **100**: 337–368, 1941–42.

129. ——, ——. The interrelation of prostigmine, adrenaline and ephedrine in skeletal muscle. J. Physiol., **101**: 224–235, 1942–43.

130. ——, ——. An action of adrenaline on transmission in sympathetic ganglia which may play a part in shock. J. Physiol., **101**: 289–303, 1942–43.

131. BÜLOW, M., HOLMES, E. G. Die Sauerstoffaufnahme und Ammoniakbildung von Gehirn bie Gegenwart narkotisch wirkender Stoffe. Biochem. Ztschr., **245**: 459–465, 1932.

132. BURK, D. The free energy of glycogen-lactic acid breakdown in muscle. Proc. Roy. Soc. London, **104B**: 153–170, 1928–29.

133. BURN, J. H. The modification of the action of insulin by pituitary extract and other substances. J. Physiol., **57**: 318–329, 1922–23.

134. ——. The relation of adrenaline to acetylcholine in the nervous system. Physiol. Rev., **25**: 377–394, 1945.

135. ——, Ling, H. W. Effect of insulin on acetonuria. J. Physiol., **65**: 191–203, 1928.

136. ——, Ling, H. W. Ketonuria in rats on a fat diet (a) after injections of pituitary (anterior lobe) extract, (b) during pregnancy. J. Physiol., **69**: p. xix, 1930.

137. ——, MARKS, H. P. The relation of the thyroid gland to the action of insulin. J. Physiol., **60**: 131–141, 1925.

138. BURROWS, M. T. The oxygen pressure necessary for tissue activity. Am. J. Physiol., **43**: 13–21, 1917.

139. BUTTS, J. S., CUTLER, C. H., DEUEL, H. J., JR. The sexual variation in carbohydrate metabolism. VI. The role of the anterior pituitary in the metabolism of diacetic acid. J. Biol. Chem., **105**: 45–58, 1934.

140. CAMERON, A. T. Temperature and life and death. Tr. Roy. Soc. Canada, **24**: 53–93, 1930.

141. CAMERON, D. E., HIMWICH, H. E., ROSEN, S. R., FAZEKAS, J. Oxygen consumption in the psychoses of the senium. Am. J. Psychiat., **97**: 566–572, 1940.

142. CAMERON, J. A. Age and species differences among rodents in resistance to CO asphyxia. J. Cell. & Comp. Physiol., **18**: 379–383, 1941.

143. CAMMERMEYER, J. Über Gehirnveränderungen, entstanden unter Sakelscher insulintherapie bei einem schizophrenen. Ztschr. f. d. ges. Neurol. u. Psychiat., **163**: 617–633, 1938.

144. CAMPBELL, A. C. P. Variation in vascularity and oxidase content in different regions of the brain of the cat. Arch. Neurol. & Psychiat., **41**: 223–242, 1939.

145. CAMPBELL, W. R., MALTBY, E. J. On the significance of respiratory quotients after administration of certain carbohydrates. J. Clin. Investigation, **6**: 303–317, 1928–29.

146. CANNON, W. B. The wisdom of the body. New York, W. W. Norton and Co., Inc., 1932.

147. ——. A law of denervation. Am. J. M. Sc., **198**: 737–750, 1939.

148. ——, McIVER, M. A., BLISS, S. W. Studies on the conditions of activity in endocrine glands. XIII. A sympathetic and adrenal mechanism for mobilizing sugar in hypoglycemia. Am. J. Physiol., **69**: 46–66, 1924.

149. CANNON, W. B., ROSENBLUETH, A. Studies on conditions of activity in endocrine organs; sympathin E. and sympathin I. Am. J. Physiol., **104**: 557–574, 1933.

150. CARLSON, H. B., GELLHORN, E., DARROW, C. W. Representation of the sympathetic and parasympathetic nervous systems in the forebrain of the cat. Arch. Neurol. & Psychiat., **45**: 105–116, 1941.

151. CERLETTI, U., BINI, L. L'elettroshock. Arch. gen. di. neurol., psichiat. e psicoanal., **19**: 266–268, 1938.

152. CHAIKOFF, I. L., SOSKIN, S. The utilization of acetoacetic acid by normal and diabetic dogs before and after evisceration. Am. J. Physiol., **87**: 58–72, 1928–29.

153. CHAMBERS, R., ZWEIFACH, B. W. Intercellular cement and capillary permeability. Physiol. Rev., **27**: 436–463, 1947.

154. CHAMBERS, W. H., SWEET, J. E., CHANDLER, J. P. Carbohydrate metabolism in the hypophysectomized depancreatized dog. Am. J. Physiol., **119**: 286–287, 1937.

155. CHARIPPER, H. A., GOLDSMITH, E. D., GORDON, A. S. Vitamin deficiency and overdosage and the resistance of rats to lowered barometric pressures. Am. J. Physiol., **145**: 130–133, 1945.

156. CHARITE, A. J., KHAUSTOV, N. W. IV. Flavin content of animal tissues under different conditions. Biochem. J., **29**: 34–37, 1935.

157. CHATFIELD, P. O., DEMPSEY, E. W. Some effects of prostigmine and acetylcholine on cortical potentials. Am. J. Physiol., **135**: 633–640, 1942.

158. CHEN, M. P., LIM, R. K. S., WANG, S. C., YI, C. L. On the question of a myelencephalic sympathetic centre. I. The effect of stimulation of the pressor area on visceral function. Chinese J. Physiol., **10**: 445–473, 1936.

159. ——, ——, ——, ——. On the question of a myelencephalic sympathetic centre. II. Experimental evidence for a reflex sympathetic centre in the medulla. Chinese J. Physiol., **11**: 355–366, 1937.

160. ——, ——, ——, ——. On the question of a myelencephalic sympathetic centre. III. Experimental location of the centre. Chinese J. Physiol., **11**: 367–384, 1937.

161. ——, ——, ——, ——. On the question of a myelencephalic sympathetic centre. IV. Experimental localization of its descending pathway with note on histology of centre and pathway. Chinese J. Physiol., **11**: 385–407, 1937.

162. CHENOWITH, M. B., ST. JOHN, E. F. Studies of the pharmacology of fluoroacetate III. Effect on the central nervous system of hogs and rabbits. J. Pharmacol. & Exper. Therap., **90**: 76–82, 1947.

163. CHERRY, I. S., CRANDALL, L. A. The absence of a significant glucose-lactic acid cycle (involving the liver) in normal unanaesthetized dogs. Am. J. Physiol., **125**: 41–47, 1939.

164. CHESLER, A. HIMWICH, H. E. The glycogen content of various parts of the central nervous system of dogs and cats at different ages. Arch. Biochem., **2**: 175–181, 1943.

165. ——, ——. Comparative studies of the rates of oxidation and glycolysis in the cerebral cortex and brain stem of the rat. Am. J. Physiol., **141**: 513–517, 1944.

166. ——, ——. Effect of insulin hypoglycemia on glycogen content of parts of the central nervous system of the dog. Arch. Neurol. & Psychiat., **52**: 114–116, 1944.

167. ——, ——. A comparison of the relationship of lactic acid and pyruvic acid in the normal and diabetic dog. J. Biol. Chem., **155**: 413–419, 1944.

168. ——, ——. Glycolysis in the parts of the central nervous system of cats and dogs during growth. Am. J. Physiol., **142**: 544–549, 1944.

169. ——, HOMBURGER, E., HIMWICH, H. E. Carbohydrate metabolism in vitamin B₁ deficiency. J. Biol. Chem., **153**: 219–225, 1944.

170. ——, LABELLE, G. C., HIMWICH, H. E. The relative effects of toxic doses of alcohol on fetal, newborn and adult rats. Quart. J. Stud. on Alcohol, **3**: 1–4, 1942–43.

171. CHIDSEY, J. L., DYE, J. A. The increase in insulin secretion following injection of epinephrine and its relation to the high liver glycogen values obtained. Am. J. Physiol., **111**: 223–229, 1935.

172. CLAMANN, H. G., BECKER-FREYSENG, H. Einwirkung des Sauerstoffs auf den Organismus bei höherem als normalem Partialdruck unter besonderer Berücksichtigung des Menschen, Luftfahrtmedizin, **4**: 1–10, 1940.

173. CLARK, D., HUGHES, J., GASSER, H. S. Afferent function in the group of nerve fibers of slowest conduction velocity. Am. J. Physiol., **114**: 69–76, 1935–36.

174. COBB, S. The cerebrospinal blood vessels. Cytology and cellular pathology of the nervous system. W. Penfield, Ed., New York, Paul B. Hoeber, 1932.

175. COHEN, R. A., GERARD, R. W. Hyperthyroidism and brain oxidations. J. Cell. & Comp. Physiol., **10**: 223–240, 1937.

176. COLLAZO, J. A., HÄNDEL, M., RUBINO, P. Über den wirkunsmechanismus des insulins. Klin. Wchnschr., **3**: 323, 1924.

177. COLLIP, J. B. The occurence of ketone bodies in the urine of normal rabbits in a condition of hypoglycemia following the administration of insulin—a condition of acute acidosis experimentally produced. J. Biol. Chem., **55**: p. xxxviii–xxxix, 1923.

178. COLOWICK, S. P., CORI, GERTY T., SLEIN, M. W. The effect of adrenal cortex and anterior pituitary extracts and insulin on the hexokinase reaction. J. Biol. Chem., **168**: 583–596, 1947.

179. ——, WELCH, M. S., CORI, C. F. Glucose oxidation and phosphorylation. J. Biol. Chem., **133**: 641–642, 1940.

180. ——, WELCH, M. S., CORI, C. F. Phosphorylation of glucose in kidney extract. J. Biol. Chem., **133**: 359–373, 1940.

181. COMROE, J. H., JR., DRIPPS, R. D., DUMKE, P. R., DEMING, M. Oxygen toxicity: the effect of inhalation of high concentrations of oxygen for twenty-four hours on normal men at sea level and at a simulated altitude of 18,000 feet. J.A.M.A., **128**: 710–717, 1945.

182. CONN, J. W .The spontaneous hypoglycemias. Importance of etiology in determining treatment. J.A.M.A., **115**: 1669–1675, 1940.

183. COPE, O., MARKS, H. P. Further experiments on the relation of the pituitary gland to the action of insulin and adrenaline. J. Physiol., **83**: 157–176, 1935.

184. CORI, C. F. Insulin and liver glycogen. J. Pharamacol. & Exper. Therap., **25**: 1–33, 1925.

185. ——. Mammalian carbohydrate metabolism. Physiol. Rev., **11**: 143–275, 1931.

186. ——. Glycogen breakdown and synthesis in animal tissues. Endocrinology, **26**: 285–296. 1940.

187. ——, CORI, G. T. The mechanism of epinephrine action. I. The influence of epinephrine on the carbohydrate metabolism of fasting rats, with a note on new formation of carbohydrates. J. Biol. Chem., **79**: 309–319, 1928.

188. ——, ——. Mechanism of epinephrine action. II. Influence of epinephrine and

insulin on carbohydrate metabolism of rats in the postabsorptive state. J Biol. Chem., **79:** 321–341, 1928.

189. CORI, G. T., CORI, C. F., BUCHWALD, K. W. The mechanism of epinephrine action. V. Changes in liver glycogen and blood lactic acid after injection of epinephrine and insulin. J. Biol. Chem., **86:** 375–388, 1930.

190. ——, CORI, C. F. The kinetics of the enzymatic synthesis of glycogen from glucose-1-phosphate. J. Biol. Chem., **135:** 733–756, 1940.

191. ——, SLEIN, M. W. Gluco- and fructokinase in mammalian tissues. Fed. Proc., **6:** 245–246, 1947.

192. CORKILL, A. B. Influence of insulin on the distribution of glycogen in normal animals. Biochem. J., **24:** 779–794, 1930.

193. ——, MARKS, H. P., WHITE, W. E. Relation of the pituitary gland to the action of insulin and adrenaline. J. Physiol., **80:** 193–205, 1933.

194. COURNAND, A., RICHARDS, D. W., MAIER, H. C. Pulmonary insufficiency. III. Cases demonstrating advanced cardiopulmonary insufficiency following artificial pneumothorax and thoracoplasty. Am. Rev. Tuberculosis, **44:** 272–287, 1941.

195. COURTICE, F. C. The effect of raised intracranial pressure on the cerebral blood flow. J. Neurol. & Psychiat., **3:** 293–305, 1940.

196. ——. The metabolism of the brain. J. Neurol. & Psychiat., **3:** 306–310, 1940.

197. ——. The gaseous tensions in the brain. J. Physiol., **100:** 192–197, 1941–42.

198. ——. The effect of oxygen lack on the cerebral circulation. J. Physiol., **100:** 198–211, 1941–42.

199. COURVILLE, C. B. Asphyxia as a consequence of nitrous oxide anesthesia. Medicine, **15:** 129–245, 1936.

200. COUTEAUX, R., NACHMANSOHN, D. Changes of choline esterase at end plates of voluntary muscle following section of sciatic nerve. Proc. Soc. Exper. Biol. & Med., **43:** 177–181, 1940.

201. CRAIG, F. N., BEECHER, H. K. The effect of oxygen tension on the metabolism of cerebral cortex, medulla and spinal cord. J. Neurophysiol., **6:** 135–141, 1943.

202. CRAIGIE, E. H. On the relative vascularity of various parts of the central nervous system of the albino rat. J. Comp. Neurol., **30–31:** 429–464, 1919–20.

203. ——. Changes in vascularity in the brain stem and cerebellum of the albino rat between birth and maturity. J. Comp. Neurol., **38:** 27–48, 1924–25.

204. ——. Postnatal changes in vascularity in the cerebral cortex of the male albino rat. J. Comp. Neurol., **39:** 301–324, 1925.

205. ——. The vascularity of the vagus nuclei and of the adjacent reticular formation in the albino rat. J. Comp. Neurol., **42:** 57–68, 1926–27.

206. ——. The vascular supply of the archicortex of the rat. II. The albino rat at birth. J. Comp. Neurol., **52:** 353–357, 1931.

207. CRANDALL, L. A., JR., CHERRY, I. S. The effects of insulin and glycine on hepatic glucose output in normal, hypophysectomized, adrenal denervated, and adrenalectomized dogs. Am. J. Physiol., **125:** 658–673, 1939.

208. CRESCITELLI, F., GILMAN, A. Electrical manifestations of the cerebellum and cerebral cortex following DDT administration in cats and monkeys. Am. J. Physiol., **147:** 127–137, 1946.

209. ——, KOELLE, G. B., GILMAN, A. Transmission of impulses in peripheral nerves treated with di-isopropyl fluorophosphate (DFP). J. Neurophysiol., **9:** 241–252, 1946.

210. CRUICKSHANK. E. W. H., STARTUP, C. W. The action of insulin on the R. Q., oxygen utilization, CO_2 production, and sugar utilization in the mammalian diabetic heart. J. Physiol., **81**: 153–161, 1934.

211. ——, STARTUP, C. W. The respiratory quotient, oxygen consumption, and glycogen content of the mammalian heart in aglycaemia. J. Physiol., **80**: 179–192, 1934.

212. CULLEN, S. C., WEIR, E. F., COOK, E. The rationale of oxygen therapy during fever therapy. Anesthesiology, **3**: 123–130, 1942.

213. CUSHING, H. Concerning a definite regulatory mechanism of the vasomotor center which controls blood pressure during cerebral compression. Bull. Johns Hopkins Hosp., **12**: 290–292, 1901.

214. ——. Some experiments and clinical observations concerning states of increased intracranial tension. Am. J. M. Sci., **124**: 375–400, 1902.

215. ——. Neurohypophysial mechanisms from a clinical standpoint. Lancet, 119–127, 175–184, 1930, Part 2.

216. CUTTING, M., McCANCE, R. A. The metabolism of kidney slices from new-born and full-grown rats. J. Physiol., **104**: 288–298, 1946.

217. DAKIN, H. D., DUDLEY, H. W. On glyoxalase. J. Biol. Chem., **14**: 423–431, 1913.

218. DALE, H. H. Nomenclature of fibers in the autonomic system and their effects. J. Physiol., **80**: 10–11, 1934.

219. DAMESHEK, W., MYERSON, A., LOMAN, J. The effects of sodium amytal on the metabolism. Am. J. Psychiat., **91**: 113–135, 1934.

220. ——, ——, STEPHENSON, C. Insulin hypoglycemia, mechanism of the neurologic symptoms. Arch. Neurol. & Psychiat., **33**: 1–18, 1935.

221. DARROW, C. W., GREEN, J. R., DAVIS, E. W., GAROL, H. W. Parasympathetic regulation of high potential in the electroencephalogram. J. Neurophysiol., **7**: 217–226, 1944.

222. DARWIN, C. The origin of species. New York, D. Appleton and Co., 1896, vol. I and II.

223. DAVENPORT, H. W. Carbonic anhydrase in the nervous system. J. Neurophysiol., **9**: 41–46, 1946.

224. DAVIDOFF, L. M. The brain in mongolian idiocy. Arch. Neurol. & Psychiat., **20**: 1229–1257, 1928.

225. DAVIES, D. R., QUASTEL, J. H. Dehydrogenations by brain tissue. The effects of narcotics. Biochem. J., **26**: 1672–1684, 1932.

226. DAVIES, P. W., RÉMOND, A. Oxygen consumption of the cerebral cortex of the cat during metrazol convulsions. A. Research Nerv. & Ment. Dis., Proc., **26**: 205–217, 1947.

227. DAVIS, E. W., McCULLOCH, W. S., ROSEMAN, E. Rapid changes in the O_2 tension of cerebral cortex during induced convulsions. Am. J. Psychiat., **100**: 825–829, 1944.

228. DAVIS, P. A., GIBBS, F. A., DAVIS, H., JETTER, W. W., TROWBRIDGE, L. S. The effects of alcohol upon the electroencephalogram (Brain waves). Quart. J. Stud. on Alcohol, **1**: 626–637, 1940–41.

229. DAVISON, C., STONE, L. Lesions of the nervous system of the rat in vitamin B deficiency. Arch. Path., **23**: 207–223, 1937.

230. DENNY-BROWN, D. Theoretical deductions from the physiology of the cerebral cortex. J. Neurol. & Psychopath., **13**: 52–67, 1932–33.

231. DERBYSHIRE, A. J., REMPEL, B., FORBES, A., LAMBERT, E. F. The effects of

anesthetics on action potentials in the cerebral cortex of the cat. Am. J. Physiol., **116:** 577–596, 1936.

232. DEWAN, J. G. Chemical steps in the metabolism of alcohol by brain in vitro. Quart. J. Stud, on Alcohol, **4:** 357–361, 1943.

233. ——. An alcohol detoxication mechanism in the central nervous system. Am. J. Psychiat., **99:** 565–568, 1942–43.

234. DICKENS, F. Oxidation of phosphohexonate and pentose phosphoric acids by yeast enzymes. I. Oxidation of phosphohexonate. II. Oxidation of pentose phosphoric acids. Biochem. J., **32:** 1626–1644, 1938.

235. ——. Yeast fermentation of pentose phosphoric acids. Biochem. J., **32:** 1645–1653, 1938.

236. ——. The toxic effects of oxygen on brain metabolism and on tissue enzymes. Biochem. J., **40:** 145–171, 1946.

237. ——, GREVILLE, G. D. Metabolism of normal and tumour tissue. XIII. Respiration in fructose and in sugar-free media. Biochem. J., **27:** 832–841, 1933.

238. ——, ——. The metabolism of normal and tumour tissue. XIII. Neutral salt effects. Biochem. J., **29:** 1468–1483, 1935.

239. ——, SIMER, F. The metabolism of normal and tumour tissue. IV. The respiratory quotient in bicarbonate-media. Biochem. J., **25:** 985–993, 1931.

240. ——, ——. The metabolism of normal and tumour tissue. II. The respiratory quotient, and the relationship of respiration to glycolysis. Biochem. J., **24:** 1301–1326, 1930.

241. DILL, D. B., EDWARDS, H. T., DE MEIO, R. H. Effects of adrenalin injection in moderate work. Am. J. Physiol., **111:** 9–20, 1935.

242. DIXON, K. C. The effect of rise in temperature on the carbohydrate catabolism of cerebral cortex. Biochem. J., **30:** 1483–1488, 1936.

243. ——. A study of cortical metabolism in relation to cerebral disease. Brain, **63:** 191–199, 1940.

244. DIXON, T. F., MEYER, A. Respiration of the brain. Biochem. J., **30:** 1577–1582, 1936.

245. DOHAN, F. C., FISH, C. A., LUKENS, F. D. W. Induction and course of permanent diabetes produced by anterior pituitary extract. Endocrinology, **28:** 341–357, 1941.

246. ——, LUKENS, F. D. W. Lesions of the pancreatic islets produced in cats by administration of glucose. Science, **105:** 183, 1947.

247. DOLIN, G., JOSEPH, S. GAUNT, R. Effect of steriod and pituitary hormones on experimental diabetes mellitus of ferrets. Endocrinology, **28:** 840–845, 1941.

248. DONALDSON, H. H., HATAI, S. On the weight of the parts of the brain and on the percentage of water in them according to brain weight and to age, in albino and in wild Norway rats. J. Comp. Neurol., **53:** 263–307, 1931.

249. DONHOFFER, C., MACLEOD, J. J. R. Studies in the nervous control of carbohydrate metabolism. I. The position of the centre. Proc. Roy. Soc. London, **110B:** 125–141, 1932.

250. DOW, R. S. The evolution and anatomy of the cerebellum. Biol. Rev., **17:** 179–220, 1942.

251. DRABKIN, D. L., SCHMIDT, C. F. Spectrophotometric studies. XII. Observation of circulating blood *in vivo*, and the direct determination of the saturation of hemoglobin in arterial blood. J. Biol. Chem., **157:** 69–83, 1945.

252. DRESEL, K. Experimentelle Untersuchungen zur Anatomie und Physiologie des peripheren und zentralen vegetativen Nervensystems. Ztschr. f. d. ges. Exper. Med., **36–37:** 373–425, 1923.

253. DRURY, A. N. The physiological activity of nucleic acid and its derivatives. Physiol. Rev., **16**: 292–325, 1936.

254. DRURY, D. R. The role of insulin in carbohydrate metabolism. Am. J. Physiol., **131**: 536–543, 1940–41.

255. ———. Control of blood sugar. J. Clin. Endocrinol., **2**: 421–430, 1942.

256. DuBois, E. F. Basal metabolism in health and disease. Philadelphia, Lea and Febiger, 1936.

257. DuBois, K. P., ALBAUM, H. G., POTTER, V. R. Adenosine triphosphate in magnesium anesthesia. J. Biol. Chem., **147**: 699–704, 1943.

258. DUMKE, P. R., SCHMIDT, C. F. Quantitative measurements of cerebral blood flow in the macacque monkey. Am. J. Physiol., **138**: 421–431, 1942–43.

259. DUNNING, H. S., WOLFF, H. G. The relative vascularity of various parts of the central and peripheral nervous system of the cat and its relation to function. J. Comp. Neurol., **67**: 433–450, 1937.

260. DUSSER DE BARENNE, J. G., McCULLOCH, W. S., NIMS, L. F. Functional activity and pH of the cerebral cortex. J. Cell. & Comp. Physiol., **10**: 277–289, 1937.

261. ———, J. G., McCULLOCH, W. S. Sensorimotor cortex, nucleus caudatus and thalamus opticus. J. Neurophysiol., **1**: 364–377, 1938.

262. ———, J. G., McCULLOCH, W. S. Suppression of motor response obtained from area 4 by stimulation of area 4s. J. Neurophysiol., **4**: 311–323, 1941.

263. DUSSIK, K. T. Three and a half years of hypoglycemic therapy of schizophrenia. Am. J. Psychiat., **94**: 269–276, 1938.

264. DWORKIN, S. Insulin and heart rate after sympathectomy and vagotomy. Am. J. Physiol., **96**: 311–320, 1931.

265. DYE, J. A. The action of thyroxin on tissue respiration. Am. J. Physiol., **105**: 518–524, 1933.

266. ———, CHIDSEY, J. L. Total carbohydrate-acetone body utilization ratios with high acetone body concentrations. Am. J. Physiol., **126**: 482–483, 1939.

267. ———, WAGGENER, R. A. Studies in tissue respiration and endocrine functions. I. The influence of thyroidectomy on the indophenol oxidase content of animal tissues. Am. J. Physiol., **85**: 1–13, 1028.

268. EDWARDS, E. A. Anatomic variations of the cranial venous sinuses. Their relation to the effect of jugular compression in lumbar manometric tests. Arch. Neurol. & Psychiat., **26**: 801–814, 1931.

269. EISENBERG, E., GORDAN, G. S. ELLIOTT, H. W. The effect of castration and of testosterone upon the respiration of rat brain. Science, **109**: 337–338, 1949.

270. ELLIOTT, K. A. C., BAKER, Z. The respiratory quotients of normal and tumor tissue. Biochem. J., **29**: 2433–2441, 1935.

271. ———, GREIG, M. E., BENOY, M. P. The metabolism of lactic and pyruvic acids in normal and tumour tissues. III. Rat liver, brain, and testis. Biochem. J., **31**: 1003–1020, 1937.

272. ———, SCOTT, D. B. M., LIBET, B. Studies on the metabolism of brain suspension. II. Carbohydrate utilization. J. Biol. Chem., **146**: 251–269, 1942.

273. ELLIOTT, W. B., KALNITSKY, G. Mechanism of fluoroacetate inhibition. Fed. Proc., **9**: 168–169, 1950.

274. ELVEHJEM, C. A. The biological action of the vitamins. Univ. Chicago Press. A symposium, Ed. by E. A. Evans, Jr. 1–16, 1942.

275. EMBDEN, G., DEUTICKE, H. J., KRAFT, G. Über die intermediären vorgänge bei der glykolyse in der muskulatur, Klin. Wchnschr., **12**: 213–215, 1933.

276. EMBDEN, G., WIRTH, J. Über Hemmung der Acetessigsäurebildung in der Leber. Biochem. Ztschr., **27**: 1–19, 1910.

277. EMERSON, H. Alcohol and Man. New York City, The Macmillan Company, p. 203, 1932.

278. ENGEL, G. L., MARGOLIN, S. G. Neuropsychiatric disturbances in internal disease. Arch. Int. Med., **70**: 236–259, 1942.

279. ——, ROMANO, J. Delirium II. Reversibility of the Electroencephalogram with Experimental Procedures. Arch. Neurol. & Psychiat., **51**: 378–392, 1944.

280. ——, ROMANO, J., FERRIS, E. B. Jr., WEBB, J. P., STEVENS, C. D. A simple method of determining frequency spectrums in the electroencephalogram. Observations on effects of physiologic variations in dextrose, oxygen, posture and acid-base balance on the normal electroencephalogram. Arch. Neurol. & Psychiat., **51**: 134–146, 1944.

282. ——, ROSENBAUM, MILTON, Delirium III. Electroencephalographic Changes Associated with Acute Alcoholic Intoxication. Arch. Neurol. & Psychiat., **53**: 44–50, 1945.

283. ENGELHARDT, W. A. Enzymatic and mechanical properties of muscle proteins. Yale J. Biol. & Med., **15**: 21–38, 1942–43. Translated by Mr. Paul Talalay of Massachusetts Institute of Technology from a review article originally published in the Russian journal, "Advances in Contemporary Biology", **14**: 177–190, 1941.

284. EPPINGER, H., HESS, L. Die vagotonie. Pt. 9 and 10 of Samml. Klin. Abhandl. u. Path. u. Therap. d. Stoffwechs. und Ernährungsstör., Berlin, 1910.

285. ERLANGER, J. The initiation of impulses in axons. J. Neurophysiol., **2**: 370–379, 1939.

286. ESMOND, W. G., JOHNS, R. J., BALES, P. D., McCAULEY, ALICE, HIMWICH, H. E. The convulsant and anticonvulsant effects of some antihistamines. EEG Clin. Neurophysiol., **2**: 115–116, 1950.

287. ESSIG, C. F., HAMPSON, J. L., HIMWICH, H. E. Biochemically induced circling behavior. J. Nerv. & Ment. Dis., in press.

288. ——, ESMOND, W., BALES, P. D., HIMWICH, H. E. Effects of caramephin and mephenesin on the convulsant action of di-isopropyl fluorophosphate (DFP). In preparation.

289. ——, HAMPSON, J. L., McCAULEY, ALICE, HIMWICH, H. E. An experimental analysis of biochemically induced circling behavior. J. Neurophysiol., **13**: 269–275, 1950.

290. ETSTEN, B., ALEXANDER, F. A. D., HIMWICH, H. E. Comparative toxicity of pentobarbital in the newborn and adult rat. J. Lab. & Clin. Med., **28**: 706–710, 1942–43.

291. ——, HIMWICH, H. E. Stages and signs of pentothal anesthesia: Physiologic basis. Anesthesiology, **7**: 536–548 1946.

292. ——, ——. Management of anoxia in pentothal anesthesia. Am. J. Surg., **76**: 268–271, 1948.

293. ——, YORK, G. E., HIMWICH, H. E. Pattern of metabolic depression induced by pentothal sodium. Arch. Neurol. & Psychiat., **56**: 171–183, 1946.,

294. EULER, H. v., GÜNTHER, G., VESTIN, R. Glykolyse und Phosphatumsatz in Zellfreien Gehirnextrakten normaler Säugetiere. Hoppe-Seyler's Ztschr. Physiol. Chem., **240**: 265–278, 1936.

295. EULER, U. S. v. A specific sympathomimetic ergone in adrenergic nerve fibres (sympathin) and its relations to adrenaline and nor-adrenaline. Acta Physiol. Scand., **12**: 73–97, 1946.

296. EVANS, C. L. Observations on cyanide anoxaemia. J. Physiol., **53**: 17–41, 1919–20.

297. EVANS, E, A., JR. Pyruvate oxidation and the citric acid cycle. Biological Symposia, **5**: 157–173, 1941.

298. ——, SLOTIN, L. Carbon dioxide utilization by pigeon liver. J. Biol. Chem., **141**: 439–450, 1941.

299. EVANS, G. Effect of adrenalectomy on carbohydrate metabolism. Endocrinology, **29**: 731–736, 1941.

300. EXTON, W. G., ROSE, A. R. The one-hour two-dose dextrose tolerance test. Am. J. Clin. Path., **4**: 381–399, 1934.

301. FABING, H. D. Induction of metrazol convulsions with the patient under nitrous oxide anesthesia. Arch. Neurol. & Psychiat., **47**: 223–233, 1942.

301a. FAY, T., HENNY, G. C. Correlation of body segmental temperature and its relation to the location of carcinomatous metastasis. Clinical observations and response to methods of refrigeration. Surg. Gyn. & Obst., **66**: 512–524, 1938.

302. FAZEKAS, J. F., ALEXANDER, F. A. D., HIMWICH, H. E. Tolerance of the newborn to anoxia. Am. J. Physiol., **134**: 281–287, 1941.

303. ——, BAKER, Z., HIMWICH, H. E. The oxidation of various substrates by the diabetic kidney. Am. J. Physiol., **123**: 62, 1938.

304. ——, COLYER, H., HIMWICH, H. E. Effect of cyanide on cerebral metabolism. Proc. Soc. Exper. Biol. & Med., **42**: 496–498, 1939.

305. ——. Cerebral metabolism of hyperthyroid, thyroid-deficient and cretinous rats. Fed. Proc., **5**: 26, 1946.

307. ——, HIMWICH, H. E. Effect of nicotine on the oxidations of the diabetic brain. Am. J. Physiol., **116**: 46–47, 1936.

308. ——, ——. Effect of hypothermia on cerebral metabolism. Proc. Soc. Exper. Biol. & Med., **42**: 537–538, 1939.

309. ——, ——. The significance of a pathway of carbohydrate breakdown not involving glycolysis. J. Biol. Chem., **139**: 971–972, 1941.

310. ——, ——. Anaerobic survival of adult animals. Am. J. Physiol., **139**: 366–370, 1943.

311. FEITELBERG, S., LAMPL, H. Über die beeinflussing der wärmebildung in den verschiedenen hirnanteilen durch narcotica, hypnotica und analeptica. Arch. internat. de pharmacol. et de thérapie, **61–62**: 255–270, 1939.

312. FELDMAN, J., CORTELL, R., GELLHORN, E. Vago-insulin and sympathetico-adrenal systems, their mutual relationship. II. Reaction to cocaine and bulbocapnine. Proc. Soc. Exper. Biol. & Med., **46**: 157–160, 1941.

313. ——, ——, GELLHORN, E. On the vago-insulin and sympathetico-adrenal systems and their mutual relationship under conditions of central excitation induced by anoxia and convulsant drugs. Am. J. Physiol., **131**: 281–289, 1940–41.

314. FERRARO, A., BARRERA, S. E. Experimental catalepsy. State Hospitals Press, Utica, New York, 1932.

315. ——, JERVIS, G. A. Brain pathology in four cases of schizophrenia treated with insulin. Psychiatric Quart., **13**: 207–228, 1939.

316. FERRIS, E. B. Objective measurement of relative intracranial blood flow in man, with observations concerning the hydrodynamics of the craniovertebral system. Arch. Neurol. & Psychiat., **46**: 377–401, 1941.

317. ——, ENGEL, G. L., STEVENS, D., LOGAN, MYRTLE. The validity of internal jugular venous blood in studies of cerebral metabolism and blood flow in man. Am. J. Physiol., **147**: 517–521, 1946.

318. FERRIS, E. B., ROSENBAUM, M., ARING, C. D., RYDER, H. W., ROSEMAN, E., HAWKINS, J. R. Intracranial blood flow in insulin coma. Arch. Neurol. & Psychiat., 46: 509–512, 1941.
319. FERRIS, S., HIMWICH, H. E. The effect of hypoglycemia and age on the glycogen content of the various parts of the feline central nervous system. Am. J. Physiol., 146: 389–393, 1946.
320. FIELD, J., 2nd, FUHRMAN, F. A., MARTIN, A. W. Effect of temperature on the oxygen consumption of brain tissue. J. Neurophysiol., 7: 117–126, 1944.
321. ——, HALL, V. E. Physiological effects of heat and cold. Ann. Rev. Physiol., 6: 69–94, 1944.
322. FINESINGER, J. E., BRAZIER, MARY A. B., TUCCI, J. H., MILES, H. H. W. A study of levels of consciousness based on electroencephalographic data in pentothal anesthesia. Tr. Am. Neurol. A., 183–185, 1947.
323. ——, COBB, S. The cerebral circulation XXXIV. The action of narcotic drugs on the pial vessels, J. Pharm. & Exper. Therap., 53: 1–33, 1935.
324. FINLEY, K. H. The capillary bed of the paraventricular and supra-optic neuclei of the hypothalamus. A. Research Nerv. & Ment. Dis. Proc., The circulation of the brain and spinal cord, 18: 94–109, 1938.
325. ——, BRENNER, C. Histologic evidence of damage to the brain in monkeys treated with metrazol and insulin. Arch. Neurol. & Psychiat., 45: 403–438, 1941.
326. FINNEY, J. M. T., FINNEY, J. M. T., JR. Resection of the pancreas. Ann. Surg., 88: 584–592, 1928.
327. FISHER, R. A. Statistical methods for research workers. Edinburgh and London, Oliver and Boyd, 1938, 7th ed., p. 177.
328. FISHER, R. E., PENCHARZ, R. I. Carbohydrate oxidation in hypophysectomized rats. Proc. Soc. Exper. Biol. & Med., 34: 106–107, 1936.
329. ——, RUSSELL, J. A., CORI, C. F. Glycogen disappearance and carbohydrate oxidation in hypophysectomized rats. J. Biol. Chem., 115: 627–634, 1936.
330. FLEXNER, L. B., FLEXNER, J. B. Succinoxidase and succinic dehydrogenase in the developing cerebral cortex of the fetal pig. Anat. Rec., 91: 274, 1945.
331. FOG, M. Cerebral circulation. I. Reaction of pial arteries to epinephrine by direct application and by intravenous injection. Arch. Neurol. & Psychiat., 41: 109–118, 1939.
332. FOGEL, E. J., GRAY, L. P. Nitrous oxide anoxia in the treatment of schizophrenia. Am. J. Psychiat., 97: 677–685, 1940.
333. FORBES, H. S. Physiologic regulation of the cerebral circulation. Arch. Neurol. & Psychiat., 43: 804–814, 1940.
334. ——, FINLEY, K. H., NASON, GLADYS. Cerebral circulation: XXIV. Action of epinephrine on pial vessels. Arch. Neurol. & Psychiat., 30: 957–968, 1933.
335. ——, NASON, GLADYS. Effect of metrazol on cerebral vessels. Proc. Soc. Exper. Biol. and Med., 43: 762–765, 1940.
336. ——, WOLFF, H. G. Cerebral circulation. III. The vasomotor control of cerebral vessels. Arch. Neurol. & Psychiat., 19: 1057–1086, 1928.
337. FORSTER, F. M. Action of acetylcholine on motor cortex: Correlation of effects of acetylcholine and epilepsy. Arch. Neurol. & Psychiat., 54: 391–394, 1946.
338. FRAENKEL-CONRAT, H. L., HERRING, V. V., SIMPSON, M. E., EVANS, H. M. Effect of purified pituitary preparations on the insulin content of the rat's pancreas. Am. J. Physiol., 135: 404–410, 1941–42.
339. FRAENKEL-CONRAT, H., HERRING, V. V., SIMPSON, M. E., EVANS, H. M. Effect

of adrenocorticotropic hormone on the insulin content of the rat's pancreas. Proc. Soc. Exper. Biol. & Med., **55:** 62–63, 1944.

340. FRANK, E., HARTMANN, E., NOTHMANN, M. Über glykogenanreicherung in der leber hungernder normaltiere unter dem einflusse des insulins. Klin. Wchnschr., **4:** 1067, 1925.

341. FREEDMAN, A. M., BALES, P. D., WILLIS, A., HIMWICH, H. E. Experimental production of electrical major convulsive patterns. Am. J. Physiol., **156:** 117–124, 1949.

342. ——, HIMWICH, H. E. Effect of age on lethality of di-isopropyl fluorophosphate. Am. J. Physiol., **153:** 121–126, 1948.

343. FREEMAN, W., WATTS, J. W. Psychosurgery. Intelligence, emotion, and social behavior following prefontal lobotomy for mental disorders. Springfield, Charles C. Thomas, 1942.

344. ——, ——. Psychosurgery during 1936–1946. Arch. Neurol. & Psychiat., **58:** 417–425, 1947.

344a. FREYHAN, F. A., WOODFORD, R. B., KETY, S. S. The blood flow, vascular resistance and oxygen consumption of the brain in the psychoses of sensility. J. Nerv. & Ment. Dis., 1950.

345. FRIEDEMANN, T. E., COTONIO, M., SHAFFER, P. A. The determination of lactic acid. J. Biol. Chem., **73:** 335–358, 1927.

346. ——. The metabolism of sodium acetoacetate intravenously injected into dogs. J. Biol. Chem., **116:** 133–161, 1936.

347. FRIEDEMANN, U. Blood-brain barrier. Physiol. Rev., **22:** 125–145, 1942.

348. FRIES, B. A., CHAIKOFF, I. L. The phosphorus metabolism of the brain as measured with radioactive phosphorus. J. Biol. Chem., **141:** 479–485, 1941.

349. ——, ENTENMAN, C., CHANGUS, G. W., CHAIKOFF, I. L. The deposition of lipids in various parts of the central nervous system of the developing rat. J. Biol. Chem., **137:** 303–310, 1941.

350. FROSTIG, J. P. Clinical observations in the insulin treatment of schizophrenia. I. The symptomatology and therapeutic factors of the insulin effect. Am. J. Psychiat., **96:** 1167–1190, 1940.

351. ——. Insulin treatment of mental disorders. In preparation.

352. ——, VAN HARREVELD, A., REZNICK, S., TYLER, D. B., WIERSMA, C. A. G. Electronarcosis in animals and in man. Arch. Neurol. & Psychiat., **51:** 232–242, 1944.

353. ——, ROSSMAN, I. M., CLINE, W. B., JR., SCHWOERER, O. Protracted shock; its cause and its prevention. Am. J. Psychiat., **98:** 192–195, 1941–42.

354. ——, SPIES, T. D. The initial nervous syndrome of pellagra and associated deficiency diseases. Am. J. M. Sc., **199:** 268–274, 1940.

355. FUHRMAN, F. A., FIELD, J., 2nd. The reversibility of the inhibition of rat brain and kidney metabolism by cold. Am. J. Physiol., **139:** 193–196, 1943.

356. ——, MARTIN, A. W., DILLE, J. M. The inhibition of brain oxidations by a convulsant barbiturate. Science, **94:** 421–422, 1941.

357. FULTON, J. F. Physiology of the nervous system. London, New York, Toronto, Oxford University Press, 1943.

358. ——, KELLER, A. D. Observations on response of same chipanzee to dial, amytal, and nembutal, used as surgical anesthetics. Surg. Gynec. & Obst., **54:** 764–770, 1932.

359. ——, ——. The sign of Babinski; a study of the evolution of cortical dominance in primates. Springfield, Ill., Charles C. Thomas, 1932.

360. FULTON, J. F., Nachmansohn, D. Acetylcholine and the physiology of the nervous system. Science, 97: 569–571, 1943.

360a. FURCHGOTT, R. F., SHORR, E. The effect of succinate on respiration and certain metabolic processes of mammalian tissues at low oxygen tensions *in vitro.* J. Biol. Chem., 175: 201–215, 1948.

361. GAGGE, A. P., ALLEN, S. C., MARBARGER, J. P. Pressure breathing. J. Aviation Med., 16: 2–8, 1945.

362. GALVAO, P. E., PEREIRA, J. Sobre a oxidacão do acido lactico no encefalo de animais normais e em avitaminose B_1. Arq. Inst. biol., São Paulo, 9: 25–37, 1938.

363. GARDNER-HILL, H., BRETT, P. C., SMITH, J. F. Carbohydrate tolerance in myxoedema. Quart. J. Med., 18: 327–334, 1924–25.

364. GARRY, R. C. Some observations on the suitability of amytal as an anesthetic for laboratory animals. J. Pharmacol. & Exper. Therap., 39: 129–136, 1930.

365. GASSER, H. S. Axons as samples of nervous tissue. J. Neurophysiol., 2: 361–369, 1939.

366. GAYET, R., GUILLAUMIE, M. La régulation de la sécrétion interne pancréatique par un processus humoral, démontrée par des transplantations de pancréas. Expériences sur des animaux normaux. Compt. rend. Soc. de biol., 97: 1613–1614, 1927.

367. ——, ——. La régulation de la sécrétion interne pancréatique par un processus humoral, démontrée par des transplantations de pancréas. Expériences sur des animaux dépancréates. Compt. rend. Soc. de biol., 97: 1615–1618, 1927.

368. ——, ——. Recherche d'une action excitatrice du nerf vague sur l'insulino-sécrétion avec de nouveaux déspositifs expérimentaux, Compt. rend. Soc. de biol., 112- 1331–1336, 1933.

369. GEBAUER, P. W., COLEMAN, F. P. Postanesthetic encephalopathy following cyclopropane. Ann. Surg., 107: 481–485, 1938.

370. GEIGER, A., MAGNES, J., TAYLOR, R., VERALLI, M. The effect of blood constituents on the permeability of the brain to glucose in perfusion experiments on the living cat. In preparation.

371. GEILING, E. M. K., DELAWDER, A. M. Metabolic changes following the intra-venous injection of posterior pituitary extracts and their correlation with the well-known pharmacodynamic action of the drugs. Bull. Johns Hopkins Hosp., 51: 1–26, 1932.

372. GELLHORN, E. The influence of carbon dioxide in combating the effect of oxygen deficiency on psychic processes with remarks on the fundamental relationship between psychic and physiologic reactions. Am. J. Psychiat., 93: 1413–1434, 1937.

373. ——. The effects of hypoglycemia and anoxia on the central nervous system; a basis for a rational therapy of schizophrenia. Arch. Neurol. & Psychiat., 40: 125–146, 1938.

374. ——, Autonomic regulations. New York City, Interscience Publishers, 1943, p. 54–70.

375. ——, BALLIN, H. M. Role of afferent impulses in experimental convulsions. Arch. Neurol. & Psychiat., 59: 718–733, 1948.

376. ——, CORTELL, R., FELDMAN, J. The effect of emotions, sham rage and hypo-thalamic stimulation on the vago-insulin system. Am. J. Physiol., 133: 532–541, 1941.

377. ——, FELDMAN, J. The influence of cold and heat on the vago-insulin and the sympathetico-adrenal systems. Am. J. Physiol., 133: 670–675, 1941.

378. ——, FELDMAN, J. The influence of the thyroid on the vago-insulin and sympathetico-adrenal systems. Endocrinology, **29**: 467–474, 1941.

379. ——, LEVIN, J. The nature of pupillary dilatation in anoxia. Am. J. Physiol., **143**: 282–289, 1945.

380. GELLHORN, E., PACKER, A. Studies on the interaction of hypoglycemia and anoxia. Am. J. Physiol., **129**: 610–617, 1940.

381. GEMMILL, C. L. The effect of insulin on the glycogen content of isolated muscles. Bull. Johns Hopkins Hosp., **66**: 232–244, 1940.

382. GEPPERT, J. Über das Wesen der Blausäurevergiftung. Ztschr. f. klin. Med., **15**: 208–242, 307–369, 1888.

383. GERARD, R. W. Brain metabolism and circulation. A. Research Nerv. Ment. Dis. Proc., The circulation of the brain and spinal cord, **18**: 316–345, 1938.

384. ——. Nerve metabolism and function. Ann. N. Y. Acad. Sci., **47**: 575–600, 1946.

385. GERMAN, W. J., PAGE, W. R., NIMS, L. Cerebral blood flow and cerebral oxygen consumption in experimental intracranial injury. Tr. Am. Neur. A. 86–88, 1947.

386. GESELL, R. On the chemical regulation of respiration 1. The regulation of respiration with special reference to the metabolism of the respiratory center and the coordination of the dual function of hemoglobin. Am. J. Physiol., **66**: 5–49, 1923.

387. ——, HANSEN, E. T. Anticholinesterase activity of acid as a biological instrument of nervous integration. Am. J. Physiol., **144**: 126–163, 1945.

388. GETTLER, A. O., TIBER, A. The quantitative determination of ethyl alcohol in human tissues. Arch. Path., **3**: 75–83, 1927.

389. GIBBS, E. L., GIBBS, F. A. The cross section areas of the vessels that form the torcular and the manner in which flow is distributed to the right and to the left lateral sinus. Anat. Rec., **59**: 419–426, 1934.

390. ——, GIBBS, F. A., LENNOX, W. G., NIMS, L. F. Regulation of cerebral carbon dioxide. Arch. Neurol. & Psychiat., **47**: 879–889, 1942.

391. ——, LENNOX, W. G., GIBBS, F. A. Variations in the carbon dioxide content of the blood in epilepsy. Arch. Neurol. & Psychiat., **43**: 223–239, 1940.

392. ——, LENNOX, W. G., NIMS, L. F., GIBBS, F. A. Arterial and cerebral venous blood, arterial-venous differences in man. J. Biol. Chem., **144**: 325–332, 1942.

393. GIBBS, F. A. A thermoelectric blood flow recorder in the form of a needle. Proc. Soc. Exper. Biol. & Med., **31**: 141–146, 1933–34.

394. ——, GIBBS, E. L., LENNOX, W. G. The cerebral blood flow in man as influenced by adrenalin, caffein, amyl nitrate and histamine. Am. Heart J., **10**: 916–924, 1934–35.

395. ——, ——, LENNOX, W. G. Changes in human cerebral blood flow consequent on alterations in blood gases. Am. J. Physiol., **111**: 557–563, 1935.

396. ——, ——. Atlas of electroencephalography. Cambridge, Mass., Lew A. Cummings, Co., 1941.

397. ——, LENNOX, W. G., NIMS, L. F. The value of carbon dioxide in counteracting the effects of low oxygen. J. Aviation Med., **14**: 250–261, 1943.

398. ——, KNOTT, J. R. Growth of the electrical activity of the cortex. EEG Clin. Neurophysiol., **1**: 223–229, 1949.

399. ——, LENNOX, W. G., GIBBS, E. L. Bilateral internal jugular blood: Comparison of A-V differences, oxygen-dextrose ratios, and respiratory quotients. Am. J. Psychiat., **102**: 184–190, 1945.

400. ——, MAXWELL, H., GIBBS, E. L. Volume flow of blood through the human brain. Arch. Neurol. and Psychiat., **57**: 137–144, 1947.

400a. GILBERT, N. C., DE TAKATS, G. Emergency treatment of apoplexy. J. A. M. A., **136:** 659–665, 1948.

401. GILDEA, E. F., COBB, S. The effects of anemia on the cerebral cortex of the cat. Arch. Neurol. & Psychiat., **23:** 876–903, 1930.

402. ——, MAILHOUSE, VIRGINIA L., MORRIS, D. L. The relationship between various emotional disturbances and the sugar content of the blood. Am. J. Psychiat., **92:** 115–130, 1935.

403. GILMAN, A., PHILIPS, F. S. Biological actions and therapeutic applications of the B-Chloroethyl amines and sulfides: Science, **103:** 409–415 and 436, 1946.

404. GLASS, H. G., SNYDER, F. F., WEBSTER, E. The rate of decline in resistance to anoxia of rabbits, dogs, and guinea pigs from the onset of viability to adult life. Am. J. Physiol., **140:** 609–615, 1943–44.

405. GOLDBLATT, M. W. The action of insulin in normal young rabbits. Biochem. J., **23:** 83–98, 1929.

406. GOLDFARB, W., BOWMAN, K. M., WORTIS, J. The effect of alcohol on cerebral metabolism. Am. J. Psychiat., **97:** 384–387, 1940.

407. ——, HIMWICH, H. E. Ketone substance production and destruction in certain tissues of diabetic dogs. J. Biol. Chem., **101:** 441–448, 1933.

408. ——, WORTIS, J. The availability of ethyl alcohol for human brain oxidations. Quart. J. Stud. on Alcohol, **1:** 268–271, 1940–41.

409. ——, ——. Availability of sodium pyruvate for human brain oxidations. Proc. Soc. Exper. Biol. & Med., **46:** 121–123, 1941.

410. GOMEZ, L., PIKE, F. H. The histological changes in nerve cells due to total temporary anaemia of the central nervous system. J. Exper. Med., **11:** 257–265, 1909.

411. GOODMAN, L., GILMAN, A. The pharmacological basis of therapeutics. New York City, The Macmillan Company, 1941. p. 85.

412. GORDON, E. S., HEMING, A. E. The effect of thyroid treatment on the respiration of various rat tissues. Endocrinology, **34:** 353–360, 1944.

413. GRANT, F. C., SPITZ, E. B., SHENKIN, H. A., SCHMIDT, C., KETY, S. S. The cerebral blood flow and metabolism in idiopathic epilepsy. Tr. Am. Neur. A. 82–86, 1940.

414. GRATTAN, J. F., JENSEN, H. The effect of the pituitary adrenocorticotropic hormone and of various adrenal cortical principles on insulin hypoglycemia and liver glycogen. J. Biol. Chem., **135:** 511–517, 1940.

415. GREELEY, P. O. Pancreatic diabetes in the rabbit. Proc. Soc. Exper. Biol. & Med., **37:** 309–312, 1937.

416. GREEN, D. E., WESTERFELD, W. W. VENNESLAND, B., KNOX, W. E. Carboxylases of animal tissues. J. Biol. Chem., **145:** 69–84, 1942.

417. GREENBERG, L. A. Acetoin not a product of the metabolism of alcohol. Quart. J. Stud. on Alcohol, **3:** 347–350, 1942–43.

418. GREGG, D. E. SHIPLEY, R. E. Experimental approaches to the study of the cerebral circulation. Fed. Proc., **3:** 144–151, 1944.

419. GREIG, MARGARET E. The site of action of narcotics on brain metabolism. J. Pharmacol. & Exper. Therap., **87:** 185–192, 1946.

420. GRENELL, R. G. Central nervous system resistance. I. The effects of temporary arrest of cerebral circulation for periods of two to ten minutes. J. Neuropath. & Exper. Neurol., **5:** 131–154, 1946.

421. GREVILLE, G. D. Fumarate and tissue respiration. I. Effect of dicarboxylic acids on the oxygen consumption. Biochem. J., **30:** 877–887, 1936.

422. ——, LEHMANN, H. Metabolism of phosphate and carbohydrate in extracts of human muscle and brain. J. Physiol., **102:** 357–361, 1943.

423. GRIFFITHS, M., MARKS, H. P., YOUNG, F. G. Influence of oestrogens and androgens on glycogen storage in the fasting rat. Nature, **147:** 359, 1941.

424. GRINKER, R. R., SPIEGEL, J. C. Men under stress. Phila. P. Blakiston's Son & Co., 1945.

425. GROB, D., HARVEY, A. M., LANGWORTHY, O. R., LILIENTHAL, J. L., JR. The administration of di-isopropyl fluorophosphate (DFP) to man. III. Effect on the central nervous system with special reference to the electrical activity of the brain. Bull. Johns Hopkins Hosp., **81:** 257–266, 1947.

426. GROLLMAN, A. Cardiac output of man in health and disease. Springfield, Ill., and Baltimore, Md. Charles C. Thomas, 1932, p. 251.

427. GRUBER, C. M., HAURY, V. G., GRUBER, C. M., JR. The depressant and paralytic actions of the barbiturates on terrapin cardiac vagus nerve. J. Pharmacol. & Exper. Therap., **63:** 229–238, 1938.

428. GUEDEL, A. E., Inhalation anesthesia. New York, The Macmillan Company, 1937.

429. GURDJIAN, E. S., WEBSTER, J. E. Experimental head injury with special reference to mechanical factors in acute trauma. Surg., Gyn. & Obstet., **76:** 623–634, 1943.

430. ——, STONE, W. E., WEBSTER, J. E. Cerebral metabolism in hypoxia. Arch. Neurol. and Psychiat., **51:** 472–477, 1944.

431. GUREVITCH, M. O., SUMSKAYA, A. M., KHACHATUREAN, A. Treatment of depressions with hypoxemia. J. Clin. Psychopathol. & Psychother., **6:** 523–533, 1944–45.

432. HAAS, E., HARRER, C. J., HOGNESS, T. R. Cytochrome reductase. II. Improved method of isolation; inhibition and inactivation; reaction with oxygen. J. Biol. Chem., **143:** 341–349, 1942.

433. ——, HORECKER, B. L., HOGNESS, T. R. The enzymatic reduction of cytochrome C. Cytochrome C reductase. J. Biol. Chem., **136:** 747–774, 1940.

434. HAFKENSCHIEL, J. H., CRUMPTON, C. W., MOYER, J. H. Blood flow and oxygen consumption of the brain in coarctation in the aorta. Proc. Soc. Exper. Biol. & Med., **71:** 165–167, 1949.

434a. ——, CRUMPTON, C. W., MOYER, J. H., JEFFERS, W. A. The effects of dihydroergocornine on the cerebral circulation of patients with essential hypertension. J. Clin. Investigation, **29:** 408–411, 1950.

434b. HAIMOVICI, H. Evidence for adrenergic sweating in man. J. Appl. Physiol., **2:** 512–521, 1950.

435. HAIST, R. E., CAMPBELL, J., BEST, C. H. The prevention of diabetes. New England J. Med., **223:** 607–615, 1940.

436. HALDANE, J. S., PRIESTLY, J. G. Respiration. New Haven, Yale Univ. Press, 1935, 2nd Ed.

437. HALPERIN, S. L., CURTIS, G. M. The genetics of gargoylism. Am. J. Ment. Def., **46:** 298–301, 1941–42.

438. HALSTRØM, FANNY, MØLLER, K. O. The content of cyanide in human organs from cases of poisoning with cyanide taken by mouth. With a contribution to the toxicology of cyanides. Acta pharmacol., **1:** 18–28, 1945.

439. HALVORSEN, C. Nitrogen gas convulsive therapy. Northwest Med., **39:** 130–132, 1940.

440. HAM, A. W., HAIST, R. E. Histological study of trophic effects of diabetogenic

anterior pituitary extracts and their relation to the pathogenesis of diabetes. Am. J. Path., **17**: 787–812, 1941.

440a. HAMILTON, W. F., WOODBURY, R. A., HARPER, H. J., JR. Arterial, cerebrospinal and venous pressures in man during cough and strain. Am. J. Physiol., **141**: 42–50, 1944.

441. HAMMAN, L., HIRSCHMAN, I. I. Studies on blood sugar. IV. Effects upon the blood sugar of the repeated ingestion of glucose. Bull. Johns Hopkins Hosp., **30**: 306–308, 1919.

442. HAMPSON, J. L., ESSIG, C. F., WILLIS, A., HIMWICH, H. E. Effects of diisopropyl fluorophosphate (DFP) on electroencephalogram and cholinesterase activity. EEG Clin. Neurophysiol., **2**: 41–48, 1950.

443. HANDLEY, C. A., SWEENEY, H. M., SCHERMAN, Q., SEVERANCE, R. Metabolism of the perfused dog's brain. Am. J. Physiol., **140**: 190–196, 1943–44.

444. HANNO, H. A., BANKS, R. W. Islet cell carcinoma of pancreas, with metastasis. Ann. Surg., **117**: 437–449, 1943.

444a. HARMEL, M. H., HAFKENSCHIEL, J. H., AUSTIN, G. M., CRUMPTON, C. W., KETY, S. S. The effect of bilateral stellate ganglion block on the cerebral circulation in normotensive and hypertensive patients. J. Clin. Investigation, **28**: 415–418, 1949.

445. VAN HARREVELD, A., MARMONT, G. The course of recovery of the spinal cord from asphyxia. J. Neurophysiol., **2**: 101–111, 1939.

446. HARRIS, A. J., HODES, M. C. R., MAGOUN, H. W. The afferent path of the pupillodilator reflex in the cat. J. Neurophysiol., **7**: 231–243, 1944.

446a. HARRIS, G. W., DE GROOT, J. Hypothalamic control of the secretion of addrenocorticotropic hormone. Fed. Proc., **9**: 57, 1950.

447. HARRIS, J. A., JACKSON, C. M., PATERSON, D. G., SCAMMON, R. E. The measurement of man. Minneapolis, The Univ. of Minnesota Press, 1930. p. 188.

448. HARRIS, M. M., BLALOCK, J. R., HORWITZ, W. A. Metabolic studies during insulin hypoglycemia therapy of the psychoses. Arch. Neurol. & Psychiat., **40**: 116–124, 1938.

449. HARRIS, S. Diagnosis and treatment of hyperinsulinism. Ann. Int. Med., **10**: 514–533, 1936.

450. HARRISON, D. C. Glucose dehydrogenase: a new oxidizing enzyme from animal tissues. Biochem. J., **25**: 1016–1027, 1931.

451. ——. The product of the oxidation of glucose by glucose dehydrogenase. Biochem. J., **26**: 1295–1299, 1932.

452. HARRISON, F. Attempt to produce sleep by diencephalic stimulation. J. Neurophysiol., **3**: 156–165, 1940.

453. HARTMAN, F. A., BROWNELL, K. A. Relation of adrenals to diabetes. Proc. Soc. Exper. Biol. & Med., **31**: 834–835, 1933–34.

454. ——, MACARTHUR, C. G., GUNN, F. D., HARTMAN, W. E., MACDONALD, J. J. Kidney function in adrenal insufficiency. Am. J. Physiol., **81**: 244–254, 1927.

455. HARTMAN, F. W. Lesions of the brain following fever therapy. Etiology and pathogenesis. J. A. M. A., **109**: 2116–2121, 1937.

456. HASSIN, G. B. Histopathology of the peripheral and central nervous systems. Baltimore, William Wood and Co., 1933. p. 308–320.

457. HASSLER, R. Zur pathologischen Anatomie des senilen und des parkinsonistischen Tremor. J. Psychol. u. Neurol., **49**: 193–230, 1937.

458. HAYASAKA, E., INAWASHIRO, R. Studies on the effect of muscular exercise in beri-beri. Tohoku J. Exper. Med., **12**: 29–61, 1928.

459. Heilbrunn, G., Liebert, E. Observations on the adrenalin level in the blood serum during insulin hypoglycemia and after metrazol convulsions. Endocrinology, **25**: 354–358, 1939.

460. Heinbecker, P., Bartley, S. H. Action of ether and nembutal on the nervous system. J. Neurophysiol., **3**: 219–236, 1940.

461. ——, Rolf, D. Hypophysial eosinophil cell and insulin sensitivity. Am. J. Physiol., **141**: 566–570, 1944.

462. Hemingway, A., Rasmussen, T., Wikoff, H., Rasmussen, A. T. Effects of heating hypothalamus of dogs by diathermy. J. Neurophysiol., **3**: 329–338, 1940.

463. Henderson, Y., Greenberg, L. A. Acidosis: Acid intoxication, or acarbia? Am. J. Physiol., **107**: 37–48, 1934.

463a. Henry, J. P., Gauer, O., Martin, E. E., Kety, S. S., Kramer, K. Factors determining cerebral oxygen supply during positive acceleration. Fed. Proc., **8**: 73, 1949.

464. Herman, M., Most, H., Jolliffe, N. Psychoses associated with pernicious anemia. Arch. Neurol. & Psychiat., **38**: 348–361, 1937.

465. Hess, W. R., Zur physiologie der vasomotoren, Schweiz. Arch. F. Neurol. u. Psychiat., **14**: 20–29, 1923.

466. Heymans, C., Bouckaert, J. J., Jourdan, F., Nowak, S. J. G., Farber, S. Survival and revival of nerve centers following acute anemia. Arch. Neurol. & Psychiat., **38**: 304–307, 1937.

467. Hill, A. V. Muscular movement in man: The factors governing speed and recovery from fatigue. New York, Mcgraw-Hill Book Co., Inc., 1927.

468. Himsworth, H. P., Scott, D. B. M. The relation of the hypophysis to changes in sugar tolerance and insulin sensitivity induced by changes of diet. J. Physiol., **91**: 447–458, 1937–38.

469. Himwich, H. E. The metabolism of fever. With special reference to diabetic hyperpyrexia. Bull. New York Acad. Med., **10**: 16–36, 1934.

470. ——. Brain metabolism. Presented at the Kansas City Academy of Medicine, Nov. 17, 1939. Reprinted from Tr. Kansas City Academy of Medicine, 31–49, 1939, '40, '41.

471. ——. The role of vitamins in brain metabolism. A. Research Nerv. & Ment. Dis., Proc., **22**: 33–41, 1943.

472. ——. Electroshock. A round table discussion. Am. J. Psychiat., **100**: 361–364, 1943.

473. ——. A review of hypoglycemia, its physiology and pathology, symptomatology and treatment. Am. J. Digest. Dis., **11**: 1–8, 1944.

474. ——, Baker, Z., Fazekas, J. F. Respiratory metabolism of infant brain. Am. J. Physiol., **125**: 601–606, 1939.

475. ——, Bernstein, A. O., Herrlich, H., Chesler, A., Fazekas, J. F. Mechanisms for the maintenance of life in the newborn during anoxia. Am. J. Physiol., **135**: 387–391, 1941–42.

476. ——, ——, Fazekas, J. F., Herrlich, H. C., Rich, E. The metabolic effects of potassium, temperature, methylene blue and paraphenylenediamine on infant and adult brain. Am. J. Physiol., **137**: 327–330, 1942.

477. ——, Bowman, K. M., Daly, C., Fazekas, J. F., Wortis, J., Goldfarb, W. Cerebral blood flow and brain metabolism during insulin hypoglycemia. Am. J. Physiol., **132**: 640–647, 1941.

478. ——, ——, Fazekas, J. F. Prolonged coma and cerebral metabolism. Arch. Neurol. & Psychiat., **44**: 1098–1101, 1940.

479. HIMWICH, H. E., BOWMAN, K. M., FAZEKAS, J. F. GOLDFARB, W. Temperature and brain metabolism. Am. J. M. Sc., **200:** 347–353, 1940.

480. ——, ——, WORTIS, J., FAZEKAS, J. F. Metabolism of the brain during insulin and metrazol treatments of schizophrenia. J.A.M.A., **112:** 1572–1573, 1939.

481. ——, ——, ——, ——. Biochemical changes occurring in the cerebral blood during the insulin treatment of schizophrenia. J. Nerv. & Ment. Dis., **89:** 273–293, 1939.

482. ——, CAMERON, D. E., HOMBURGER, E., FELDMAN, F. Cerebral metabolism in patients with depression. Am. J. Psychiat., **101:** 453–454, 1945.

483. ——, CASTLE, W. B. Studies in the metabolism of muscle. I. The respiratory quotient of resting muscle. Am. J. Physiol., **83:** 92–114, 1927–28.

484. ——, CHAMBERS, W. H., KOSKOFF, Y. D., NAHUM, L. H. Studies in carbohydrate metabolism. II. Glucose-lactic acid cycle in diabetes. J. Biol. Chem., **90:** 417–426, 1931.

485. ——, DALY, C., FAZEKAS, J. F. Effect of neosynephrin on gaseous exchange of the brain. Proc. Soc. Exper. Biol. & Med., **53:** 78–79, 1943.

486. ——, ——, ——, HERRLICH, H. E. Effect of thyroid medication on brain metabolism of cretins. Am. J. Psychiat., **98:** 489–493, 1942.

487. ——, ESSIG, C. F., HAMPSON, J. L., BALES, P. D., FREEDMAN, A. M. Effect of trimethadione (tridione) and other drugs on convulsions caused by diisopropyl fluorophosphate (DFP). Am. J. Psychiat., **106:** 816–820, 1950.

488. ——, ETSTEN, B. Criteria for the stages of pentothal anesthesia. J. Nerv. & Ment. Dis., **104:** 407–413, 1946.

489. ——, FAZEKAS, J. F. Respiratory quotient of various parts of the brain. Proc. Soc. Exper. Biol. & Med., **30:** 366, 1932–33.

490. ——, ——. The effect of nicotine on oxidations in the brain. Am. J. Physiol., **113:** 63–64, 1935.

491. ——, ——. Protamine-insulin and infection. Am. J. M. Sc., **194:** 345–351, 1937.

492. ——, ——. The effect of hypoglycemia on the metabolism of the brain. Endocrinology, **21:** 800–807, 1937.

493. ——, ——. Respiratory quotient of diabetic liver. Proc. Soc. Exper. Biol. & Med., **38:** 137–139, 1938.

494. ——, ——. Cerebral metabolism in mongolian idiocy and phenylpyruvic oligophrenia. Arch. Neurol. & Psychiat., **44:** 1213–1218, 1940.

495. ——, ——. Comparative studies of the metabolism of the brain of infant and adult dogs. Am. J. Physiol., **132:** 454–459, 1941.

496. ——, ——. Factor of hypoxia in the shock therapies of schizophrenia. Arch. Neurol. & Psychiat., **47:** 800–807, 1942.

497. ——, ——. Cerebral arterio-venous oxygen difference. I. Effect of age and mental deficiency. Arch. Neurol. & Psychiat., **50:** 546–551, 1943.

498. ——, ——. Cerebral arterio-venous oxygen difference II. Mental deficiency. Arch. Neurol. & Psychiat., **51:** 73–77, 1944.

499. ——, ——. The oxygen content of cerebral blood in patients with acute symptomatic psychoses and acute destructive brain lesions. Am. J. Psychiat., **100:** 648–651, 1944.

500. ——, ——, BERNSTEIN, A. O., CAMPBELL, E. H., MARTIN, S. J. Syndromes secondary to prolonged hypoglycemia. Proc. Soc. Exper. Biol. & Med., **39:** 244–245, 1938.

501. ——, ——, HERRLICH, H., JOHNSON, A. E., BARACH, A. L. Studies on the effects of adding carbon dioxide to oxygen-enriched atmospheres in low pressure

chambers. II. The oxygen and carbon dioxide tensions of cerebral blood. J. Aviation Med., **13:** 177–181, 1942.

502. ——, ——, HOMBURGER, E. Effect of hypoglycemia and anoxia on the survival period of infant and adult rats and cats. Endocrinology, **33:** 96–101, 1943.

503. ——, ——, HURLBURT, M. H. Effect of methylene blue and cyanide on respiration of cerebral cortex, testicle, liver and kidney. Proc. Soc. Exper. Biol. & Med., **30:** 904–906, 1932–33.

504. ——, ——, MARTIN, S. J. The effect of bilateral ligation of the lumbo-adrenal veins on the course of pancreas diabetes. Am. J. Physiol., **123:** 725–731, 1938.

505. ——, ——, NAHUM, L. H., DuBois, D., GREENBURG, L., GILMAN, A. Diabetic hyperpyrexia. Am. J. Physiol., **110:** 19–27, 1934–35.

506. ——, ——, NESIN, S. The glucose and lactic acid exchanges during hypoglycemia. Am. J. Physiol., **127:** 685–688, 1939.

507. ——, ——, RAKIETEN, N., SANDERS, R. Respiratory quotient of cerebral cortex in B_1 avitaminosis. Proc. Soc. Exper. Biol. & Med., **30:** 903–904, 1932–33.

508. ——, FROSTIG, J. P., FAZEKAS, J. F., HADIDIAN, Z. The mechanism of the symptoms of insulin hypoglycemia. Am. J. Psychiat., **96:** 371–385, 1939.

509. ——, GOLDFARB, W., FAZEKAS, J. F. The carbohydrate metabolism of the heart during pancreas diabetes. Am. J. Physiol., **114:** 273–277, 1935–36.

510. ——, ——, RAKIETEN, N., NAHUM, L. H., DuBois, D. The respiratory quotient of muscle of depancreatized dogs. Am. J. Physiol., **110:** 352–356, 1934–35.

511. ——, ——, WELLER, A. The effect of various organs on the acetone content of the blood in phlorhizin and pancreatic diabetes. J. Biol. Chem., **93:** 337–342, 1931.

512. ——, HADIDIAN, Z., FAZEKAS, J. F., HOAGLAND, H. Cerebral metabolism and electrical activity during insulin hypoglycemia in man. Am. J. Physiol., **125:** 578–585, 1939.

513. ——, HAYNES, F. W. Effects of posterior pituitary extracts on basal metabolism. Am. J. Physiol., **96:** 640–646, 1931.

514. ——, HAYNES, F. W., FAZEKAS, J. F. Effect of posterior pituitary extracts on the constituents of the blood. Am. J. Physiol., **101:** 711–714, 1932.

515. ——, KELLER, A. D. Effect of stimulation of hypothalamus on blood glucose. Am. J. Physiol., **93:** 658, 1930.

516. ——, KOSKOFF, Y. D., NAHUM, L. H. Studies in carbohydrate metabolism. I. A glucose lactic acid cycle involving muscle and liver. J. Biol. Chem., **85:** 571–584, 1929–30.

517. ——, LOEBEL, R. O., BARR, D. P. Studies on the effect of exercise in diabetes. I. Changes in acid-base equilibrium and their relation to the accumulation of lactic acid and acetone. J. Biol. Chem., **59:** 265–293, 1924.

518. ——, MARTIN, S. J., ALEXANDER, F. A. D., FAZEKAS, J. F. Electrocardiographic changes during hypoglycemia and anoxemia. Endocrinology, **24:** 536–541, 1939.

519. ——, NAHUM, L. H. The respiratory quotient of brain. Am. J. Physiol., **90:** 389–390, 1929. *Ibid*, **101:** 446–453, 1932.

520. ——, ——, RAKIETEN, N., FAZEKAS, J. F., DuBois, D., GILDEA, E. F. The metabolism of alcohol. J.A.M.A., **100:** 651–654, 1933.

521. ——, ROSE, M. I. Studies in the metabolism of muscle. II. The respiratory quotient of exercising muscle. Am. J. Physiol., **88:** 663–679, 1929.

522. ——, SPIES, T. D., FAZEKAS, J. F., NESIN, S. Cerebral carbohydrate metabolism during deficiency of various members of the vitamin B complex. Am. J. M. Sc., **199:** 849–853, 1940.

523. HIMWICH, H. E., SYKOWSKI, P., FAZEKAS, J. F. A comparative study of excised cerebral tissues of adult and infant rats. Am. J. Physiol., **132**: 293–296, 1941.

524. HIMWICH, WILLIAMINA A., HIMWICH, H. E. Pyruvic acid exchange of the brain. J. Neurophysiol., **9**: 133–136, 1946.

525. ——, ——. Organic phosphates and insulin. Fed. Proc., **5**: 47–48, 1946.

526. ——, ——. Pyruvic acid in exercising depancreatized dogs and diabetic patients. J. Biol. Chem., **165**: 513–519, 1946.

527. ——, ——. The influence of some organs on the pyruvate level in the blood. Am. J. Physiol., **148**: 323–326, 1947.

528. ——, HOMBURGER, E., MARESCA, R., HIMWICH, H. E. Brain metabolism in man: unanesthetized and in pentothal narcosis. Am. J. Psychiat., **103**: 689–696, 1947.

528a. HINES, M. The "motor" cortex. Johns Hopkins Hosp. Bull., **60**: 313–336, 1937.

529. HOAGLAND, H., HIMWICH, H. E., CAMPBELL, E., FAZEKAS, J. F., HADIDIAN, Z. Effects of hypoglycemia and pentobarbital sodium on electrical activity of cerebral cortex and hypothalamus (dogs). J. Neurophysiol., **2**: 276–288, 1939.

530. ——, RUBIN, M. A., CAMERON, D. E. The electroencephalogram of schizophrenics during insulin hypoglycemia and recovery. Am. J. Physiol., **120**: 559–570, 1937.

531. HÖBER, R. Beiträge zur physikalischen Chemie der Erregung und der Narkose. Pflüger's Arch. f. d. ges. Physiol., **120**: 492–516, 1907.

532. HOET, J., ERNOULD, H. On the nervous control of insulin secretion. J. Physiol., **70**: i–ii, 1930.

533. HOFF, E. C., GREEN, H. D. Cardiovascular reactions induced by electrical stimulation of the cerebral cortex. Am. J. Physiol., **117**: 411–422, 1936.

534. VAN'T HOFF, J. H. Studies in chemical dynamics. Translated by T. Ewan. London, Williams and Norgate, 1896.

535. HOLMES, E. G. Oxidations in central and peripheral nervous tissue. Biochem. J., **24**: 914–925, 1930.

536. ——. The metabolic activity of the cells of the trigeminal ganglion. Biochem. J., **26**: 2005–2009, 1932.

537. HOMBURGER, E., ETSTEN, B., HIMWICH, H. E. Some factors affecting the susceptibility of rats to various barbiturates. J. Lab. & Clin. Med., **32**: 540–547, 1947.

538. ——, HIMWICH, WILLIAMINA A., ETSTEN, B., YORK, G., MARESCA, R., HIMWICH, H. E. Effect of pentothal anesthesia on canine cerebral cortex. Am. J. Physiol., **147**: 343–345, 1946.

539. HOOKER, D. A preliminary atlas of early human fetal activity. Published by the author, 1939.

540. HORECKER, B. L., KORNBERG, A. The cytochrome C-cyanide complex. J. Biol. Chem., **165**: 11–20, 1946.

540a. ——. Phosphogluconic acid metabolism. Fed. Proc., **9**: 185–186, 1950.

541. HORTON, B. T., ZIEGLER, L. H., ADSON, A. W. Intracranial arterio-venous fistula. III. Diagnosis by discovery of arterial blood in jugular veins. Arch. Neurol. & Psychiat., **33**: 1232–1234, 1935.

541a. HOSKINS, R. G. The biology of schizophrenia. New York, W. W. Norton & Co. 1946.

542. HOUGH, H. B., WOLFF, H. G. The relative vascularity of subcortical ganglia

of the cat's brain; the putamen, globus pallidus, substantia nigra, red nucleus and geniculate bodies. J. Comp. Neurol., **71:** 427–436, 1939.

543. Houssay, B. A. The hypophysis and metabolism. New England J. Med., **214:** 961–971, 1936.

544. ——, Lewis, J. T., Molinelli, E. A. Role de la sécrétion d'adrénaline pendant l'hypoglycémie produite par l'insuline. Compt. rend. Soc. de biol., **91:** 1011–1013, 1924.

545. ——, Molinelli, E. A. Sécrétion d'adrénaline produite par la piqûre ou l'excitation électrique du bulbe. Compt. rend. Soc. de biol., **91:** 1045–1049, 1924.

546. Huggett, A. St. G. Foetal blood-gas tensions and gas transfusion through the placenta of the goat. J. Physiol., **62:** 373–384, 1926–27.

547. Huszák, I., Über den Kohlenhydratabbau im Zentral-nervensystem, Biochem. Zeit., **312:** 315–329, 1942.

548. Hutchens, T. O., McMahon, T. Effect of sodium fluoroacetate on oxidative steps of carbohydrate metabolism. Fed. Proc., **6:** 264, 1947.

549. Hutchinson, M. C., Stotz, E. Observations on inhibition of brain respiration and narcosis. J. Biol. Chem., **140:** lxv–lxvi, 1941.

550. Hydén, H., and Hartelius, H. Stimulation of the nucleoprotein-production in the nerve cells by malononitrile and the effect on psychic functions in mental disorders. Acta. Psychiat. et Neurol. Suppl., **48:** Lund, 1948.

551. Ingle, D. J. The production of glycosuria in the normal rat by means of stilbestrol. Am. J. M. Sc., **201:** 153–154, 1941.

552. ——. Diabetogenic effect of stilbestrol in force-fed normal and partially depancreatized rats. Endocrinology, **29:** 838–848, 1941.

553. ——. The production of glycosuria in the normal rat by means of 17-hydroxy-11-dehydrocortosterone. Endocrinology, **29:** 649–652, 1941.

554. ——. The diabetogenic effect of diethylstilbestrol in adrenalectomized-hypophysectomized-partially depancreatized rats. Endocrinology, **34:** 361–369, 1944.

555. ——, Evans, J. S., Sheppard, Ruth. The effect of insulin on the urinary excretion of sodium, chloride, nitrogen and glucose in normal rats. Endocrinology, **35:** 370–379, 1944.

556. ——, Thorn, G. W. A comparison of the effects of 11-desoxycorticosterone acetate and 17-hydroxy-11-dehydrocorticosterone in partially depancreatized rats. Am. J. Physiol., **132:** 670–678, 1941.

557. Irving, L., Welch, M. S. The effect of the composition of the inspired air on the circulation through the brain. Quart. J. Exper. Physiol., **25:** 121–129, 1935.

558. Jackson, J. H. The Croonian lectures on evolution and dissolution of the nervous system. Brit. M. J., **1:** 591–593, 660–663, 703–707, 1884.

559. Janes, R. G. Effect of sex hormones on the endocrine glands and carbohydrate metabolism in the rat. Anat. Rec., **79:** Supplement, 34–35, 1941.

560. ——, Nelson, W. O. Effect of stilbestrol on certain phases of carbohydrate metabolism. Proc. Soc. Exper. Biol. & Med., **43:** 340–342, 1940.

561. ——, ——. The relation of diethyl-stilbestrol to carbohydrate metabolism in adrenalectomized and hypophysectomized rats. Am. J. Physiol., **137:** 557–563, 1942.

562. Jervis, G. A. Phenylpyruvic oligophrenia. Introductory study of 50 cases of mental deficiency associated with excretion of phenylpyruvic acid. Arch. Neurol. & Psychiat., **38:** 944–963, 1937.

563. JERVIS, G. A. Recent progress in the study of mental deficiency mongolism. Am. J. Ment. Def., **46**: 467–481, 1941–42.

564. ——. Familial mental deficiency akin to amaurotic idiocy and gargoylism. Arch. Neurol. & Psychiat., **47**: 943–961, 1942.

564a. JOHNS, R. J., HIMWICH, H. E. A central action of some antihistamines: correction of forced circling movements and of seizure brain waves produced by the intracarotid injection of di-isopropyl fluorophosphate (DFP). Am. J. Psychiat. **107**, 367–372, 1950.

565. JOHNSON, R. E. a-Glycerophosphoric acid and brain metabolism. Biochem. J., **30**: 33–42, 1936.

566. JOHNSON, W. A. Aconitase. Biochem. J., **33**: 1046–1053, 1939.

567. JOLLIFFE, N., BOWMAN, K. M., ROSENBLUM, L. A., FEIN, H. D. Nicotinic acid deficiency encephalopathy. J.A.M.A., **114**: 307–312, 1940.

568. JOSLIN, E. P., ROOT, H. F., WHITE, P., MARBLE, A. The treatment of diabetes mellitus. Philadelphia, Lea and Febiger, 1940, 7th ed.

569. JOWETT, M., QUASTEL, J. H. Studies in fat metabolism. III. The formation and breakdown of acetoacetic acid in animal tissues. Biochem. J., **29**: 2181–2191, 1935.

570. ——, ——. Effects of narcotics on tissue oxidations. Biochem. J., **31**: 565–578, 1937.

571. ——, ——. The effects of ether on brain oxidations. Biochem. J., **31**: 1101–1112, 1937.

572. KABAT, H. The greater resistance of very young animals to arrest of the brain circulation. Am. J. Physiol., **130**: 588–599, 1940.

573. KALCKAR, H. M. The nature of energetic coupling in biological syntheses. Chem. Rev., **28**: 71–178, 1941.

574. KALINOWSKY, L. B. Convulsions in nonepileptic patients on withdrawal of barbiturates, alcohol and other drugs. Arch. Neurol. & Psychiat., **48**: 946–956, 1942.

575. ——, WORTHING, H. J. Results with electric convulsive therapy in 200 cases of schizophrenia. Psychiatric Quart., **17**: 144–153, 1943.

576. KAPLAN, N., GREENBERG, D. M. Observations with P^{32} of the changes in the acid-soluble phosphates in the liver coincident to alterations in carbohydrate metabolism. J. Biol. Chem., **150**: 479–480, 1943.

577. KATZENELBOGEN, S. A critical appraisal of the "Shock Therapies" in the major psychoses. II. Insulin. Psychiatry, **3**: 211–228, 1940.

578. KATZIN, B., LONG, C. N. H. The effect of adrenal cortical extract on the carbohydrate and protein metabolism of the rat. Am. J. Physiol., **126**: 551, 1939.

579. KEESER, E. Über die Verteilung der Diäthylbarbitursäure im Gehirn. Arch. f. exper. Path. u. Pharmakol., **186**: 449–450, 1937.

580. ——, KEESER, J. Über die Lokalisation des Veronals, der Phenyläthyl- und Diallylbarbitursäure im Gehirn. Arch. f. exper. Path. u. Pharmakol., **125**: 251–256, 1927.

581. KEILIN, D. On cytochrome, a respiratory pigment, common to animals, yeast and higher plants. Proc. Roy. Soc. London, **98B**: 312–339, 1925.

582. ——. Cytochrome and respiratory enzymes. Proc. Roy. Soc. London, **104B**: 206–252, 1928–29.

583. ——, HARTREE, E. F. Prosthetic group of glucose oxidase (Notatin). Nature, **157**: 801, 1946.

584. ——, HARTREE, E. F. Properties of glucose oxidase (notatin). Biochem. J., **42**: 221–229, 1948.

585. KENNARD, M. A. Focal autonomic representation in the cortex and its relation to sham rage. J. Neuropath. & Exper. Neurol. 4: 295–304, 1945.

586. ——, NIMS, L. F. Changes in normal electroencephalogram of *macaca mulatta* with growth. J. Neurophysiol., 5: 325–333, 1942.

587. KENNEDY, A. Hypoglycaemic shock and the grasp-reflex. The effect of insulin shock on bulbocapnine catalepsy in the monkey. J. Neurol. & Psychiat. 3: 27–36, 1940.

588. KENNEDY, E. P., LEHNINGER, A. L. Oxidation of fatty acids and tricarboxylic acid cycle intermediates by isolated rat liver mitochondria. J. Biol. Chem. 179: 957–972, 1949.

589. KERR, S. E., GHANTUS, M. The carbohydrate metabolism of the brain. II. The effect of varying the carbohydrate and insulin supply on the glycogen, free-sugar, and lactic acid in mammalian brain. J. Biol. Chem., 116: 9–20, 1936.

590. ——, HAMPEL, C. W., GHANTUS, M. The carbohydrate metabolism of brain. IV. Brain glycogen, free sugar, and lactic acid as affected by insulin in normal and adrenal-inactivated cats, and by epinephrine in normal rabbits. J. Biol. Chem., 119: 405–421, 1937.

591. KESSLER, M., GELLHORN, E. The effect of anoxia on brain potentials of hyperthyroid animals. Am. J. Physiol., 137: 703–705, 1942.

592. KETTRINGHAM, R. C., AUSTIN, B. R. Blood sugar during labor, at delivery and postpartum, with observations on newborns. Am. J. M. Sc., 195: 318–329, 1938.

592a. KETY, S. S. Circulation and metabolism of the human brain in health and disease. Am. J. Med., 8: 205–217, 1950.

592b. ——, DRIPPS, R. D., WECHSLER, R. L., KLOTZ, H., KLEISS, L. The effects of intravenous thiopental anesthesia on cerebral metabolism and blood flow in man.

593. ——, HAFKENSCHIEL, J. H., JEFFERS, W. A., LEOPOLD, I. H., SHENKIN, H. A. The blood flow, vascular resistance, and oxygen consumption of the brain in essential hypertension. J. Clin. Investigation, 27: 511–514, 1948.

593a. ——, ——, KING, B. D., HORVATH, S. H., JEFFERS, W. A. The effects of an acute reduction in blood pressure by means of differential spinal sympathetic block on the cerebral circulation of hypertensive patients. J. Clin. Investigation, 29: 402–407, 1950.

594. ——, HARMEL, M. H., BROOMELL, HANNAH, T., RHODE, C. B. The solubility of nitrous oxide in blood and brain. J. Biol. Chem., 173: 487–496, 1948.

595. ——, POLIS, B. D., NADLER, C. S., SCHMIDT, C. F. The blood flow and oxygen consumption of the human brain in diabetic acidosis and coma. J. Clin. Investigation, 27: 500–510, 1948.

596. ——, SCHMIDT, C. F. The determination of cerebral blood flow in man by the use of nitrous oxide in low concentrations. Am. J. Physiol. 143: 53–66, 1945.

597. ——, ——. The effects of altered arterial tensions of carbon dioxide and oxygen on cerebral blood flow and cerebral oxygen consumption of normal young men. J. Clin. Investigation, 27: 484–492, 1948.

598. ——, ——. The nitrous oxide method for the quantitative determination of cerebral blood flow in man: theory, procedure and normal values. J. Clin. Investigation, 27: 476–483, 1948.

599. ——, SHENKIN, H. A., SCHMIDT, C. F. The effects of increased intracranial pressure on cerebral circulatory functions in man. J. Clin. Investigation, 27: 493–499, 1948.

600. KETY, S. S., WOODFORD, R. B., HARMEL, M. H., FREYHAN, F. A., APPEL, K. E., SCHMIDT, C. F. Cerebral blood flow metabolism in schizophrenia. The effects of barbiturate semi-narcosis, insulin coma and electroshock. Am. J. Psychiat., **104**: 765–770, 1948.

601. KEYS, A., STAPP, J. P., VIOLANTE, A. Responses in size, output and efficiency of the human heart to acute alteration in the composition of inspired air. Am. J. Physiol., **138**: 763–771, 1942–43.

602. KIBLER, H. H., BRODY, S. Metabolism and growth rate of rats. J. Nutrition, **24**: 461–468, 1942.

603. KING, C. G., BICKERMAN, H. A., BOUVET, W., HARRER, C. J., OYLER, J. R., SEITZ, C. P. Aviation Nutrition Studies 1. Effects of pre-flight and in-flight meals of varying composition with respect to carbohydrate, protein and fat. J. Aviation Med. **16**: 69–84, 1945.

604. KLEIN, D. The effects of administration of glucose and insulin on blood pyruvate and lactate in diabetes mellitus. J. Biol. Chem., **145**: 35–43, 1942.

605. KLEIN, J. R. Nature of the increase in activity of the d-amino acid oxidase of rat liver produced by thyroid feeding. J. Biol. Chem., **131**: 139–147, 1939.

606. ——. Inhibition of brain respiration by picrotoxin. J. Biol. Chem. **151**: 651–657, 1943.

607. ——. Oxidation of fructose by brain in vitro. J. Biol. Chem., **153**: 295–300, 1944.

608. ——. Phosphorylation of glucose induced by oxidation of L(+)-glutamate by brain *in vitro*. Fed. Proc., **4**: 94, 1945.

609. ——, HURWITZ, RUTH, OLSEN, N. S. Distribution of intravenously injected fructose and glucose between blood and brain. J. Biol. Chem. **164**: 509–512, 1946.

610. ——, OLSEN, N. S. Distribution of intravenously injected glutamate, lactate, pyruvate, and succinate between blood and brain. J. Biol. Chem., **167**: 1–5, 1947.

611. ——, OLSEN, N. S. Effect of convulsive activity upon the concentration of brain glucose, glycogen, lactate, and phosphates. J. Biol. Chem., **167**: 747–756, 1947.

612. KLEITMAN, N. Sleep. Physiol. Rev., **9**: 624–665, 1929.

613. KLENK, E. Beiträge zur Chemie der Lipoidosen, Niemann-Picksche Krankheit und amaurotische Idiotie. Hoppe-Seyler's Ztschr. f. physiol. Chem., **262**: 128–143, 1939.

614. ——. Beiträge zur Chemie der Lipoidosen. 4. Mitteilung. Hoppe-Seyler's Ztschr. f. physiol. Chem., **267**: 128–144, 1940.

615. KOCH, W., KOCH, M. L. Contributions to the chemical differentiation of the central nervous system. III. The chemical differentiation of the brain of the albino rat during growth. J. Biol. Chem., **15**: 423–448, 1913.

616. KOELLE, G. B. Protection of cholinesterase against irreversible inactivation by di-isopropyl fluorophosphate *in vitro*. J. Pharmacol. & Exper. Therap., **88**: 232–237, 1946.

617. KOHN, H. I., KLEIN, J. R., DANN, W. J. The V-factor content and oxygen consumption of tissues of the normal and black-tongue dog. Biochem. J., **33**: 1432–1442, 1939.

618. KON, S. K., DRUMMOND, J. C. Physiological role of vitamin B: Part III. Study of vitamin B deficiency in pigeons. Biochem. J., **21**: 632–652, 1927.

619. KOPELOFF, L. M., BARRERA, S. E., KOPELOFF, N. Recurrent convulsive sei-

zures in animals produced by immunologic and chemical means. Am. J. Psychiat., **98:** 881–902, 1941–42.

620. KOPPANYI, T., DILLE, J. M., KROP, S. Studies of barbiturates. VIII. Distribution of barbiturates in the brain. J. Pharmacol. & Exper. Therap., **52:** 121–128, 1934.

621. ——, LINEGAR, C. R., DILLE, J. M. Peripheral action of barbiturates. Science, **82:** 232, 1935.

622. KOSTER, R. Synergisms and antagonisms between physostigmine and diisopropyl fluorophosphate in cats. J. Pharmacol. & Exper. Therap., **88:** 39–46, 1946.

622a. KOUGH, R. H., COOPER, D. Y., JR., EMMEL, G. L., LOESCHCKE, H. H., LAMBERTSEN, C. J., SCHMIDT, C. F. Effect of inhalation of oxygen at high partial pressure upon cerebral circulation and cerebral oxygen consumption in man. Fed. Proc., **9:** 72, 1950.

623. KREBS, H. A. Metabolism of amino acids. III. Deamination of amino-acids. Biochem. J., **29:** 1620–1644, 1935.

624. ——. Metabolism of amino acids. IV. The synthesis of glutamine from glutamic acid and ammonia, and the enzymic hydrolysis of glutamine in animal tissues. Biochem. J., **29:** 1951–1969, 1935.

625. ——. The citric acid cycle and the Szent-Györgyi cycle in pigeon breast muscle. Biochem. J., **34:** 775–779, 1940.

626. ——. Modified citric acid cycle. Biochem. J., **36:** ix, 1942.

627. ——, EGGLESTON, L. V. Biological synthesis of oxaloacetic acid from pyruvic acid and carbon dioxide. Biochem. J., **34:** 1383–1395, 1940.

628. ——, JOHNSON, W. A. Acetopyruvic acid ($\alpha\gamma$-diketovaleric acid) as intermediate metabolite in animal tissues. Biochem. J., **31:** 772–779, 1937.

629. ——, JOHNSON, W. A. Metabolism of ketonic acids in animal tissues. Biochem. J., **31:** 645–660, 1937.

630. KROGH, A. The active and passive exchanges of inorganic ions through the surfaces of living cells and through living membranes generally. Proc. Roy. Soc. Ser. B., **133:** 140–200, 1946.

631. KUBIE, L. S., MARGOLIN, S. The therapeutic role of drugs in the process of repression, dissociation and synthesis. Psychosomat. Med., **7:** 147–151, 1945.

632. KUNDE, M. M. Studies on metabolism. VI. Experimental hyperthyroidism. Am. J. Physiol., **82:** 195–215, 1927.

633. KUNTZ, A., RICHINS, C. A. Reflex pupillodilator mechanisms. An experimental analysis. J. Neurophysiol., **9:** 1–7, 1946.

634. LA BARRE, J. Sur l'augmentation de la teneur en insuline du sang veineux pancreatique apres excitation du nerf vague. Compt. rend. Soc. de biol., **96:** 193–196, 1927.

635. ——, SARIC, R. Sur les causes de l'augmentation postinsulinque de la teneur en adrenaline de sang veineux surrenal. Compt. rend. Soc. de biol., **124:** 287–289, 1937.

635a. LAMSON, P. D., GREIG, M. E., ROBBINS, B. H. Potentiating effect of glucose and its metabolic products on barbiturate anesthesia. Fed. Proc., **9:** 293–294, 1950.

636. LANGWORTHY, O. R. General principles of autonomic innervation. Arch. Neurol. & Psychiat., **50:** 590–602, 1943.

637. LARDY, H. A., HANSEN, R. G., PHILLIPS, P. H. Ineffectiveness of sodium

succinate in control of duration of barbiturate anesthesia. Proc. Soc. Exper. Biol. & Med., **55**: 277–278, 1944.

638. ——, HANSEN, R. G., PHILLIPS, P. H. The metabolism of bovine epididymal spermatozoa. Arch. Biochem., **6**: 41–51, 1945.

639. ——, ZIEGLER, J. A. The enzymatic synthesis of phosphopyruvate from pyruvate. J. Biol. Chem., **159**: 343–351, 1945.

639a. LARRABEE, M. G., RAMOS, J. G., BULBRING, E. Do anesthetics depress nerve cells by depressing oxygen consumption? Fed. Proc., **9**: 75, 1950.

640. LAWRENCE, R. D., MEYER, A., NEVIN, S. The pathological changes in the brain in fatal hypoglycemia. Quart. J. Med., **11**: 181–201, 1942.

641. LEGALLOIS, J. J. C. Experiments on the principle of life, and particularly on the principle of the motions of the heart, and on the seat of this principle. Transl. by N. C. and J. G. Nancrede, Philadelphia, M. Thomas, 1813.

642. LEHMANN, H., BOS, C. The advantages of nitrous oxide inhalation in psychiatric treatment. Am. J. Psychiat., **104**: 164–170, 1947.

643. LEHNINGER, A. L. The metabolism of acetopyruvic acid. J. Biol. Chem., **148**: 393–404, 1943.

644. ——. Fatty acid oxidation and the Krebs tricarboxylic acid cycle. J. Biol. Chem., **161**: 413–414, 1945.

645. ——. On the activation of fatty acid oxidation. J. Biol. Chem., **161**: 437–451, 1945.

646. LEIBEL, B. S., HALL, G. E. Cerebral blood flow changes during insulin and metrazol (pentamethylenetetrazol) shock. Proc. Soc. Exper. Biol. & Med., **38**: 894–896, 1938.

647. LEIBSON, R. G., LIKHNITZKY, I. I., SAX, M. G. Oxygen transport of the foetal and maternal blood during pregnancy. J. Physiol., **87**: 97–112, 1936.

648. LEITER, L., GRINKER, R. R. Role of the hypothalamus in regulation of blood pressure; experimental studies, with observations on respiration. Arch. Neurol. & Psychiat., **31**: 54–86, 1934.

649. LENNOX, W. G. The oxygen and carbon dioxide content of blood from the internal jugular and other veins. Arch. Int. Med., **46**: 630–636, 1930.

650. ——. The cerebral circulation. XIV. The respiratory quotient of the brain and of the extremities in man. Arch. Neurol. & Psychiat., **26**: 719–724, 1931.

651. ——. Alcohol and epilepsy. Quart. J. Stud. on Alcohol, **2**: 1–11, 1941–42.

652. ——. The petit mal epilepsies, their treatment with tridione. J. A. M. A., **129**: 1069–1074, 1945.

653. ——, GIBBS, E. L. The blood flow in the brain and the leg of man, and the changes induced by alteration of blood gases. J. Clin. Investigation, **11**: 1155–1177, 1932.

654. ——, GIBBS, F. A., GIBBS, E. L. Relationship of unconsciousness to cerebral blood flow and to anoxemia. Arch. Neurol. & Psychiat., **34**: 1001–1013, 1935.

655. ——, ——, ——. Effect on the electro-encephalogram of drugs and conditions which influence seizures. Arch. Neurol. & Psychiat., **36**: 1236–1245, 1936.

656. ——, ——, ——. The relationship in man of cerebral activity to blood flow and to blood constituents. A. Research Nerv. & Ment. Dis. Proc. The circulation of the brain and spinal cord, **18**: 277–297, 1938.

656a. LEPAGE, G. A. Biological energy transformations during shock as shown by tissue analyses. Am. J. Physiol., **146**: 267–281, 1946.

657. LEPPIEN, R., PETERS, G. Todesfall infolge Insulinshock-behandlung bei einem Schizophrenen. (Klinische und pathologisch-anatomische Beschreibung.) Ztschr. f. d. ges. Neurol. u. Psychiat., **160**: 444–454, 1937–38.

658. LEWIS, L. A., McCULLAGH, E. P. Carbohydrate metabolism of animals treated with methyl testosterone and testosterone propionate. J. Clin. Endocrinol., **2:** 502–506, 1942.

659. LEWIS, N. D. C. The present status of shock therapy of mental disorders. Bull. New York Acad. Med., **19:** 227–244, 1943.

660. LEWIS, R. A., KUHLMAN, D., DELBUE, C., KOEPF, G. F., THORN, G. W. The effect of the adrenal cortex on carbohydrate metabolism. Endocrinology, **27:** 971–982, 1940.

661. LEWIS, R. C., KINSMAN, G. M., ILIFF, A. The basal metabolism of normal boys and girls from 2 to 12 years old, inclusive. Am. J. Dis. Child., **53:** 348–428, 1937.

662. LEWY, F. H. Die Lehre vom Tonus und der Bewegung. Berlin, Springer, 1923. p. 375–377.

663. LIBET, B., FAZEKAS, J. F., HIMWICH, H. E. A study of the central action of metrazol. Am. J. Psychiat., **97:** 366–371, 1940.

664. LIBET, B., FAZEKAS, J. F., HIMWICH, H. E. The electrical response of the kitten and adult cat brain to cerebral anemia and analeptics. Am. J. Physiol., **132:** 232–238, 1941.

665. LIEB, C. C., MULINOS, M. G. Some further observations on sodium iso-amylethyl-barbiturate as a laboratory anesthetic. Proc. Soc. Exper. Biol. & Med., **26:** 709–711, 1928–29.

666. LIEBERMEISTER, C. Untersuchungen über die quantitativen Veränderungen der Kohlensäureproduction beim Menschen. Deutsch. Arch. f. klin. Med., **8:** 153–205, 1871.

667. LINDSLEY, D. B., SCHREINER, L. H., MAGOUN, H. W. An electromyographic study of spasticity. J. Neurophysiol., **12:** 197–205, 1949.

668. LIPETZ, B. Preliminary report on the results of the treatment of schizophrenia by nitrogen inhalation. Psychiatric Quart., **14:** 496–503, 1940.

669. LIPMANN, F. Fermentation of phosphogluconic acid. Nature, **138:** 588–589, 1936.

670. ——. Metabolic generation and utilization of phosphate bond energy. Advances Enzymol., **1:** 99–162, 1941.

671. LIPSCHITZ, M. A., POTTER, V. R., ELVEHJEM, C. A. The metabolism of pyruvic acid in vitamin B_1 deficiency and inanition. J. Biol. Chem., **123:** 267–281, 1938.

672. LIPTON, B. S. Case Report: Blocking of chemical decerebration by pontile pathology. J. Nerv. & Ment. Dis., **106:** 537–539, 1947.

673. LIPTON, M. A., ELVEHJEM, C. A. Chemical reaction of thiamin and cocarboxylase in vivo. Symposia on Quantitative Biology, **7:** 184–194, 1939.

674. LOEBEL, R. O. Beiträge zur Atmung und Glykolyse tierischer Gewebe. Biochem. Ztschr., **161:** 219–239, 1925.

675. LOEVENHART, A. S., LORENZ, W. F., MARTIN, H. G., MALONE, J. Y. Stimulation of the respiration by sodium cyanide and its clinical application. Arch. Int. Med., **21:** 109–129, 1918.

676. LOEWI, O. Über humorale Übertragbarkeit der Herznervenwirkung. I. Mitteilung. Pflüger's Arch. f.d.ges. Physiol., **189:** 239–242, 1921; and Mitteilung II., **193:** 201–213, 1921.

677. ——. Aspects of the transmission of the nervous impulse, J. Mt. Sinai Hosp., **12:** 803–865, 1945.

678. LOGAN, MYRTLE, FERRIS, E. B., ENGEL, G. L., EVANS, J. P. Arterialization

of internal jugular blood during hyperventilation as an aid in the diagnosis of intracranial vascular tumors. An. Int. Med., **27**: 220–224, 1947.

679. LOHMANN, K. Über Phosphorylierung und Dephosphorylierung. Bildung der natürlichen Hexosemonophosphorsäure aus ihren Komponenten. Biochem. Ztschr., **262**: 137–151, 1933.

680. ——, SCHUSTER, P. Untersuchungen über die Cocarboxylase. Biochem. Ztschr., **294**: 188–214, 1937.

681. LOMAN, J., MYERSON, A. Studies in the dynamics of the human craniovertebral cavity. Am. J. Psychiat., **92**: 791–815, 1936.

682. ——, ——. Alcohol and cerebral vasodilatation. New England J. Med., **227**: 439–441, 1942.

683. LONG, C. N. H. Influence of pituitary and adrenal glands upon pancreatic diabetes. Medicine, **16**: 215–247, 1937.

684. ——. A discussion of the mechanism of action of adrenal cortical hormones on carbohydrate and protein metabolism. Endocrinology, **30**: 870–883, 1942.

684a. ——. The conditions associated with the secretion of the adrenal cortex. Fed. Proc., **6**: 461–471, 1947.

685. ——, KATZIN, B., FRY, E. G. The adrenal cortex and carbohydrate metabolism. Endocrinology, **26**: 309–344, 1940.

686. ——, LUKENS, F. D. W. The effects of adrenalectomy and hypophysectomy upon experimental diabetes in cat. J. Exper. Med., **63**: 465–490, 1936.

687. LOONEY, J. M., BORKOVIC, E. J. The changes produced on the oxygen and carbon dioxide content of arterial and venous blood of the brain during diathermy therapy for general paresis. Am. J. Physiol., **136**: 177–181, 1942.

688. ——, CAMERON, D. E. Effect of prolonged insulin therapy on glucose tolerance in schizophrenic patients. Proc. Soc. Exper. Biol. & Med., **37**: 253–257, 1937–38.

689. LORBER, V., EVANS, G. T. Mechanical response of the isolated mammalian heart to anoxia. Proc. Soc. Exper. Biol. & Med., **54**: 1–4, 1943.

690. LORENTE DE NO, R. Liberation of acetylcholine by the superior cervical sympathetic ganglion and the nodosum ganglion of the vagus. Am. J. Physiol.' **121**: 331–349, 1938.

691. ——. A study of nerve physiology. New York. Studies from the Rockefeller Institute for Medical Research, **131**: 1947.

692. LOWENBERG, K., WAGGONER, R., ZBINDEN, TH. Destruction of the cerebral cortex following nitrous oxide-oxygen anesthesia. Ann. Surg., **104**: 801–810, 1936.

693. LU, G. D., PLATT, B. S. Studies on the metabolism of pyruvic acid in normal and vitamin B_1-deficient states. V. The effect of exercise on blood pyruvate in vitamin B_1 deficiency in man. Biochem. J., **33**: 1538–1543, 1939.

694. LUBIN, M., WESTERFELD, W. The metabolism of acetaldehyde. J. Biol. Chem., **161**: 503–512, 1945.

695. LUKENS, F. D. W. Pancreatectomy in the goat. Am. J. Physiol., **122**: 729–733, 1938.

696. ——, DOHAN, F. C. Pituitary-diabetes in the cat; recovery following insulin or dietary treatment. Endocrinology, **30**: 175–202, 1942.

697. MACARTHUR, C. G., DOISY, E. A. Quantitative chemical changes in the human brain during growth. J. Comp. Neurol., **30–31**: 445–486, 1918–20.

698. ——, JONES, O. C. Some factors influencing the respiration of ground nervous tissue. J. Biol. Chem., **32**: 259–274, 1917.

699. MACLEOD, J. J. R. The control of carbohydrate metabolism. Bull. Johns Hopkins Hosp., **54:** 79–139, 1934.
700. MACLEOD, L. D., REISS, M. Tissue metabolism of brain cortex and liver after hypophysectomy and treatment with thyrotrophic hormone. Biochem. J., **34:** 820–822, 1940.
701. MADDOCK, S., HAWKINS, J. E., JR., HOLMES, E. The inadequacy of substances of the "glucose cycle" for maintenance of normal cortical potentials during hypoglycemia produced by hepatectomy with abdominal evisceration. Am. J. Physiol., **125:** 551–565, 1939.
702. MAGNUS, R., DE KLEIJN, A. Die Abhängigkeit des Tonus der Extremitätenmuskeln von der Kopfstellung. Pflüger's Arch. ges Physiol., **145:** 455–548, 1912.
703. MAGOUN, H. W., RHINES, R. An inhibitory mechanism in the bulbar reticular formation. J. Neurophysiol., **9:** 165–171, 1946.
704. MALAMUD, N., GROSH, L. C., JR. Hyperinsulinism and cerebral changes. Arch. Int. Med., **61:** 579–599, 1938.
705. MANN, F. C. The effects of complete and of partial removal of the liver. Medicine, **6:** 419–511, 1927.
706. ——, MAGATH, T. B. Studies on the physiology of liver. III. The effect of administration of glucose in the condition following total extirpation of the liver. Arch. Int. Med., **30:** 171–181, 1922.
707. MANN, P. J. G., QUASTEL, J. H. Toxic effects of oxygen and of hydrogen peroxide in brain metabolism. Biochem. J., **40:** 137–144, 1946.
708. MARRAZZI, A. S. Electrical studies on the pharmacology of autonomic synapses II. The action of a sympathomimetic drug (epinephrine) on sympathetic ganglia. J. Pharmacol. & Exper. Therap., **65:** 395–404, 1939.
709. ——. Chapter V. Pharmacology of the nervous system. 85–114. New York, Progress in Neurology and Psychiatry. Grune & Stratton. Edited by E. A. Spiegel, 1949.
710. MARKS, H. P., YOUNG, F. G. The hypophysis and pancreatic insulin. Lancet, Part **1:** 493–497, 1940.
711. MARSHALL, W. H. Observations on subcortical somatic sensory mechanisms of cats under nembutal anesthesia. J. Neurophysiol., **4:** 25–43., 1941.
712. ——, WOOLSEY, C. N., BARD, P. Observations on cortical somatic sensory mechanisms of cat and monkey. J. Neurophysiol., **4:** 1–24, 1941.
713. MARTIUS, C., KNOOP, F. Der physiologische Abbau der Citronensäure. Vorläufige Mitteilung. Hoppe-Seyler's Ztschr. f. physiol. Chem., **246:** p. I–II (supplementary pages following p. 114), 1937.
714. MASSERMAN, J. H. Effects of sodium amytal and other drugs on the reactivity of the hypothalamus of the cat. Arch. Neurol. & Psychiat., **37:** 617–628, 1937.
715. MAYER-GROSS, W., BERLINER, F. Observations in hypoglycemia: IV. Body temperature and coma. J. Ment. Sc., **88:** 419–427, 1942.
716. ——, WALKER, J. W. Effect of L-glutamic acid and other amino-acids in hypoglycaemia. Biochem. J., **44:** 92–97, 1949.
717. MAZZA, F. P., LENTI, C. Über die Glykolyse im Nervengewebe, Ber. u.d. Wissenschaftliche Biol., **50:** 630–631, 1939. Condensed from Sulla glicolisi nel tessuto nervoso. Arch. di sc. biol., **24:** 203–228, 1938.
718. ——, MALAGUZZI VALERI, C. Sulla glicolisi nel tessuto nervoso. Arch. di sc. biol., **21:** 443–465, 1935.

719. McCALL, M. L. Cerebral blood flow and metabolism in normal and toxemic pregnancy. Am. J. M. Sc., **216**: 596–597, 1948.

720. McCULLAGH, E. P., LEWIS, L. A. Carbohydrate metabolism of patients treated with methyl testosterone. J. Clin. Endocrinol., **2**: 507–510, 1942.

720a. McCULLOCH, W. S. Quart. Report. Apr. 3–July 3, 1946. Contract No. W-49-057-cws-29.

721. McCULLOCH, W. S., GRAF, C., MAGOUN, H. W. A cortico bulbo-reticular pathway from area 4-S J. Neurophysiol., **9**: 127–132, 1946.

721a. McELROY, W. D. The mechanism of inhibition of cellular activity by narcotics. Quart. Rev. Biol., **22**: 25–58, 1947.

722. McFARLAND, R. A., HALPERIN, M. H., NIVEN, J. I. Visual thresholds as an index of the modification of the effects of anoxia by glucose. Am. J. Physiol., **144**: 378–388, 1945.

723. ——, HALPERIN, M. H., NIVEN, J. I. Visual thresholds as an index of physiological imbalance during insulin hypoglycemia. Am. J. Physiol., **145**: 299–313 1946.

724. McGINTY, D. A. The regulation of respiration. XXV. Variations in the lactic acid metabolism in the intact brain. Am. J. Physiol., **88**: 312–325, 1929.

725. McGOWAN, G. K. Pyruvate oxidation in brain. II. Oxygen pyruvate ratio and R. Q. Biochem. J., **31**: 1627–1636, 1937.

725a. McLENNAN, H., ELLIOTT, K. A. C. Factors affecting synthesis of acetylcholine (ACH) by rat brain cortex slices. Fed. Proc., **9**: 202–203, 1950.

726. McNAMARA, B. P., KROP, S. Observations on the pharmacology of the isomers of hexachlorocyclohexane. J. Pharmacol. & Exper. Therap., **92**: 140–146, 1948.

727. ——, KOELLE, G. B., GILMAN, A. The treatment of di-isopropyl fluorophosphate (DFP) poisoning in rabbits. J. Pharmacol. & Exper. Therap., **88**: 27–33, 1946.

728. McQUARRIE, I., JOHNSON, R. M., ZIEGLER, M. R. Plasma electrolyte disturbance in patient with hypercorticoadrenal syndrome contrasted with that found in Addison's Disease. Endocrinology, **21**: 762–772, 1937.

729. MEDUNA, L. J. Pharmaco-dynamic treatment of psychoneuroses. Dis. Nerv. System, **8**: 37–40, 1947.

730. MEDUNA, L. J., FRIEDMAN, E. The convulsive-irritative therapy of the psychoses. J.A.M.A., **112**: 501–509, 1939.

731. MEIKLEJOHN, A. P., PASSMORE, R., PETERS, R. A. The independence of vitamin B_1 deficiency and inanition. Proc. Roy. Soc. London, **111B**: 391–395, 1932.

732. METTLER, F. A., ADES, H. W., LIPMAN, E., CULLER, E. A. The extrapyramidal system. An experimental demonstration of function. Arch. Neurol. & Psychiat., **41**: 984–995, 1939.

733. MEYER, A., JONES, T. B. Histological changes in the brain in mongolism. J. Ment. Sc., **85**: 206–221, 1939.

734. MEYER, K. H. Contributions to the theory of narcosis. Tr. Faraday Soc., **33**: 1062–1068, 1937.

735. MEYERHOF, O. Über die Synthese der Kreatinphosphorsäure im Muskel und die "Reaktionsform" des Zuckers. Naturwissenschaften, **25**: 443–446, 1937.

736. ——. Oxidoreductions in carbohydrate breakdown. Biological Symposia, **5**: 141–156, 1941.

737. ——, HIMWICH, H. E. Beiträge zum Kohlehydratstoffwechsel des Warmblüter-

muskels, insbesondere nach einseitiger Fetternährung. Pflüger's Arch. f.d.ges. Physiol., **205:** 415–437, 1924.

738. ——, Lohmann, K. Über Atmung und Kohlehydratumsatz tierischer Gewebe. I. Mitteilung. Biochem. Ztschr., **171:** 381–402, 1926.

739. ——, ——. Über Atmung und Kohlehydratumsatz tierischer Gewebe. III. Mitteilung. Biochem. Ztschr., **171:** 421–435, 1926.

740. ——, ——. Über den Nachweis von Triosephosphorsäure als Zwischenprodukt bei der enzymatischen Kohlehydratspaltung. Naturwissenschaften, **22:** 134–135, 1934.

741. ——, Wilson, Jean R. Studies on glycolysis of brain preparations. V. Affinity of hexokinase for glucose and fructose. Arch. Biochem., **19:** 502–508, 1948.

742. Michaelis, M., Quastel, J. H. The site of action of narcotics in respiratory processes. Biochem. J., **35:** 518–533, 1941.

743. Milhorat, A. T., Chambers, W. H. The effect of insulin on protein metabolism. J. Biol. Chem., **77:** 595–602, 1928.

744. Miller, F. R., Stavraky, G. W., Woonton, G. A. Effects of eserine, acetylcholine and atropine on electrocorticogram. J. Neurophysiol., **3:** 131–138, 1940.

745. Miller, J. A. Factors in neonatal resistance to anoxia I. Temperature and survival of newborn guinea pigs under anoxia. Science., **110:** 113–117, 1949.

746. Minkowski, M. Neurobiologische Studien am menschlichen Foetus. Abderhalden's Handb. biol. Arbeitsmeth., Abt. V., Teil 5B, 511–618, 1938.

747. Minot, A. S., Cutler, J. T. Quanidine retention and calcium reserve as antagonistic factors in carbon tetrachloride and chloroform poisoning. J. Clin. Investigation, **6:** 369–402, 1928–29.

748. Mirsky, I. A. The influence of insulin on the protein metabolism of nephrectomized dogs. Am. J. Physiol., **124:** 569–575, 1938.

749. ——, Broh-Kahn, R. H. The influence of dextrose administration on the utilization of B-hydroxybutyric acid by the normal and eviscerated rabbit. Am. J. Physiol., **119:** 734–739, 1937.

750. ——, Nelson, N., Grayman, I., Korenberg, M. Studies on normal and depancreatized domestic ducks. Am. J. Physiol., **135:** 223–229, 1941.

750a. Mitchell, S. Observations on the physiological action of nitrous oxide. The West Riding Lunatic Asylum Medical Reports, **1:** 27–57, 1871.

751. Modell, W., Krop, S. Antidotes to poisoning by di-isopropyl fluorophosphate in cats. J. Pharmacol. & Exper. Therap., **88:** 34–38, 1946.

752. Mogensen, E. Spontaneous hypoglycemia in Simmonds' Disease. Endocrinology **27:** 194–199, 1940.

753. Morrison, L. R. Histopathologic effect of anoxia on the cerebral nervous system. Arch. Neurol. & Psychiat., **55:** 1–34, 1946.

754. Moulton, C. R. Units of reference for basal metabolism and their interrelations. J. Biol. Chem., **24:** 299–320, 1916.

755. Mulder, A. G., Crandall, L. A. The metabolism of the brain in the ketotic state. Am. J. Physiol., **133:** P392–393, 1941.

756. Myerson, A., Halloran, R. D., Hirsch, H. L. Technic for obtaining blood from the internal jugular vein and internal carotid artery. Arch. Neurol. & Psychiat., **17:** 807–808, 1927.

757. Nachmansohn, D. Choline esterase in brain and spinal cord of sheep embryos. J. Neurophysiol., **3:** 396–402, 1940.

758. NACHMANSOHN, D. The role of acetylcholine in conduction. Bull. Johns Hopkins Hosp., **83**: 463–493, 1948.

759. ——, Cox, R. T., COATES, C. W., MACHADO, A. L. Action potential and enzyme activity in the electric organ of *electrophorus electricus*. II. Phosphocreatine as energy source of the action potential. J. Neurophysiol., **6**: 383–396, 1943.

760. ——, HESTRIN, S., VORIPAIEFF, HELEN. Enzymatic synthesis of a compound with acetylcholine-like biological activity. J. Biol. Chem., **180**: 875–877, 1949.

761. ——, JOHN, HEDDA M. Studies on choline acetylase 1. Effect of amino acids on the dialyzed enzyme. Inhibition by a-Keto acids. J. Biol. Chem., **158**: 157–171, 1945.

762. ——, MACHADO, A. L. The formation of acetylcholine. A new enzyme: "choline acetylase". J. Neurophysiol., **6**: 397–403, 1943.

763. ——, STEINBACH, H. B., MACHADO, A. L., SPIEGELMAN, S. Localization of enzymes in nerves. II. Respiratory enzymes. J. Neurophysiol., **6**: 203–211, 1943.

764. NAHUM, L. H., HIMWICH, H. E. Effect of adrenalin on the glucose and lactic acid exchange of the brain. Proc. Soc. Exper. Biol. & Med., **29**: 72–73, 1931–32.

765. NEEDHAM, J. Chemical embryology. Vol. III. New York, Cambridge, London, The Macmillan Company, 1931.

766. NEGELEIN, E. Über die glykolytische Wirkung des embryonalen Gewebes. Biochem. Ztschr., **165**: 122–133, 1925.

767. ——, HAAS, E. Über die Wirkungsweise des Zwischenferments. Biochem. Ztschr., **282**: 206–220, 1935.

767a. NELSON, D. H., REICH, H., SAMUELS, L. T. Isolation of a steroid hormone from the adrenal-vein blood of dogs. Science, **111**: 578–579, 1950.

768. NELSON, N., ELGART, S., MIRSKY, I. A. Pancreatic diabetes in the owl. Endocrinology, **31**: 119–123, 1942.

769. NEUBERG, C. Über die Zerstörung von Milchsäurealdehyd und Methyl-glyoxal durch tierische Organe. Biochem. Ztschr., **49**: 502–506, 1913.

770. NIMS, L. F., GIBBS, E. L., LENNOX, W. G. Arterial and cerebral venous blood. Changes produced by altering arterial carbon dioxide. J. Biol. Chem., **145**: 189–195, 1942.

771. NOVELLI, G. D., LIPMANN, F. Bacterial conversion of pantothenic acid into coenzyme A (Acetylation) and its relation to pyruvic oxidation. Arch. Biochem., **14**: 23–27, 1947.

772. OCHOA, S. "Coupling" of phosphorylation with oxidation of pyruvic acid in brain. J. Biol. Chem., **138**: 751–773, 1941.

773. ——. Glycolysis and phosphorylation in brain extracts. J. Biol. Chem., **141**: 245–251, 1941.

774. ——, PETERS, R. A. Vitamin B₁ and cocarboxylase in animal tissues. Biochem. J., **32**: 1501–1515, 1938.

774a. OGSTON, A. G. Interpretation of experiments on metabolic processes using isotopic tracer elements. Nature, **142**: 763, 1948.

775. O'LEARY, P. Methods for estimating the outcome of neurosyphilis. Am. Assoc. Adv. Sci., No. 6: Syphilis. The Science Press, 93–100, 1938.

776. OLSEN, N. S., KLEIN, J. R. Effect of insulin hypoglycemia on brain glucose, glycogen, lactate and phosphates. Arch. Biochem., **13**: 343–347, 1947.

777. ——, KLEIN, J. R. Effect of cyanide on the concentration of lactate and phosphates in brain. J. Biol. Chem., **167**: 739–746, 1947.

778. OLSON, R. E., KAPLAN, N. O. The effect of pantothenic acid deficiency upon the coenzyme A content and pyruvate utilization of rat and duck tissues. J. Biol. Chem., **175:** 515–529, 1948.

779. ——, MILLER, O. N., TOPPER, Y. J., STARE, F. J. The effect of vitamin deficiencies upon the metabolism of cardiac muscle *in vitro*. II. The effect of biotin deficiency in ducks with observations on the metabolism of radioactive carbon-labeled succinate. J. Biol. Chem., **175:** 503–514.

779a. OLSON, R. O., ROBSON, J. S., RICHARDS, H., HIRSCH, E. G. Comparative metabolism of radioactive glucose in heart, brain, kidney and liver slices. Fed. Proc., **9:** 211, 1950.

780. OSTER, R. H., TOMAN, J. E. P., SMITH, D. C. Recovery of the cerebral cortex of the cat following hypoxia. Am. J. Physiol., **141:** 410–414, 1944.

781. PACELLA, B. L., BARRERA, S. E., KALINOWSKY, L. Variations in electroencephalogram associated with electric shock therapy of patients with mental disorders. Arch. Neurol. & Psychiat., **47:** 367–384, 1942.

781a. PALADINI, A. C., CAPUTTO, R., LELOIR, L. F., TRUCCO, R. E., CARDINI, C. E. The enzymatic synthesis of glucose-1,6-diphosphate. Arch. Biochem., **23:** 55–66, 1949.

782. PARKER, C. S. Observations on the autonomic functions during the hypoglycemic treatment of schizophrenics. J. Ment. Sc., **86:** 645–659, 1940.

783. PARNAS, J. K. Über die enzymatischen Phosphorylierungen in der alkoholischen Gärung und in der Muskelglykogenolyse. Enzymologia, **5:** 166–184, 1938.

783a. PATTERSON, J. L., JR., HEYMAN, A., NICHOLS, F. T., JR. Cerebral blood flow and oxygen consumption in neurosyphilis. J. Clin. Investigation, **28:** 803, 1949.

783b. PEARSON, H. E., WINZLER, R. J. Oxidative and glycolytic metabolism of minced day-old mouse brain in relation to propagation of Theiler's GD VII virus. J. Biol. Chem., **181:** 577–582, 1949.

784. PEMBRY, M. S. The effect of variations in external temperature upon the output of carbonic acid and the temperature of young animals. J. Physiol., **18:** 363–379, 1895.

785. PENFIELD, W. Circulation of the epileptic brain. A. Research Nerv. & Ment. Dis. Proc. The circulation of the brain and spinal cord, **18:** 605–637, 1938.

786. PETERS, J. P., VAN SLYKE, D. D. Quantitative clinical chemistry. Vol. II: Interpretations. Baltimore, The Williams and Wilkins Co., 1931.

787. PETERS, R. A. Biochemistry of brain tissue. Chem. and Industry, **59:** 373–378, 1940.

788. ——, SINCLAIR, H. M. Studies in avian carbohydrate metabolism. IV. Factors nfluencing the maintenance of respiration in surviving brain tissue of the normal pigeon. Biochem. J., **27:** 1677–1686, 1933.

789. ——, ——, THOMPSON, R. H. S. An analysis of inhibition of pyruvate oxidation by arsenicals in relation to the enzyme theory of vesication. Biochem. J., **40:** 516–524, 1946.

790. ——, THOMPSON, R. H. S. Pyruvic acid as an intermediary metabolite in the brain tissue of avitaminous and normal pigeons. Biochem. J., **28:** 916–925, 1934.

791. PFEIFER, R. A. Die Angioarchitektonik der Grosshirnrinde. Berlin, J. Springer, 1928.

792. PICK, E. P. Über neue Schlaf- und Narkose-Versuche. Cong. internat. de l'Union thérap., **1:** 225–239, 1937.

792a. PILCHER, C., THUSS, C. Cerebral blood flow: cerebral effects of occlusion of the common and internal carotid arteries. Arch. Surg., **29:** 1024–1038, 1934.

793. PITTS, R. F. The function of components of the respiratory complex. J. Neurophysiol., **5:** 403–413, 1942.

794. POOL, J. L., NASON, GLADYS I. Cerebral circulation: XXXV. The comparative effect of ergotamine tartrate on the arteries in the Pia, Dura and skin of cats. Arch. Neurol. & Psychiat., **33:** 276–282, 1935.

794a. POPE, A., MORRIS, A. A., JASPER, H., ELLIOTT, K. A. C., PENFIELD, W. Histochemical and action potential studies on epileptogenic areas of cerebral cortex in man and the monkey. A. Research Nerv. & Ment. Dis. Proc., **26:** 218–233, 1947.

795. PORTER, R. R., DOWNS, R. S. Some physiological observations on the circulation during recovery from vitamin B₁ deficiency. Ann. Int. Med., **17:** 645–658, 1942.

796. POTTER, V. R. The mechanism of hydrogen transport in animal tissues. Medicine, **19:** 441–474, 1940.

796a. ——, BUSCH, H. Effect of fluoroacetate on reactions in the Krebs oxidative cycle. Fed. Proc., **9:** 215, 1950.

797. ——, DuBOIS, K. P. The quantitative determination of cytochrome C. J. Biol. Chem., **142:** 417–426, 1942.

797a. ——, HEIDELBERGER, C. Biosynthesis of 'asymmetric' citric acid: a substantiation of the Ogston concept. Nature, **164:** 180–181, 1944.

797b. ——, RECKNAGEL, R. O. Alternative metabolic pathways in rat liver homogenates. Fed. Proc., **9:** 215–216, 1950.

798. ——, SCHNEIDER, B. S., LIEBL, G. J. Enzyme changes during growth and differentiation in the tissues of the newborn rat. Cancer Research, **5:** 21–24 1945.

799. PRICE, J. C., WAELSCH, H., PUTNAM, T. J. dl-Glutamic Acid Hydrochloride in treatment of Petit Mal and Psychomotor Seizures. J. A. M. A., **122:** 1153–1156, 1943.

800. PRICE, W. H., CORI, C. F., COLOWICK, S. P. The effect of anterior pituitary extract and of insulin on the hexokinase reaction. J. Biol. Chem., **160:** 633–634, 1945.

801. ——, SLEIN, M. W., COLOWICK, S. P., CORI, GERTY, T. Effect of adrenal cortex extract on the hexokinase reaction. Fed. Proc., **5:** 150, 1946.

802. PÜTTER, VON A. Die Atmung der Protozoen. Ztschr. f. Allg. Physiol., **5:** 566–612, 1905.

803. QUASTEL, J. H. Respiration in the central nervous system. Physiol. Rev., **19:** 135–183, 1939.

804. ——, TENNENBAUM, M., WHEATLEY, A. H. M. Choline ester formation in, and choline esterase activities of, tissues *in vitro*. Biochem. J., **30:** 1668–1681, 1936.

805. ——, WHEATLEY, A. H. M. Oxidation by the brain. Biochem. J., **26:** 725–744, 1932.

806. ——, ——. Anaerobic oxidations. On ferricyanide as a reagent for the manometric investigation of dehydrogenase systems. Biochem. J., **32:** 936–943, 1938.

807. Queries and Minor Notes. Resuscitation of submerged persons. J. A. M. A., **114:** 2585–2586, 1940.

808. RAAB, W. Das hormonal-nervöse Regulationssystem des Fettstoffwechsels. Ztschr. f.d.ges. exper. Med., **49:** 179–269, 1926.

809. ——. Wirkung der blutfettsenkenden Hypophysensubstanz ("Lipoitrin") am menschen. Ztschr. f.d.ges. exper. Med., **89**: 588–615, 1933.

810. ——, KERSCHBAUM, E. Die blutfettsenkende Hypophysensubstanz "Lipoitrin" (Tier experimentelle untersuchungen). Ztschr. f.d.ges. exper. Med., **90**: 729–749, 1933.

811. RABINOWITCH, I. M. Biochemical findings in a rare case of acute yellow atrophy of the liver. With particular reference to the origin of urea in the body. J. Biol. Chem., **83**: 333–335, 1929.

812. RACKER, E. Observations on the metabolism of human fetal brain in vitro. Fed. Proc., **1**: 69, 1942.

813. ——, KRIMSKY, I. Inhibition of phosphorylation of glucose in mouse brains by viruses and its prevention by preparations of diphosphopyridine nucelotide. J. Exper. & Med., **84**: 191–203, 1946.

814. RAKIETEN, N., NAHUM, L. H., DuBOIS, D., GILDEA, E. F., HIMWICH, H. E. The effect of some compounds of barbituric acid and of urethane. J. Pharmacol. & Exper. Therap., **50**: 328–335, 1934.

815. RANDLES, F. S., HIMWICH, WILLIAMINA A., HOMBURGER, E., HIMWICH, H. E. The influence of vitamin B₁ deficiency on the pyruvate exchange of the heart. Am. Heart J., **33**: 341–345, 1947

816. RANSON, S. W. Somnolence caused by hypothalamic lesions in the monkey. Arch. Neurol. & Psychiat., **41**: 1–23, 1939.

817. ——, FISHER, C., INGRAM, W. R. Hypothalamic regulation of temperature in the monkey. Arch. Neurol. & Psychiat., **38**: 445–466, 1937.

818. REINECKE, R. M. The kidney as a source of glucose in the eviscerated rat. Am. J. Physiol., **140**: 276–285, 1943–44.

819. REINER, J. M. The effect of age on the carbohydrate metabolism of tissue homogenates. J. Gerontol., **2**: 315–320, 1947.

819a. REINER, L., MISANI, F., CORDASCO, M. G., FAIR, T. W. Nitrogen trichloride-treated prolamines. VII. Further characterization of toxic factor. Fed. Proc., **9**: 218, 1950.

820. RHINES, R., MAGOUN, H. W. Brain stem facilitation of cortical motor response. J. Neurophysiol., **9**: 219–229, 1946.

821. RICHARDSON, H. B., SHORR, E., LOEBEL, R. O. Tissue metabolism. II. The respiratory quotient of normal and diabetic tissue. J. Biol. Chem., **86**: 551–569, 1930.

822. RICHARDSON, K. C. The influence of diabetogenic anterior pituitary extracts on the islets of Langerhans in dogs. Proc. Roy. Soc. London, **128B**: 153–169, 1939–40.

823. RICKETTS, H. T., BRUNSCHWIG, A., KNOWLTON, K. Diabetes in a totally depancreatized man. Proc. Soc. Exper. Biol. & Med., **58**: 254–255, 1945.

824. ROBB, G. P., WEISS, S. A method for the measurement of the velocity of the pulmonary and peripheral venous blood flow in man. Am. Heart J., **8**: 650–670, 1932–33.

825. ROBERTS, S., SAMUELS, L. T., REINECKE, R. M. Previous diet and the apparent utilization of fat in the absence of the liver. Am. J. Physiol., **140**: 639–644, 1943–44.

826. ROBERTSON, J. D., STEWART, C. P. The effect of alcohol on the oxygen uptake of brain tissue. Biochem. J., **26**: 65–74, 1932.

827. ROGERS, L. The function of the circulus arteriosus of Willis. Brain, **70**: 171–178, 1948.

828. ROGOFF, J. M., STEWART, G. N. Studies on adrenal insufficiency. IV. The in-

fluence of intravenous injections of Ringer's solution upon the survival period in adrenalectomized dogs. Am. J. Physiol., **84:** 649–659, 1928.

829. Romano, J., Engel, G. L. Delirium I. Electroencephalographic Data. Arch. Neurol. & Psychiat., **51:** 356–377, 1944.

830. Roos, J., Romijn, C. Some conditions of foetal respiration in the cow. J. Physiol., **92:** 249–267, 1938.

831. Root, H. F., Carpenter, T. M. The effect of glucose administration in diabetic acidosis. Am. J. M. Sc., **206:** 234–243, 1943.

832. Rose, W. C. The nutritive significance of the amino acids. Physiol. Rev., **18:** 109–136, 1938.

833. Rosen, S. R., Cameron, D. E., Ziegler, J. B. The prevention of metrazol fractures by beta-erythroidin hydrochloride. Psychiatric Quart., **14:** 477–480, 1940.

834. Rosenbaum, M., Roseman, E., Aring, C. D., Ferris, E. B. Intracranial blood flow in dementia paralytica, cerebral atrophy and schizophrenia. Arch. Neurol. & Psychiat., **47:** 793–799, 1942.

835. Ross, A. T., Dickerson, W. W. Tuberous sclerosis. Arch. Neurol. & Psychiat., **50:** 233–257, 1943.

836. Rossen, R., Kabat, H., Anderson, J. P. Acute arrest of cerebral circulation in man. Arch. Neurol. & Psychiat., **50:** 510–528, 1943.

837. Russell, J. A. The relation of the anterior pituitary to carbohydrate metabolism. Physiol. Rev., **18:** 1–27, 1938.

838. ——. The relationship of the anterior pituitary and the adrenal cortex in the metabolism of carbohydrate. Am. J. Physiol., **128:** 552–561, 1939–40.

839. ——. The relationship of the anterior pituitary to the thyroid and the adrenal cortex in the control of carbohydrate metabolism. Taken from Essays in Biology; in honor of Herbert M. Evans, Univ. of California Press, Berkeley and Los Angeles, 1943. p. 509–527.

840. ——, Cori, G. T. A comparison of the metabolic effects of subcutaneous and intravenous epinephrine injections in normal and hypophysectomized rats. Am. J. Physiol., **119:** 167–174, 1937.

841. ——, Wilhelmi, A. E. Glyconeogenesis in kidney tissue of the adrenalectomized rat. J. Biol. Chem., **140:** 747–754, 1941.

842. Sachs, E., Jr., Brendler, S. J. Some effects of stimulation of the orbital surface of the frontal lobe in the dog and monkey. Fed. Proc., **7:** 107, 1948.

843. Sachs, E., MacDonald, M. E. Blood sugar studies in experimental pituitary and hypothalamic lesions. Arch. Neurol. & Psychiat., **13:** 335–368, 1925.

844. Sacks, J. On the mechanism of insulin action: observations with radioactive phosphorus. Science, **98:** 388–389, 1943.

845. Sakel, M. Pharmacological treatment of schizophrenia. Nervous and Mental Disease, Monograph series, no. 62, New York and Washington, 1938. Authorized translation by Joseph Wortis, M.D.

846. von Sántha, K., Cipriani, A. Focal alterations in subcortical circulation resulting from stimulation of the cerebral cortex: an experimental demonstration of cortico-subcortico connections. A. Research Nerv. and Ment. Dis. Proc. The circulation of the brain and spinal cord, **18:** 346–362, 1938.

847. Sayhun, M., Luck, J. M. The influence of epinephrine and insulin on the distribution of glycogen in rabbits. J. Biol. Chem., **85:** 1–20, 1929–30.

848. Schachner, H., Fries, B. A., Chaikoff, I. L. The effect of hexoses and pentoses on the formation in vitro of phospholipid by brain tissue as measured with radioactive phosphorus. J. Biol. Chem., **146:** 95–103, 1942.

848a. SCHEINBERG, P., STEAD, E. A., JR. The cerebral blood flow in male subjects as measured by the nitrous oxide technique. Normal values for blood flow, oxygen utilization, glucose utilization, and peripheral resistance, with observations on the effect of tilting and anxiety. J. Clin. Investigation, **28:** 1163–1171, 1949.

848b. ——, ——. Cerebral metabolism in hyperthyroidism and myxedema. Fed. Proc., **9:** 113, 1950.

848c. ——. The effects of postural changes, stellate ganglion block, and anemia on the cerebral circulation. J. Clin. Investigation, **28:** 808–809, 1949.

848d. ——. Cerebral circulation in heart failure. Am. J. Med., **8:** 148–152, 1950.

849. SCHILLER, J., COHN, SALLY, ASHBY, WINIFRED. Carbonic anhydrase content in the brain of rats with thiouracil induced cretinism. Fed. Proc., **5:** 253, 1946.

850. SCHLOSSMANN, H. The carbohydrate metabolism of the foetal dog under the influence of insulin. J. Physiol., **92:** 219–227, 1938.

851. SCHMIDT, C. F. The influence of cerebral blood-flow on respiration. 1. The respiratory responses to changes in cerebral blood-flow. Am. J. Physiol., **84:** 202–222, 1928.

852. ——. The influence of cerebral blood-flow on respiration. 2. The gaseous metabolism of the brain. Am. J. Physiol., **84:** 223–241, 1928.

853. ——. The mechanism and probable significance of the convulsions produced by cyanide. Science, **93:** 465, 1941.

854. ——. The present status of knowledge concerning the intrinsic control of the cerebral circulation and the effects of functional derangements in it. Fed. Proc., **3:** 131–139, 1944.

855. ——, HENDRIX, J. P. The action of chemical substances on cerebral blood-vessels. A. Research Nerv. & Ment. Dis. Proc., **18:** 229–276, 1938.

856. ——, KETY, S. S., PENNES, H. H. The gaseous metabolism of the brain of the monkey. Am. J. Physiol., **143:** 33–52, 1945.

857. SCHMID, H. Zur Histopathologie der Sakel'schen Hypoglykämieschockbehandlung der Schizophrenie. Vorläüfige Mitteilung. Schweiz. med. Wchnschr., **66:** 960–961, 1936.

858. SCHNEIDER, M., SCHNEIDER, D. Untersuchungen über die Regulierung der Gehirndurchblutung. Mitteilung 1. Arch. f. Exper. Path., **175:** 606–639, 1934.

859. SCHNEIDER, R., DROLLER, H. The relative importance of ketosis and acidosis in the production of diabetic coma. Quart. J. Exper. Physiol., **28:** 323–333, 1938.

860. SCHREIBER, F. Apnea of the newborn and associated cerebral injury. J. A. M. A., **111:** 1263–1269, 1938.

861. SELLE, W. A. Influence of glucose on the gasping pattern of young animals subjected to acute anoxia. Am. J. Physiol., **141:** 297–302, 1944.

862. ——, WITTEN, T. A. Survival of the respiratory (gasping) mechanism in young animals. Am. J. Physiol., **133:** P441, 1941.

863. SEROTA, H. M. Temperature changes in the cortex and hypothalamus during sleep. J. Neurophysiol., **2:** 42–47, 1939.

864. SHAPIRO, B., WERTHEIMER, E. Phosphorolysis and synthesis of glycogen in animal tissues. Biochem. J., **37:** 397–403, 1943.

865. SHAW, L. A., BEHNKE, A. R., MESSER, A. C. The role of carbon dioxide in producing the symptoms of oxygen poisoning. Am. J. Physiol., **108:** 652–661, 1934.

865a. SHENKIN, H. A., HAFKENSCHIEL, J. H., KETY, S. S. The effects of sympathectomy on the cerebral circulation of hypertensive patients. Arch. Surg. 1950.

866. ——, HARMEL, M. H., KETY, S. S. Dynamic anatomy of the cerebral circulation. Arch. Neurol. & Psychiat., **60:** 240–252, 1948.

867. ——, SPITZ, E. B., GRANT, F. C., KETY, S. S. The acute effects on the cerebral
circulation of the reduction of increased intracranial pressure by means of
intravenous glucose or ventricular drainage. J. Neurosurg., **5:** 466–470, 1948.

868. ——, ——, ——, ——. Physiologic studies of arterio-venous anomalies of the
brain. J. Neurosurg., **5:** 165–172, 1948.

869. ——, WOODFORD, R. B., FREYHAN, F. A., KETY, S. S. The effect of frontal lobotomy on the cerebral blood flow and metabolism. A. Research Nerv. & Ment.
Dis. Proc., 823–831, 1948.

870. ——, YASKIN, J. C. The cerebral circulation and metabolism in postencephalitic
Parkinson's disease. Tr. Am. Neur. A., 70–72, 1949.

871. SHERIF, M., HOLMES, E. G. A note on oxygen consumption of nerve in presence of glucose and galactose. Biochem. J., **24:** 400–401, 1930.

872. SHERMAN, W. C., ELVEHJEM, C. A. *In vitro* studies on lactic acid metabolism
in tissues from polyneuritic chicks. Biochem. J., **30:** 785–793, 1936.

873. ——, ——. In vitro action of crystalline vitamin B_1 on pyruvic acid metabolism
in tissues from polyneuritic chicks. Am. J. Physiol., **117:** 142–150, 1936.

874. SHERRINGTON, C. S. Decerebrate rigidity and reflex coordination of movements. J. Physiol., **22:** 319–332, 1897–98.

875. ——. The integrative action of the nervous system. New Haven, Yale Univ.
Press, 1911.

876. ——. The brain and its mechanism. The Rede lecture delivered Dec. 5, 1933.
Cambridge, England. The University Press, 1933.

877. SHIPLEY, R. A. The metabolism of acetone bodies and glucose *in vitro* and the
effect of anterior pituitary extract. Am. J. Physiol., **141:** 662–668, 1944.

878. SHORR, E. The relation of hormones to carbohydrate metabolism *in vitro*.
Cold Spring Harbor Sympos. on Quant. Biol., **7:** 323–348, 1939.

879. ——, BARKER, S. B. *In vitro* action of insulin on minced avian and mammalian
muscle. Biochem. J., **33:** 1798–1809, 1939.

880. ——, LOEBEL, R. O., RICHARDSON, H. B. Tissue metabolism. I. The nature of
phlorhizin diabetes. J. Biol. Chem., **86:** 529–549, 1930.

881. SILVER, M. L., POLLOCK, G. H. Role of carbon dioxide and of the hindbrain
in agene-induced canine epilepsy. Am. J. Physiol., **154:** 439–442, 1948.

882. SINGAL, S. A., SYDENSTRICKER, V. P., LITTLEJOHN, J. M. The nicotinic acid
content of tissues of rats on corn rations. J. Biol. Chem., **176:** 1069, 1073,
1948.

883. SIRKIN, J. Acrocephalosyndactylia: Report of a case. Am. J. Ment. Def., **48:**
335–338, 1944.

883a. SLEIN, M. W. Competitive effects of substrates for hexokinase. Fed. Proc., **9:**
229–230, 1950.

884. SMITH, C. A., KAPLAN, E. Adjustment of blood oxygen levels in neonatal life.
Am. J. Dis. Child., **64:** 843–859, 1942.

885. SMITH, D. C., OSTER, R. H. Influence of blood sugar levels on resistance to low
oxygen tension in the cat. Am. J. Physiol., **146:** 26–32, 1946.

886. SMITH, W. K. The functional significance of the rostral cingular cortex as
revealed by its responses to electrical excitation. J. Neurophysiol., **8:** 241–
255, 1945.

887. SMYTH, D. H. Vitamin B₁ and the synthesis of oxaloacetate by *staphylococcus*. Biochem. J., **34**: 1598–1604, 1940.

888. SNAPPER, I., GRÜNBAUM, A. Über den abbau von diacetsäure und B-oxybuttersäure in den musklen. Biochem. Ztschr., **201**: 464–472, 1928.

889. SNIDER, R. S., MAGOUN, H. W., McCULLOCH, W. S. A suppressor cerebello-bulbo-reticular pathway from anterior lobe and paramedian lobules. Fed. Proc., **6**: 207, 1947.

890. SNYDER, F. F., ROSENFELD, M. Direct observation of intrauterine respiratory movements of the fetus and the role of carbon dioxide and oxygen in their regulation. Am. J. Physiol., **119**: 153–166, 1937.

891. SOMOGYI, M. Ketosis caused by overdoses of insulin. J. Biol. Chem., **133**: p. xciii, 1940.

892. ——. Effects of insulin upon the production of ketone bodies. J. Biol. Chem., **141**: 219–227, 1941.

893. SOONG, H. Y. Assay of insulin content of pancreas in rats receiving anterior pituitary extract. Chinese J. Physiol., **15**: 335–341, 1940.

894. SOSKIN, S., ALLWEISS, M. D., COHN, D. J. Influence of the pancreas and the liver upon the dextrose tolerance curve. Am. J. Physiol., **109**: 155–165, 1934.

895. ——, ——. The hypoglycemic phase of the dextrose tolerance curve. Am. J. Physiol., **110**: 4–7, 1934–35.

896. ——, LEVINE, R. Carbohydrate Metabolism. Correlation of physiological, biochemical, and clinical aspects. Chicago, Univ. of Chicago Press, 1946.

897. ——, MIRSKY, I. A., ZIMMERMAN, L. M., CROHN, N. Influence of hypophysectomy on gluconeogenesis in the normal and depancreatized dog. Am. J. Physiol., **114**: 110–118, 1935–36.

898. ——, TAUBENHAUS, M. Sodium succinate as an antidote for barbiturate poisoning and in the control of the duration of barbiturate anesthesia. J. Pharmacol. & Exper. Therap., **78**: 49–55, 1943.

899. SPATZ, H. Über den Eisennachweis im Gehirn, besonders in Zentren des extrapyramidalmotorischen Systems. Ztschr. f.d.ges. Neurol. u. Psychiat., **77**: 261–390, 1922.

900. SPIEGEL-ADOLF, M., FREED, H. Effects of insulin treatment on the cerebro-spinal fluids of schizophrenics. Proc. Soc. Exper. Biol. & Med., **40**: 398–400, 1939.

901. ——. Cerebrospinal fluid in convulsive disorders. Proc. Soc. Exper. Biol. & Med., **37**: 92–93, 1937–38.

902. SPIEGELMAN, S., STEINBACH, H. B. Substrate-Enzyme orientation during embryonic development. Biol. Bull., **88**: 254–268, 1945.

903. SPIRTES, M. A. Oxygen consumption of brain cortex in thyrotoxic guinea pigs Proc. Soc. Exper. Biol. & Med., **46**: 279–280, 1941.

904. SPRAGUE, R. G., PRIESTLEY, J. T., DOCKERTY, M. B. Diabetes mellitus without other endocrine manifestations in a case of tumor of the adrenal cortex. J. Clin. Endocrinol., **3**: 28–32, 1943.

905. STADIE, W. C. Fat metabolism in diabetes mellitus. J. Clin. Investigation, **19**: 843–861, 1940.

906. ——, RIGGS, B. C., HAUGAARD, N. Oxygen poisoning. Am. J. Med. Sc., **207**: 84–114, 1944.

907. ——, ——, ——. Oxygen poisoning III. The effect of high oxygen pressures upon the metabolism of brain. J. Biol. Chem., **160**: 191–208, 1945

908. STANDER, H. J. A chemical study of a case of chloroform poisoning. Bull. Johns Hopkins Hosp., **35**: 46–49, 1924.

909. STANNARD, J. N. Additional evidence of qualitative differences between the resting and activity oxygen consumptions of frog muscle. Am. J. Physiol., **135:** 238–248, 1941–42.

910. STARE, F. J., LIPTON, M. A., GOLDINGER, J. M. Studies on biological oxidations. XVIII. The citric acid cycle in pigeon muscle respiration. J. Biol. Chem., **141:** 981–987, 1941.

911. STARLING'S principles of human physiology. Philadelphia, Lea and Febiger, 1936.

912. STAUB, H. Bahnung im intermediären zuckerstoffwechsel. Biochem. Ztschr., **118:** 93–102, 1921.

912a. STERN, J. R., OCHOA, S. Enzymatic synthesis of citric acid. Fed. Proc., **9:** 234–235, 1950.

913. STIEF, A., TOKAY, L. Weitere experimentelle Untersuchungen über die cerebrale Wirkung des Insulins. Ztschr. f.d.ges. Neurol. u. Psychiat., **153:** 561–572, 1935.

914. STOCKEN, L. A., THOMPSON, R. H. S. British Anti-Lewisite. 2. Dithiol compounds as antidotes for arsenic. Biochem. J., **40:** 535–548, 1946.

915. STONE, W. E. The effects of anaesthetics and of convulsants on the lactic acid content of the brain. Biochem. J., **32:** 1908–1918, 1938.

916. ——, MARSHALL, C., NIMS, L. F. Chemical changes in the brain produced by injury and by anoxia. Am. J. Physiol., **132:** 770–775, 1941.

917. ——, WEBSTER, J. E., GURDJIAN, E. S. Chemical changes in the cerebral cortex associated with convulsive activity. J. Neurophysiol., **8:** 233–240, 1945.

918. ——, ——, KOPALA, J., GURDJIAN, E. S. Effects of carbon dioxide administration on cerebral metabolism in hypoxia. Fed. Proc., **5:** 101–102, 1946.

919. STORMONT, R. T., HATHAWAY, H. R., SHIDEMAN, F. E., SEEVERS, M. H. The acid-base balance during cyclopropane anesthesia. Anesthesiology, **3:** 369–378, 1942.

920. STOTZ, E. The estimation and distribution of cytochrome oxidase and cytochrome C in rat tissues. J. Biol. Chem., **131:** 555–565, 1939.

921. ——, ALTSCHUL, A. M., HOGNESS, T. R. The cytochrome C-cytochrome oxidase complex. J. Biol. Chem., **124:** 745–754, 1938.

922. STOTZ, E., WESTERFELD, W. W., BERG, R. L. The metabolism of acetaldehyde with acetoin formation. J. Biol. Chem., **152:** 41–50, 1944.

923. STRAUSS, H. Strangulationsfolgen und Hirnstamm. Ztschr. f.d.ges. Neurol. u. Psychiat., **131:** 363–374, 1930–31.

924. STREET, H. R., ZIMMERMAN, H. M., COWGILL, G. R., HOFF, H. E., FOX, J. C., JR. Some effects produced by long-continued subminimal intakes of vitamin B₁. Yale J. Biol. & Med., **13:** 293–308, 1940–41.

925. STRONG, O. S., ELWYN, A. Human Neuroanatomy. The Williams and Wilkins Company, Baltimore, 1943.

926. SUGAR, O., GERARD, R. W. Anoxia and brain potentials. J. Neurophysiol., **1:** 558–572, 1938.

926a. SUTHERLAND, E. W. Activation of phosphoglucomutase by metal-binding agents. J. Biol. Chem., **180:** 1279–1284, 1949.

927. SUTHERLAND, E. W., COLOWICK, S. P., CORI, C. F. The enzymatic conversion of glucose-6-phosphate to glycogen. J. Biol. Chem., **140:** 309–310, 1941.

928. SUTHERLAND, E. W., CORI, C. F. Influence of insulin on glycogen synthesis and breakdown in liver slices. Fed. Proc., **6:** 297, 1947.

929. SUTHERLAND, E. W., DE DUVE, C. Origin and distribution of the hyperglycemic-glycogenolytic factor of the pancreas. J. Biol. Chem., **175:** 663–674, 1948.

930. SWANK, R. L. Avian thiamin deficiency. A correlation of the pathology and clinical behavior. J. Exper. Med., **71:** 683–702, 1940.

931. SWANK, R. L., FOLEY, J. M. Respiratory, electrocenephalographic, and blood gas changes in progressive barbiturate narcosis in dogs. J. Pharmacol. & Exper. Therap., **92:** 381–396, 1948.

931a. SWEET, W. H., BENNETT, H. S. Changes in internal carotid pressure during carotid and jugular occlusion and their clinical significance. J. Neurosurg., **5:** 178–195, 1948.

932. SWINGLE, W. W. Studies on the functional significance of the suprarenal cortex. I. Blood changes following bilateral epinephrectomy in cats. Am. J. Physiol., **79:** 666–678, 1926–27.

933. SYM, E., NILSSON, R., EULER, H. v. Co-Zymasegehalt verschiedener tierischer Gewebe. Hoppe-Seyler's Ztschr. f. physiol. Chem., **190:** 228–246, 1930.

934. Szent-Györgyi, A. Oxidation and fermentation. Perspectives in biochemistry. Cambridge, The University Press, 1938. p. 165–174.

935. TANNENBERG, J. Comparative experimental studies on symptomatology and anatomical changes produced by anoxic and insulin shock. Proc. Soc. Exper. Biol. & Med., **40:** 94–96, 1939.

936. Taylor's principles and practise of medical jurisprudence. London, J. and A. Churchill, 1920. Revised by Fred J. Smith. Vol. I, p. 647.

937 TAYLOR, J. F. The purification of phosphofructokinase from rabbit muscle. Fed. Proc., **6:** 297–298, 1947.

938. TAYLOR, J., HOLMES, G., WALSHE, F. M. R. Selected writings of John Hughlings Jackson, London, Hodder & Stoughton, Ltd., 1931.

939. TEITZ, E. B., DORNHEGGEN, H., GOLDMAN, D. Blood adrenalin levels during insulin shock treatments for schizophrenia. Endocrinology, **26:** 641–644, 1940.

940. THOMAS, C. B., COBB, S. Cerebral circulation: constriction of pial vessels in the unanesthetized cat produced by stimulation of the cervical sympathetic chain. J. Clin. Investigation, **14:** 713, 1935.

941. ——. The cerebral circulation. XXXI. Effect of alcohol on cerebral vessels. Arch. Neurol. & Psychiat., **38:** 321–339, 1937.

942. THOMPSON, W. R. On confidence ranges for the median and other expectation distributions for populations of unknown distribution form. Ann. Math. Stat., **7:** 122–128, 1936.

943. THORN, G. W., KEOPF, G. F., LEWIS, R. A., OLSEN, E. F. Carbohydrate metabolism in Addison's Disease. J. Clin. Investigation, **19:** 813–832, 1940.

944. TILNEY, F., RILEY, H. A. The form and functions of the central nervous system. New York, Paul B. Hoeber, Inc., 1928.

945. TIPTON, S. R., LEATH, MARTHA J., TIPTON, ISABEL H., NIXON, W. L. The effects of feeding thyroid substance and of adrenalectomy on the activities of succinoxidase and cytochrome oxidase in the liver tissue of rats. Am. J. Physiol., **145:** 693–698, 1946.

946. TORDA, C., WOLFF, H. G. Effect of epinephrine on the synthesis of acetylcholine. Fed. Proc., **3:** 48, 1944.

947. TORRES, I. Über die Restatmung von Säugetiergeweben in Blausäure. Biochem. Ztschr., **280:** 114–117, 1935.

948. TOWER, D. B., McEACHERN, D. Acetylcholine and neuronal activity. II. Acetylcholine and cholinesterase activity in the cerebrospinal fluids of patients with epilepsy. Canad. J. Research, E, **27:** 120–131, 1949.

949. TRAUBE, J. Theorie der Osmose und Narkose. Pflüger's Arch. f.d.ges. Physiol., **105**: 541–558, 1904.

950. TRAUGOTT, K. Über das verhalten des blutzuckerspiegels bei wiederholter und verschiedener art enteraler zuckerzufuhr und dessen bedeutung für die leberfunktion. Klin. Wchnschr., **1**: 892–894, 1922.

951. TYLER, D. B. The mechanism of the production of brain damage during insulin shock. Am. J. Physiol., **131**: 554–560, 1941.

952. ——. Effect of malonate and iodoacetate on respiration of brains of rats of various ages. Proc. Soc. Exper. Biol. & Med., **49**: 537–539, 1942.

953. ——, VAN HARREVELD, A. The respiration of the developing brain. Am. J. Physiol., **136**: 600–603, 1942.

954. VAN MIDDLESWORTH, L. Metabolism of I^{131} in severe anoxic anoxia. Science, **110**: 120–121, 1949.

955. ——, KLINE, R. F., BRITTON, S. W. Carbohydrate regulation under severe anoxic conditions. Am. J. Physiol., **140**: 474–482, 1944.

956. VAN SLYKE, D. D., NEILL, J. M. The determination of gases in the blood and other solutions by vacuum extraction and manometric measurement. J. Biol. Chem., **61**: 523–573, 1924.

957. VENNESLAND, B., SOLOMON, A. K., BUCHANAN, J. M., CRAMER, R. D., HASTINGS, A. B. Metabolism of lactic acid containing radioactive carbon in the α or β position. J. Biol. Chem., **142**: 371–377, 1942.

958. VOGT, MARTHE. Die Verteilung von Arzneistoffen auf verschiedene Regionen des Zeutralnervensystems, zugleid ein Beitrag zu ihrer quantitativen Mikrobestimmung in Gewebe, Mitteilung: Barbitursaurederivate. Arch. Exper. Path. u. Pharm., **178**: 603–627, 1935.

959. VOGT, O. Der Begriff der Pathoklise. J. Psychol. et Neurol., **31**: 245–255, 1925.

960. VOLLAND, W. Beitrag zur Frage der Herkunft des "Paralyseeisens". Virchow's Arch. f. Path. Anat., **303**: 611–622, 1938–39.

961. VONDERAHE, A. R. Central nervous system and sugar metabolism. Clinical, pathologic and theoretical considerations, with special reference to diabetes mellitus. Arch. Int. Med., **60**: 694–704, 1937.

962. WAELSCH, H., RACKOW, H. Natural and synthetic inhibitors of choline esterase. Science, **96**: 386, 1942.

963. ——, SPERRY, W. M., STOYANOFF, V. A. Lipid metabolism in brain during myclination. J. Biol. Chem., **135**: 297–302, 1940.

964. WAGNER-JAUREGG, J. The treatment of general paresis by inoculation of malaria. J. Nerv. & Ment. Dis., **55**: 369–375, 1922.

965. WAKEMAN, A. M., MORRELL, C. A. Chemistry and metabolism in experimental yellow fever in Macacus rhesus monkeys; concentration of nonprotein nitrogenous constituents in blood. Arch. Int. Med., **46**: 290–305, 1930.

966. WALKER, A. E. Central representation of pain. Res. Publ. Ass. Nerv. Ment. Dis. Baltimore, The Williams and Wilkins Co., **23**: 63–85, 1943.

967. WARBURG, O. Über die katalytischen wirkungen der lebendigen substanz. Berlin, J. Springer, 1928.

968. ——, CHRISTIAN, W. Über Aktivierung der Robinsonschen Hexose-Mono-Phosphorsäure in roten Blutzellen und die Gewinnung aktivierender Fermentlösungen. Biochem. Ztschr., **242**: 206–227, 1931.

969. ——, ——. Über ein neues Oxydationsferment und sein Absorptionsspektrum. Biochem. Ztschr., **254**: 438–458, 1932.

970. ——, ——. Verbrennung von Robison-Ester durch Triphospho-Pyridin-Nucleotid. Biochem. Ztschr., **287**: 440–441, 1936.
971. ——, ——. Abbau von Robisonester durch Triphospho-Pyridin-Nucleotid. Biochem. Ztschr., **292**: 287–295, 1937.
972. ——, Negelein, E. Sammelreferate. Fermentproblem und oxydation in der lebendigen substanz. Ztschr. Electrochem., **35**: 928–935, 1929.
973. ——, Posener, K., Negelein, E. Über den Stoffwechsel der Carcinomzelle. Biochem. Ztschr., **152**: 309–344, 1924.
974. Ward, A. A., Jr. Decerebrate rigidity. J. Neurophysiol., **10**: 89–103, 1947.
975. ——. Convulsive activity induced by fluoroacetate, J. Neurophysiol., **10**: 105–111, 1947.
976. ——. The anterior cingular gyrus and personality. A. Research Nerv. & Ment. Dis. Proc., **27**: 438–445, 1948.
977. ——, Wheatley, M. D. Sodium cyanide: Sequence of changes of activity induced at various levels of the central nervous system. J. Neuropath. & Exper. Neurol., **6**: 292–294, 1947.
978. Warkany, J., Nelson, R. C. Skeletal abnormalities in the offspring of rats reared on deficient diets. Anat. Rec., **79**: 83–100, 1941.
979. Waters, E. T., Fletcher, J. P., Mirsky, I. A. The relation between carbohydrate and β-hydroxybutyric acid utilization by the heart-lung preparation. Am. J. Physiol., **122**: 542–546, 1938.
979a. Wechsler, R. L., Kleiss, L. M., Kety, S. S. The effects of intravenously administered aminophylline on cerebral circulation and metabolism in man. J. Clin. Investigation, **29**: 28–30, 1950.
980. Weil, A. The phospholipids of the brain, kidneys and heart of white rats in experimental hyperthyroidism. Endocrinology, **21**: 101–108 1937.
981. ——. The chemical constitution of brain, kidneys and heart of white rats in experimental hypothyroidism. Endocrinology, **29**: 919–926, 1941.
982. ——. The influence of sex hormones upon the chemical growth of the brain of white rats. Growth, **8**: 107–115, 1944.
983. ——, Groat, R. A. The effect of adrenalectomy upon the brain of white rats. J. Neuropath. & Exper. Neurol. **3**: 374–378. 1944.
984. ——, Liebert E., Heilbrunn, G. Histopathologic changes in the brain in experimental hyperinsulinism. Arch. Neurol. & Psychiat., **39**: 467–481, 1938.
985. Weil-Malherbe, H. Studies on brain metabolism. I. The metabolism of glutamic acid in brain. Biochem. J., **30**: 665–676, 1936.
985a. ——. The action of glutamic acid in hypoglycemia coma. J. Ment. Sc., **95**: 930–944, 1949.
986. Weinberger, L. M., Gibbon, M. H., Gibbon, J. H., Jr. Temporary arrest of the circulation to the central nervous system. I. Physiologic effects. Arch. Neurol. & Psychiat., **43**: 615–634, 1940.
987. ——, ——, ——. Temporary arrest of the circulation to the central nervous system. II. Pathologic effects. Arch. Neurol. & Psychiat., **43**: 961–986, 1940.
988. Weiss, S., Wilkins, R. W. The nature of the cardiovascular disturbances in nutritional deficiency states (beri-beri). Ann. Int. Med., **11**: 104–148, 1937.
989. Wells, B. B. The influence of crystalline compounds separated from the adrenal cortex on gluconeogenesis. Proc. Staff Meetings Mayo Clinic, **15**: 294–297, 1940.
990. Welsh, J. H., Hyde, J. E. The distribution of acetylcholine in brains of rats of different ages. J. Neurophysiol., **7**: 41–49, 1944.

991. WELTY, J. W., ROBERTSON, H. F. Hypoglycemia in Addison's Disease. Am. J. M. Sc., **192**: 760–764, 1936.

992. WERKMAN, C. H. Bacterial dissimilation of carbohydrates. Bact. Rev., **3–4**; 187–227, 1939–40.

993. WERTHEIMER, E. Glycogen in adipose tissue. J. Physiol., **103**: 359–366, 1945.

994. WESTFAL, A. Pyruvic acid antagonism to barbiturate depression. J. Pharmacol. & Exper. Therap., **87**: 32–36, 1946.

995. WHITE, W. H. The effect upon the bodily temperature of lesions of the corpus striatum and optic thalamus. J. Physiol., **11**: 1–24, 1890.

996. WIELAND, H. Über den Mechanismus der Oxydationsvorgänge. Ber. d. Deutschen Chem. Gesellschaft, **46**: 3327–3342, 1913.

997. WIENER, N. Cybernetics, or control and communication in the animal and the machine. New York: John Wiley; Paris: Hermann et Cie, 1948.

998. WIERZUCHOWSKI, M. Animal calorimetry. Respiratory metabolism in phlorhizin diabetes after glucose ingestion. J. Biol. Chem., **68**: 385–397, 1926.

999. ——. Outflow diabetes and toxic phenomena due to the infusion of glucose in normal dogs. J. Physiol., **87**: 85P–86P, 1936.

1000. WILDER, J. Ein neues hypophysäres Krankheitsbild: Die hypophysäre Spontanhypoglykämie. Deutsche Ztschr. f. Nervenh., **112**: 192–250, 1930.

1001. ——. Problems of criminal psychology related to hypoglycemic states. J. Crim. Psychopath., **1**: 219–233, 1940.

1002. ——. Psychological problems in hypoglycemia. Am. J. Digest. Dis., **10**: 428–435, 1943.

1003. WILLIAMS, D. The effect of cholin-like substances on the cerebral electrical discharges in epilepsy. J. Neurol. & Psychiat., **4**: 32–47, 1941.

1004. ——, LENNOX, W. G. The cerebral blood-flow in arterial hypertension, arteriosclerosis, and high intracranial pressure. Quart. J. Med., **8**: 185–194, 1939.

1005. WILLIAMS, R. D., MASON, H. L., POWER, M. H., WILDER, R. M. Induced thiamine (vitamin B₁) deficiency in man. Relation of depletion of thiamine to development of biochemical defect and of polyneuropathy. Arch. Int. Med., **71**: 38–53, 1943.

1006. ——, ——, WILDER, R. M., SMITH, B. F. Observations on induced thiamine (vitamin B₁) deficiency in man. Arch. Int. Med., **66**: 785–799, 1940.

1007. ——, ——, SMITH, B. F., WILDER, R. M. Induced thiamine (vitamin B₁) deficiency and the thiamine requirement of man. Arch. Int. Med., **69**: 721–738, 1942.

1008. WILLIAMS, R. R., SPIES, T. D. Vitamin B₁ and its use in medicine. New York, The Macmillan Company, 1939.

1009. WILLIAMSON, C. S., MANN, F. C. Studies on the physiology of the liver. V. The hepatic factor in chloroform and phosphorous poisoning. Am. J. Physiol., **65**: 267–276, 1923.

1010. WINDLE, W. F. Physiology of the fetus, Philadelphia and London, W. B. Saunders Co., 1940. Chapter VI.

1011. ——, BECKER, R. F. Asphyxia neonatorum. Am. J. Obst. & Gynec., **45**: 183–200, 1943.

1012. WINKELMAN, N. W., MOORE, M. T. Neurohistopathologic changes with metrazol and insulin shock therapy. An experimental study of the cat. Arch. Neurol. & Psychiat., **43**: 1108–1137, 1940.

1013. WINTROBE, M. M., STEIN, H. J., MILLER, M. H., FOLLIS, R. H., JR., NAJJAR, V., HUMPHREYS, S. A study of thiamine deficiency in swine together with a comparison of methods of assay. Bull. Johns Hopkins Hosp., **71**: 141–162 1942.

1014. WINZLER, R. J. A comparative study of the effects of cyanide, azide and carbon monoxide on the respiration of bakers' yeast. J. Cell. & Comp. Physiol., **21**: 229–252, 1943.

1015. WISLICKI, L. The antagonism between the posterior pituitary lobe and insulin. J. Physiol., **102**: 274–280, 1943.

1016. WOLFF, H. G. The cerebral circulation. Physiol. Rev., **16**: 545–596, 1936.

1017. ——, LENNOX, W. G. Cerebral circulation. XII. The effect on pial vessels of variations in the oxygen and carbon dioxide content of the blood. Arch. Neurol. & Psychiat., **23**: 1097–1120, 1930.

1018. WOOD, H. G., WERKMAN, C. H., HEMINGWAY, A., NIER, A. O. Mechanism of fixation of carbon dioxide in the Krebs cycle. J. Biol. Chem., **139**: 483–484, 1941.

1019. ——, WERKMAN, C. H., HEMINGWAY, A., NIER, A. O. Fixation of carbon dioxide by pigeon liver in the dissimilation of pyruvic acid. J. Biol. Chem., **142**: 31–45, 1942.

1020. WOODBURY, R. A., ROBINOW, M., HAMILTON, W. F. Blood pressure studies on infants. Am. J. Physiol., **122**: 472–479, 1938.

1021. WORTIS, H., BUEDING, E., JOLLIFFE, N. Pyruvic acid studies in the peripheral neuropathy of alcohol addicts. New England J. Med., **226**: 376–379, 1942.

1022. ——, ——, STEIN, M. H., JOLLIFFE, N. Pyruvic acid studies in the Wernicke syndrome. Arch. Neurol. & Psychiat., **47**: 215–222, 1942.

1023. ——, MAURER, W. S. "Sham rage" in man: report of cases. Am. J. Psychiat., **98**: 638–644, 1942.

1024. WORTIS, J. Cardiac psychosis and the symptom of anxiety. Am. Heart J., **13**: 394–412, 1937.

1025. ——, BOWMAN, K. M., GOLDFARB, W. Human brain metabolism. Normal values and values in certain clinical states. Am. J. Psychiat., **97**: 552–565, 1940.

1026. ——, GOLDFARB, W. A method of studying the availability of various substrates for human brain metabolism during therapeutic insulin shock. Science, **91**: 270–271, 1940.

1027. ——, ——. Schizophrenic brain metabolism in the course of insulin shock treatment. New York State J. Med., **42**: 1053–1059, 1942.

1028. ——, BOWMAN, K. M., GOLDFARB, W., FAZEKAS, J. F., HIMWICH, H. E. Availability of lactic acid for brain oxidations. J. Neurophysiol., **4**: 243–249, 1941.

1029. WORTIS, S. B. Respiratory metabolism of excised brain tissue. II. The effects of some drugs on brain oxidations. Arch. Neurol. & Psychiat., **33**: 1022–1029, 1935.

1030. WRIGHT, E. B. A comparative study of the effects of oxygen lack on peripheral nerve. Am. J. Physiol. **147**: 78–89, 1946.

1031. YANNET, H. The etiology of congenital cerebral palsy. J. Pediat., **24**: 38–45, 1944.

1032. YORK, G. E., HOMBURGER, E., HIMWICH, H. E. The similarity of the cerebral arterio-venous oxygen differences on the right and left sides in resting man. Arch. Neurol. & Psychiat., **55**: 578–582, 1946.

1033. YOUNG, F. G. Permanent experimental diabetes produced by pituitary (anterior lobe) injections. Lancet, Part I: 372–374, 1937.

1034. ——. The pituitary gland and carbohydrate metabolism. Endocrinology, **26**: 345–351, 1940.

1035. YOUNGSTROM, K. A. Acetylcholine esterase concentration during the development of the human fetus. J. Neurophysiol., **4**: 473–477, 1941.

1036. ZUNZ, E., LA BARRE, J. Sur l'augmentation de la teneur en insuline du sang veineux parcreatique après l'hyperglycémie provoquée par injection de glucose. Compt. Rend. Soc. de Biol., **96**: 421–423, 1927.

1037. ——, ——. Sur les causes de l'augmentation de la teneur en insuline du sang veineux pancreatique lors de l'hyperglycémie provoquée par injection de dextrose. Compt. Rend. Soc. de Biol., **96**: 708–710, 1927.

1038. ZWEMER, R. L., SULLIVAN, R. C. Corticoadrenal influence on blood sugar mobilization. Endocrinology., **18**: 730–738, 1934.

1039. COLFER, H. F. Studies of the relationship between electrolytes of the cerebral cortex and the mechanism of convulsions. A. Research Nerv. & Ment. Dis. Proc., **26**: 98–117, 1947.

1040. STARK, W., BARRERA, S. E. Use of potassium in protracted insulin coma. Arch. Neurol. & Psychiat., **62**: 280–286, 1949.

1041. YANNET, H. Effects of prolonged insulin hypoglycemia on distribution of water and electrolyte in brain and in muscle. Arch. Neurol. & Psychiat., **42**: 237–247, 1939.

1042. SLOAN, N., JASPER, H. The identity of spreading depression and "suppression." EEG Clin. Neurophysiol., **11**: 59–78, 1950.

AUTHOR INDEX

Abdon, N. O., 317
Adler, E., 74, 84, 85
Abreu, B. E., 192
Adolph, E. F., 147
Albaum, H. G., 155, 156, 357
Aldersberg, D., 258
Alexander, F. A. D., 125, 127, 130, 147, 168, 172, 244, 245, 273, 283, 313, 320, 355
Allweiss, M. D., 298
Anderson, E., 31, 37
Angyal, L. v., 259
Appel, K. E., 180, 181, 194, 214, 333, 345, 362
Aring, C. D., 121, 180, 181, 189, 190, 191, 197, 220, 362
Armstrong, H. G., 215, 216, 221, 243
Ashby, W., 171, 214, 239
Ashford, C. A., 11, 17, 20, 85, 87, 123, 300
Ask-Upmark, E., 95, 185
Augustinsson, K. B., 171, 317

Babinski, J., 261
Bacon, J. S. D., 152
Baker, A. B., 295, 296
Baker, Z., 23, 65, 85, 86, 88, 89, 140, 156
Bales, P. D., 110, 251, 252, 364
Ball, E. G., 9
Banga, I., 11, 80, 84, 85, 204
Banting, F. G., 26, 32, 33, 48, 88, 258
Barach, A. L., 146, 221
Barcroft, J., 152, 154, 192, 215
Bard, P., 308, 346
Barker, S. B., 40, 45, 65, 82, 83, 85, 86
Barr, D. P., 82
Barrera, S. E., 123, 250, 251, 362
Barron, D. H., 79, 84, 172
Barron, E. S. G., 64, 67, 252
Bartlett, G. R., 78, 79, 252
Batson, O. V., 92, 179, 332
Bean, J. W., 222, 223, 243, 274
Beecher, H. K., 289, 346
Behnke, A. R., 222, 243
Bell, D. J., 152
Bellinger, C. H., 243, 273
Benda, C. E., 212, 213, 214
Bender, M. B., 316, 317, 318
Benedict, F. G., 202

Bennett, A. E., 240, 246
Berger, H., 106, 360
Bernard, C., 33
Bernstein, A. O., 87, 112, 114, 131, 132, 133, 135, 136, 139, 140, 157, 123, 234, 267
Bert, P., 125
Best, C. H., 26, 32, 33, 37, 42, 43, 44, 48, 49, 58, 88, 103, 258
Biasotti, A., 36, 44, 56
Bini, L., 240, 247
Bissinger, E., 32
Blixenkrone-Møller, N., 58
Bodansky, O., 42
Bond, D. D., 321
Booth, V. H., 156
Bouckaert, J. J., 114, 292
Bowman, K. M., 12, 16, 17, 18, 21, 22, 23, 24, 52, 53, 56, 120, 178, 180, 181, 189, 190, 191, 194, 197, 203, 208, 218, 229, 232, 234, 275, 345, 352, 360, 362, 363, 367
Braceland, F. J., 29
Brazier, Mary, A. B., 344
Bremer, F., 346
Brenner, C., 110, 295, 300, 318
Breusch, F. L., 77, 79, 84
Brink, F., 96
Britton, S. W., 30, 38, 128, 130, 149, 150
Brody, S., 140, 201, 348
Bronk, D. W., 96
Brooks, C. M., 33
Brown-Séquard, E., 292
Buchanan, J. M., 26, 71, 79
Buchwald, K. W., 26, 28, 32, 48, 50
Bueding, E., 36, 65, 82, 205, 206, 207
Bülbring, E., 317, 324, 346
Burk, D., 141
Burn, J. H., 35, 40, 56, 317, 323, 324
Butts, J. S., 56

Cameron, A. T., 147
Cameron, D. E., 59, 121, 189, 197, 246, 250, 278, 362
Cameron, J. A., 128
Campbell, E. H., 97, 267, 290, 291
Cannon, W. B., 26, 30, 33, 285, 313, 317
Caputto, R., 68

421

SUBJECT INDEX

Acetaldyhyde, 79, footnote 12

Acetic acid
oxidation inhibited by fluoracetate, 78, footnote
unavailability in blood for brain, 20

Acetoacetic acid, 58
oxidation by brain, 11

Acetoin, 79, footnote 12

Acetopyruvic acid,
availability for brain *in situ*, 19, footnote 9

Acetylation, 72

Acetylcholine
cerebrospinal fluid in, 318
concentration in brain, 101, 168–169
effect of acid-base equilibrium on, 110
effect on C.B.F., 100, 101, 113
formation, 11, footnote 1; 72; 101; 317, footnote
poisoning, effect of age, 170, footnote 16
present status in nerve conduction, 317, footnote

Acetyl group, 77, 81

Acetyl phosphate, 77, footnote 11

Acid-base equilibrium
effect on acetylcholine, 101, 110
effect on C.B.F., 101, 103, 113
on cholinesterase, 110
in anoxia, effect of breathing carbon dioxide, 113
in relation to epilepsy, 109–110

Acidosis, *see* Acid-base equilibrium

Aconitase, 84

ACTH—*see* Adrenocorticotrophic hormone

Addison's disease, carbohydrate metabolism in, 38

Adenosine, as vasodilator, 113, footnote 10

Adenosine diphosphate, 55, 69
effect of cyanide on, 243

Adenosine monophosphate, as vasodilator, 113, footnote 10

Adenosine triphosphate, 69; 71, footnote 6; 72

Adenosine triphosphate—*continued*
concentration in brain, effect of cyanide on, 243
effect of electroshock on, 249–250
in convulsions, 138
in injury, 139, footnote 4
in insulin hypoglycemia, 55
synthesis, 66, footnote 1

Adenosine triphosphatase, concentration, 157

Adenylic acid, 76

Adrenal gland, hormonal connections between medulla and cortex, 151

Adrenocortical hormones
effect on brain constituents, 32, footnote 5
on carbohydrate metabolism, 38, 82–83
on survival in anoxia, 150
on transformation of protein to carbohydrate, 38

Adrenalemia, 50

Adrenaline, as a neurohormone, 30; 261, footnote 5; 317, footnote 2
effect, comparison with amphetamine, 192, footnote
on blood sugar level in hypoglycemia, 52
on carbohydrate metabolism, 34, 83
on C.B.F., 100
on survival time in anoxia, 150
relation to hypothalmus, 41, footnote 9
to other hormones, 34

Adreno cortical hormones, relation to other hormones, 39, 319

Adrenocorticotrophic hormone, effects, 35, footnote 7; 36

Adrenergic fibers, to sweat glands, 261, footnote 5

Adrenergic substances, in blood, 316–320

Adult
human, resistance to anoxia, 299
resistance to anoxia, 129–130, 299

Age
effect on barbiturate susceptibility, 348, footnote

430

Calories, supplied to brain
by anaerobic metabolism, 141
by aerobic metabolism, 141
Camphor, in convulsive therapy, 246
Caramiphen, as antagonist to DFP, 365
Carbohydrate meals for aviators, 223
Carbon dioxide, *see also* Hyperventilation
Carbon dioxide, 71, footnote 4; 78, footnote
as a means of producing anoxia, 128
effect on electroencephalogram, 106, 109
during anoxia, 112
on cerebral AVO₂ difference, 182–183
on C.B.F., 101, 103–110, 182–183
on C.M.R., 182–183, 224
in blood, relation to epileptic seizures, 109
in treatment of psychoneurosis, 274
pressure, cerebral circulation, 96
Carbon, isotopic, 77
Carbon monoxide, 87
poisoning, effect on cerebral metabolism, 209
lesions in brain, 298, 308
Carbon tetrachloride poisoning, hypoglycemia due to, 269
Carbonic anhydrase
content in various parts of the brain, 170
function of, 171, footnote, 18, 19
effect of thyroxin on concentration, 238
Cardiac decompensation, effect on C.M.R., 218–219, 224
Cardiac output
in arterio-venous aneurysm, 97
in fever therapy, 231
Carotid artery, therapeutic ligation of, 94
Carotid sinus, 99
syndrome, 100
Cats, depancreatized, 89
Caudate nucleus, *see* also Basal ganglia
Caudate nucleus
cholinesterase content, 170
glycolysis in, 166, 289
glycogen content, 53, 167, 168, 169, 287

Caudate nucleus—*continued*
lesions in, following fatal hypoglycemia, 297
oxygen consumption, 141, 289
resistance to cerebral anemia, 293
C.B.F., *see* Cerebral blood flow
Central nervous system
effect of cold on, 147, footnote 9
functional organization of, 270–276
patterns of activity, 300, 303–360
somatic division, definition, 257, footnote 1
Cerebellum, 92
acetylcholine content, 168
effect of anoxia, 295
glycogen content, 53, 167–169, 287
lesions in, following fatal hypoglycemia, 297
myelinization in, 175
oxygen consumption, 140–141, 161, 164–165, 288
Purkinje cells effects of cerebral anemia, 294
Cerebral activity
and oxygen consumption, 96, footnote 2
and oxygen pressure, 97
Cerebral anemia, resistance to, 293
Cerebral arteries, mixing of blood in, 94
Cerebral arteriosclerosis
effect on cerebral AVO₂ difference, 121, 191
on CMR, 191, 224
Cerebral arterio-venous oxygen differences
comparison of left and right, 94, 95, 329, 331
constancy, 120–121
effect of age, 197, 198, 199, 200
of carbon dioxide, 182–183
of drugs and therapeutic procedures, 191, 228–252, 353, 355
of electroshock, 246, 250
light and deep barbiturate anesthesia, 332
of oxygen, 182–183
in normal adults, 178
in relation to cerebral blood flow, 119–122

Cerebral arterio-venous oxygen differences—*continued*
in relation to C.M.R., 121
in various conditions, 121, 180-224
Cerebral blood pressure, effect of cerebrospinal fluid pressure, 102
Cerebral blood flow
comparison of right and left, 95
during insulin hypoglycemia, 12, 14,
150, 181, 224
effect of carbon dioxide, 182-183
of cerebral vascular resistance, 187
of cerebrospinal fluid pressure, 102
of drugs, 100, 113, 114, 191, 192, 332,
353-355
of oxygen, 182-183
evaluation of methods, 360
in normal adults, 178-179
in relation to metabolism, 114
in various conditions, 95, 99, 100, 101,
102, 105, 113, 119, 139, 180, 184, 185,
187-192, 193
measurement, 12, 179
measurement, with thermocouples, cri-
tique of, 14, footnote 8
regulation, 97-114
effect of carbon dioxide, 103-110
of systemic arterial pressure, 99
of systemic blood pressure, 98
values, 98
ways of altering, 98
Cerebral circulation
anatomy, 91
regulation, 98
time, 230, 232
venous drainage, 94
Cerebral hemispheres
cholinesterase in, 301
cortex, acetylcholine content, 168
autonomic representation in, 304
cholinesterase content, 170
effect of cerebral anemia, 294
electroencephalogram in insulin hypoglycemia, 291
glycogen content, 53, 167
glycolysis, 166, 289
injury, in fatal cyclopropane anesthesia, 355
in nitrous oxide fatality, 308-309
integrative activity, 284

Cerebral hemispheres—*continued*
cortex—*continued*
lesions in, following fatal hypoglycemia, 297
metabolic rate, 50
in humans, 289
of dogs with black tongue, utilization of oxygen, 203
oxygen consumption, 141; 161; 164-
165; 201, footnote 9; 289
effect of anoxia on, 295
lesions in, following death in nitrous
oxides anesthesia, 297
oxygen consumption, 288-289
venous drainage, 94
Cerebral metabolic rate determined
definition, 177
effect of carbon dioxide, 182-183
of drugs on, 191, 236
of oxygen on, 182-183
in insulin hypoglycemia, 181
in normal adults, 178
in various conditions, 178-196, 217-
218-219, 236-237, 224
estimated, in various conditions, 196-
211, 224, 229
requirement for environmental contact, 196
Cerebral metabolism, *see also* Oxygen
consumption and Cerebral metabolic
rate
Cerebral metabolism, 95
analysis of place in cerebral disease,
366
calculated from in vitro observations,
180, footnote 3
carbohydrate utilization, in normal, 23
in schizophrenics, 23
effect of convulsions on, 250
of drugs, 160, 241-252, 332, 353
of glucose deprivation, 257-273
effect of injury, 139, footnote 4
of metabolism, 147, footnote 10, 159,
240
of oxygen deprivation, 131, 215-216,
240
of temperature, 146, 159, 232
in relation to mental disturbances, 220
in relation to neurophylogenesis, 163-
175
in relation to vascularity of brain, 114

Sympathetic—*continued*
  control of C.B.F., 100
  -parasympathetic balance—various interactions, 322–324
    as related to levels of activity, 307–311
    in insulin hypoglycemia, 260, 305, 306, 311, 314
    predominance, analysis of, 312, 313
    stellectomy, effect on C. B. F., 193
Sympatho-adrenaline activity, effect of hypothalamus, 61
  activity, in insulin hypoglycemia, 51
  apparatus, 33, 270
  anatomy, 33
Syncopy, 99
Syphilis, destruction *see also* General paresis
  effect on C.M.R., 209, 224
Systemic blood pressure, fall in various conditions, 99–100
Szent-Györgyi cycle, 74, footnote 8; 81

Temperature
  effect of cold on C.N.S., 147, footnote 9
  on C.B.F., 159
  on C.M.R., 146
Temporal lobes, effect of anoxia on, 295
Testes *see* Testosterone
Testosterone
  effect on brain constituents, 32, footnote 5
  on carbohydrate metabolism, 39
  on C.M.R., 32, footnote 5
  relation to other hormones, 32, footnote 5
Thalamus, glycogen content, 53, 168, 169
  glycogen content in hypoglycemia, 287
  glycolysis in, 166, 288
  oxygen consumption, 141, 164–165, 288
  release in insulin hypoglycemia, 260
  ventrolateral nucleus, resistance to cerebral anemia, 293
Theiler's F. A. virus of experimental poliomylitus, 85, footnote 15
  G. B. VII virus, 85, footnote 15
Theophylline ethylenediamine *see* Aminophylline
Thiamin *see* Vitamin B₁, *see also* Diphosphothiamin

Thiopental anesthesia, 95, 332–335
  clinical signs, effect of premedication on, 345
  analysis, 335–339, 345
  stage, one, clouding of consciousness, 336–337
  stage, two, delirium, 336–337
  stage, three, surgical anesthesia 336, 339
  stage, four, impending failure, 336 339
  during recovery from 344
  C.M.R. in, 332
  comparison with hypoglycemia, 347
  effect on cortex, 95
    on cerebral AVO₂ difference, 120, 332
    on C.B.F., 114, 332
    on respiration, 342
  electroencephalagram in, 344
  inhibition of energy turnover, 252
  oxygen saturation of hemoglobin in 342–343
Thiophene-2-sulphanilamide, as enzyme inhibitor, 171, footnote 19
Thiouracil, effect on enzyme concentration, 238
Thyroid *see* Thyroxin
Thyroxin
  see also Hyperthyroidism
Thyroxin
  and anoxia, effect on E.E.G., 146, 238
  effect on brain constituents, 32, footnote 5
    on brain metabolism, in vitro, 236
    on carbohydrate metabolism, 32, footnote; 40; 83;
    on C.M.R., 32, footnote 5; 146; 236–238
    on cretins, 236–238
    on enzyme concentration, 239
  in relation to other hormones, 32, footnote 5; 40, 270
  lack, as protection against anoxia, 146, footnote 8
  physiological effects, 239–240
  production during anoxia, 146, footnote 8
Tilting, effect on C.B.F., 100
Torcular, 92
Tridione, as antagonist to D.F.P., 251